D1474335

Fundamentals of Motor Control

Fundamentals of Motor Control

Mark L. Latash

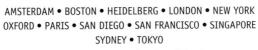

AMSTERDAM • BOSTON • HEIDELBERG • LONDON • NEW YORK
OXFORD • PARIS • SAN DIEGO • SAN FRANCISCO • SINGAPORE
SYDNEY • TOKYO

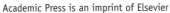

Academic Press is an imprint of Elsevier

ELSEVIER

Academic Press is an imprint of Elsevier
32 Jamestown Road, London NW1 7BY, UK
225 Wyman Street, Waltham, MA 02451, USA
525 B Street, Suite 1800, San Diego, CA 92101-4495, USA

First edition 2012

Notice

No responsibility is assumed by the publisher for any injury and/or damage to persons or property as
a matter of products liability, negligence or otherwise, or from any use or operation of any methods,
products, instructions or ideas contained in the material herein.

Because of rapid advances in the medical sciences, in particular, independent verification
of diagnoses and drug dosages should be made

British Library Cataloguing-in-Publication Data
A catalogue record for this book is available from the British Library

Library of Congress Cataloging-in-Publication Data
A catalog record for this book is available from the Library of Congress

ISBN : 978-0-12-415956-3

For information on all Academic Press publications visit our
website at elsevierdirect.com

Typeset by TNQ Books and Journals Pvt Ltd.
www.tnq.co.in

Printed and bound in United States of America

12 13 14 15 16   10 9 8 7 6 5 4 3 2 1

Working together to grow
libraries in developing countries

www.elsevier.com | www.bookaid.org | www.sabre.org

ELSEVIER   BOOK AID
             International   Sabre Foundation

Contents

Preface

Motor control is a relatively young field of research. It can be defined as an area of science exploring how the nervous system interacts with the rest of the body and the environment in order to produce purposeful, coordinated movements. Over the past 25 years, the field of motor control has developed rapidly, resulting in the formation of the International Society of Motor Control, publication of an international journal *Motor Control*, a series of biennial conferences *Progress in Motor Control*, and an annual Motor Control Summer School. Today, motor control is an established area of natural science.

Many universities offer both undergraduate and graduate courses in motor control in various departments, such as kinesiology, movement science, exercise and sport science, psychology, physiology, neuroscience, engineering, physical therapy, etc. Surprisingly, there is no comprehensive book on motor control. There are a few books with the expression "motor control" in the title, but these books touch on aspects of the field without offering a comprehensive overview. Frequently, a particular perspective is emphasized, behavioral, biomechanical, neurophysiological, clinical, control–theoretical, cognitive–psychological, dynamical systems, etc.

This book attempts to cover all the major perspectives in motor control, and is appropriate both as a reference and overview to the field and/or as an upper-level undergraduate text. Since motor control is a young field, established knowledge is scarce and one can hardly name a hypothesis that would be acceptable to all researchers. So, this book is subjective: It reflects the author's personal opinion on what motor control is and how it should be taught. The book is designed to present a balanced approach based on both physics and neurophysiology.

One of my undergraduate students once asked me: "What is physics? Is it about how things work?" I like this non-scientific definition. Physics is indeed about "how things work" in our Universe. Over the past few hundred years, physics of the inanimate world has achieved fantastic progress and set an example for other areas of research. This has been due to the development of its two important components—mathematics and experimental observations. The development of mathematics provided physics with an adequate language to describe the laws of nature in a compact way. The development of sophisticated methods of observation allowed acquiring information about a variety of ways "things work" in the Universe and also guided the development of the mathematical language of physics.

Is biology a "complex physics"? In other words, can the development of physics be expected to lead to a qualitative jump in our understanding of biological objects? I do not know the answer but hope that it is yes.

Even at the time of Ancient Greece, the philosophers understood the great complexity of living objects as compared to objects in the inanimate world. Indeed, functions of the human body were commonly described using such terms as "soul" and "spirits," which reflected the inability of the science of inanimate nature to handle aspects of behavior of living systems. Many brilliant scientists of the past, including the great Isaac Newton, thought of human movements as being produced by the soul. Only over the past century have scientists attempted to approach the exactness and rigor of classical physics in biological sciences.

The complexity of biological objects seems to be a good excuse for the relatively slow progress in biology. Indeed, the human body consists of about 10^{16} cells, while each cell is a living being of its own consisting of about 10^{12} atoms. The cells contain giant molecules that may themselves be viewed as living systems; they consist of $10^{8}–10^{10}$ atoms each. However, the numbers themselves are not the main source of biological complexity: Planets consist of many more atoms than typical biological objects, while behavior of the planets is rather well described by the laws of classical physics. The problem, or rather the main source of excitement in studying biological objects, is that these objects are active. This means that, for an inanimate object, knowing its initial state, physical properties and external forces acting on the object is sufficient to predict its behavior. This is not true for biological objects that commonly generate forces to satisfy their needs. If you leave a tennis ball on the top of a table, you may be certain that you will find it there tomorrow (unless an earthquake strikes, or a biological object—for example, your friend—takes the ball). If you leave a dog (cat, gerbil, even worm) on the same table, the chances that it will wait for you there the next day are next to nil.

Many years ago the author graduated from a program called Physics of Living Systems in the Moscow Physics-Technical Institute (known also as FizTekh). The name of the program suggested that there was such a field of study as physics of living systems at that time. However, now it seems that the name was a promise for a future discipline, which is still unavailable. In that program physics was presented as the cornerstone of any science about the Universe, biology being no exception.

Although the emphasis of this book is on physics and neurophysiology, this does not mean that other approaches are not covered. There are sections explicitly dedicated to control theory, dynamical systems, biomechanics, motor learning, different behaviors, and even a few pathological cases are briefly reviewed. The only underrepresented field is psychology. This is partly due to my lack of knowledge in the field and partly to the fact that a very nice book dedicated to psychological aspects of motor control has been written by David Rosenbaum.

My personal experience with teaching motor control-related courses at Penn State has taught me that there is little common background among students who register for such courses, even at the 300 or 400 level. Even if all the prerequisites are enforced, there will be students in the class who have never solved a single equation, do not know what a vector is, and cannot name a single reflex. Therefore, I tried to present all the necessary background information in the textbook, certainly very briefly. In particular, Chapter 3 reviews the basic peripheral elements and features of the system for movement production, while elements of basic physics and mathematics are scattered throughout other chapters, as they become necessary.

The structure of the book follows certain logic. First, there is an introductory chapter (Chapter 1) that presents a somewhat philosophical overview on motor control. In a way, it prepares the reader for the style and contents of the rest of the book. It is followed by a review on the history of movement studies that ultimately led to the emergence of motor control (Chapter 2). As already mentioned, Chapter 3 presents a brief review of the very basic information about the system for movement production. Chapter 4 is rather unusual. It presents several "instructive examples." The purpose of this chapter is to whet the appetite of the reader and nudge him or her towards making his or her own decisions on how such a system could be organized.

The next five chapters (Chapters 5–9) form the core of the book. They discuss different theoretical approaches to the main issues of motor control and coordination. I am confident that many of my colleagues (maybe even all of them) will be dissatisfied with the way I present their favorite theories. I say *mea culpa* and offer sincere apologies: The book reflects my understanding of those theories and the field in general. This book is not "objective," because this word is inapplicable to a field of science that consists mostly of white spots and guesses, with only a few established facts and no universally accepted theoretical viewpoints.

Then, there is a relatively large Chapter 10 dedicated to the spinal cord and several brain structures such as the motor cortex, the cerebellum, and the basal ganglia. It would be logical to study the material presented in this chapter immediately after Chapter 3. However, I wanted the reader to have basic information about the main motor control theories before looking into structures within the central nervous system. Chapter 10 also presents brief descriptions of several major motor pathologies associated with injuries to or dysfunction of particular neural structures.

Chapter 11 is also rather large. It tries to apply the information from the earlier chapters to a number of typical behaviors such as standing, walking, reaching, and grasping. This chapter (as well as the following Chapter 12 dedicated to motor learning and adaptation) is written in a much more traditional way: The material follows experimental observations much more than theoretical views. However, in all sections of Chapters 11 and 12, I tried to relate the experimental facts to theories described in Chapters 5–9.

Finally, Chapter 13 describes some of the commonly used methods in the field of motor control, from methods of biomechanics to electrophysiological methods and brain imaging techniques. This material may be viewed as auxiliary. On the other hand, if a course on motor control involves laboratories (to me this sounds like a good idea), Chapter 13 may become useful.

Individual chapters are relatively independent. This means that, depending on the level of expertise of the audience, the reader can skip some chapters and/or jump from chapter to chapter, not necessarily in the order they are presented in the book. Each chapter ends with a list of self-test questions and recommended future readings, ranging from original classical papers to review articles and books. I would recommend any instructors who plan to adopt this book as a text to begin with going through the self-test questions themselves.

The book ends with a Glossary. It is purposefully very long and detailed. I strongly believe that all the terms and expressions have to be defined clearly and unambiguously to be useful in a scientific discourse.

I am very much grateful to my colleagues, Greg Anson, Natalia Dounskaia, Anatol Feldman, Robert Sainburg, and John Scholz who took the time to read earlier drafts of individual chapters and provided me with invaluable—often strongly negative!—feedback. My dear friend and colleague, Professor Vladimir Zatsiorsky read earlier drafts of all the chapters. His critique was truly invaluable! The imperfection of the final text is only due to the stubbornness of the author, not to the lack of good advice. I would also like to express deep gratitude to my colleagues who offered highly valuable advice on illustrations from their papers that are used in the book: Daniel Corcos, Yuri Ivanenko, David Ostry, Monica Perez, Robert Peterka, Robert Sainburg, and Lena Ting.

Teaching is probably the best way to learn. I learned a lot from my students, both undergraduate and graduate, who took classes on different aspects of motor control. I am very much grateful to them all, particularly to those who were not afraid to ask questions and challenge my statements.

Teaching in a major university is inseparable from research. I would like to thank all the graduate and postdoctoral students who worked in the Motor Control Laboratory at Penn State over the past 15 years or so. Our discussions during the laboratory meetings have been very helpful in the pursuit of clarity and exactness in formulating motor control problems and approaches to those problems.

Finally, I am what I am only thanks to my parents Lev and Sara, my wife Irina, and my children Liza Jr., Liza Sr., and Samvel.

1 A philosophical introduction

Chapter Outline

1.1   Adequate language

The Ancient Egyptians built pyramids, perfect geometrical structures. However, we associate the birth of the science of geometry not with those anonymous Egyptian architects but with the name of Euclid. Why? This name was not selected by pure chance. Euclid did turn a set of rules that had been known for hundreds of years before him into a science. This required making a very bold step: Introducing a definition for an object that did not exist—a point. Euclid defined a point as an object that had no length, no width, and no height (look around and you will find no such objects). Despite the fact that points did not exist, this was a crucial step that later allowed for the introduction of definitions for a line, a plane, and a sphere, and geometry became a science. The step made by Euclid may be called "introducing an adequate language" for spatial relations among objects. This language permitted questions to be formulated in a way that allowed rigorous, exact scientific inquiry.

For any area of science, questions have to be formulated in an adequate language. As of now, unfortunately, no such language has been introduced for biology.

Motor control is a relatively young field of research in biology. Let me define it as an area of science exploring natural laws that define how the nervous system interacts with other body parts and the environment to produce purposeful, coordinated movements. It is very hard to look for an adequate set of notions in an area that does not have them, but it is also very challenging and exciting! It is much more simple and tempting to borrow one of the developed approaches from another field that shares "key words" with motor control, for example basic mechanics, control theory, or engineering. One should keep in mind, however, that such an approach has strict limitations. It can provide tools that help find answers to questions after the questions have been formulated. As of now, the main problems of motor control are not in finding answers but in formulating questions.

Fundamentals of Motor Control. DOI: 10.1016/B978-0-12-415956-3.00001-4

To achieve a scientific, physical understanding of the system for movement production, researchers have to use adequate methods. Using methods developed for systems that have very little in common with the human body (for example, control theory was developed for ballistic missiles and other human-built objects) may lead to important progress in building artificial systems that imitate aspects of human behavior, with substantial impact in such areas as prosthetics and robotics. But this is not motor control as defined above. Such approaches cannot offer an adequate formulation of questions in a field that differs from the area for which those approaches have been developed.

1.2   Specific features of biological objects

Let us start with a few basic features of biological objects. Such objects belong to the physical world and they are alive. So, help with formulating questions may be expected to come from natural sciences such as physics, chemistry, and biology (physiology).

Consider the following major difference between living and inanimate (including man-made) objects. The behavior of living objects is intentional, that is, typically it has a purpose. This is a major difference from the inanimate world. If one knows the initial state of an inanimate object and the forces acting on the object, its behavior can be predicted using the laws of classical mechanics. For example, a stone never rolls uphill unless an external force pushes it up. In contrast, animals can run uphill using forces that they themselves bring about. Sophisticated man-made systems, for example cars, can also move uphill, but they are designed by humans to behave in this way. So, we can view them as extensions of biological objects for as long as they are able to perform their programmed functions. A car that has run out of gas or had one of its major components broken immediately starts to behave as a member of the class of inanimate objects.

The fact that biological objects are intentional does not mean that they violate the laws of physics. Living beings differ from the inanimate in their ability to turn the laws of physics to their advantage.

If we now turn to the system for movement production, there are a few features in this system that would make an engineer think that it was designed by someone with no knowledge of basic engineering (which is very likely true!). Certain features of the neuro-sensory-motor system look, to put it mildly, suboptimal, particularly when considered by an expert in designing artificial moving systems. We will consider basic properties of the system for movement production in one of the next sections; here, let me emphasize only a few important points.

Slow muscles produce forces that depend on muscle length and velocity

Consider our motors, the muscles. Motors built by engineers are powerful, quick, and can produce pre-computed forces and/or moments of force. In contrast, muscles are sluggish, not very powerful, and generate forces that depend on muscle length and its rate of change (velocity). Let me focus on this last feature. It means that when you send a neural command to a muscle, the force transmitted by its tendons to the points of their attachment to bones will depend not only on the magnitude of the command but also on the actual muscle length and velocity. Since motion of body segments depends not only on muscle forces but also on forces from the environment, actual muscle forces become unpredictable, unless the central nervous system possesses an ability to predict changes in the environment perfectly, with 100% confidence. The environment is typically unpredictable (at least, not predictable perfectly). This means that the central nervous system is in principle unable to prescribe time patterns of muscle forces, except in very special laboratory conditions with perfectly reproducible external force fields (actually, this is impossible even in the best laboratory environments). This feature of the system for movement production was emphasized by Nikolai Bernstein, a great Russian physiologist who is sometimes considered the father of contemporary motor control.

Confusing sensory receptors

To produce coordinated purposeful movements it is necessary for animals to get information on the environment and on the current state of body segments. This information is used for planning actions as well as for correcting ongoing movements if they happen to be inaccurate or if a major perturbation acts on the body from the environment. Our body is equipped with a large number of sensors that supply such information. In particular, we have sensors of muscle length and velocity (muscle spindles), of tendon force (Golgi tendon organs), of the state of joints (articular receptors), and of pressure on and motion of the skin (cutaneous and subcutaneous receptors). At first glance, these sensors are sufficient to provide all the necessary information. However, when one starts to consider their design and properties, a few apparent problems emerge. The sensors seem to be noisy and information from them can be confusing, at least as compared to nearly perfect sensors that measure the variables of interest in artificial moving systems.

For example, muscle spindles produce signals related to muscle length and velocity, but their gain is modulated by a special system of neurons in the spinal cord, the gamma-motoneurons. So, one and the same signal may be generated at different positions and velocities depending on the gamma-motoneuronal activity.

Golgi tendon organs are accurate tendon force sensors. Note, however, that our joint movements are rotations. This means that adequate mechanical variables for joint motion are moments of force, not forces. One and the same tendon force produces different moments of force with respect to a joint at different joint positions because the moment arm of the force changes with joint position. So, information from Golgi tendon organs is by itself insufficient to know moments of force. Articular receptors look even less reliable in providing information about variables that seem to be most relevant for joint action: Joint angle, its angular velocity, and moment of force. More information on the features of different sensors will be presented in Chapter 3.

Long conduction delays

As already mentioned, unexpected changes in the environment happen rather commonly. To avoid movement disruptions by such changes, commands to muscles have to be corrected appropriately. Such corrections are made based on sensory signals reporting that something unexpected has happened. A major problem is that conduction pathways in our bodies are relatively long (typical distances are on the order of 1 m), and the speed of conduction is relatively low (at best, about 100 m/s, but frequently much lower). As a result, delays of a few tens of milliseconds are common even for the quickest motor reactions to peripheral signals, and such delays can easily reach 0.1 s and more, if they are computed from a peripheral signal to a useful motor reaction produced by muscles. This is a very long time for some of the quickest voluntary movements. A top-level sprinter covers 1 m over this time, while a well-served tennis ball flies over 5 m. So, the central nervous system always deals with outdated information on the state of the peripheral organs, and this information becomes even more outdated when signals generated by the neural controller reach their target muscles.

Neurons—threshold elements

The main element of the central nervous system is the neural cell, the neuron. Individual neurons and neural networks are commonly assumed to perform all the necessary computations to allow the organism to function adequately. Neurons possess a feature that looks like a source of major computational problems: They are threshold elements. This means that small changes in the input signals into a neuron, that is, changes in the potential on its membrane, do not lead to any changes in its output until these changes reach a certain threshold value. Then, the neuron generates a standard signal, an action potential, with characteristics that do not depend on the strength of the input. So, if one knows the output of a neuron (a time series of its action potentials), it is in principle impossible to reconstruct the input into the neuron. For example, if someone turned on the light in a room, you would have no idea with what force that person pressed on the switch, only that the force was sufficiently high. In other words, if you want a neuron to generate a particular output signal, there are an infinite number of combinations of input signals into the neuron that can achieve this result. This feature of neurons creates an insurmountable problem for so-called inverse problems (see Section 5.1), that is, problems of computing a neural command (somewhere in the brain) that would produce a desired motor output. As we will see further in the book, this is a problem for scientists, not for the system for movement production.

   To summarize this section, our bodies were definitely not designed by well-educated twenty-first century engineers or experts in control theory. So, engineering and control theory will not help us understand how the structures within the body interact among themselves and with the environment to bring about purposeful, coordinated movements. We have to take a closer look at specific features of human (and animal) movements and at the physiology of the main structures that participate in movement production. First, however, let us consider the history of movement science, a few facts about the system for movement production, and a few examples from everyday life and laboratory experiments that emphasize several basic features of typical human movements and suggest principles of their construction.

2 Elements of history

Chapter Outline

2.1 From Ancient Greece to the early twentieth century

Classical Greek philosophers: body vs. soul

The great Greek philosophers of the past did not know the expression "motor control"; they were interested, however, in the origins of purposeful biological movements and focused on the relation between the *body* (that moves) and the *soul* (that controls). The following three questions were commonly discussed: What is the origin of movement in the world? What makes the soul command the body to move? How does the soul induce body movement?

The great philosopher Pythagoras (571?–497? B.C.), best known for his famous theorem about the relations among the sides of a right triangle, viewed movement as evolution of metaphysical numbers. Soul was defined as a number with an ability to move by itself. Movement of the soul was produced by movement of heavenly

Fundamentals of Motor Control. DOI: 10.1016/B978-0-12-415956-3.00002-6

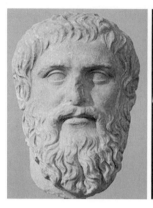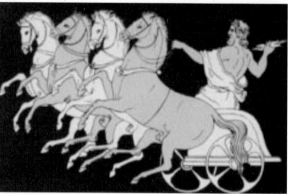

Figure 2.1 Left: Copy of the portrait of Plato made by Silanion, ca. 370 B.C. © Marie-Lan Nguyen/Wikimedia Commons. Right: An illustration of Plato's idea of the Soul (the charioteer) controlling the Body (the chariot). The Chariot of Zeus–Project Gutenberg eText 14994.png from the 1879 Stories from the Greek Tragedians by Alfred Church; Wikimedia Commons.

spheres. The issue of how movement of the soul induced body movement remained unexplored. Heracletius of Ephesus (540–??? B.C.) started a school known as "those who believe in movement." According to philosophers of that school, objects were beyond the human knowledge, only their trajectories could be observed. About a century later, Democritus (460–370? B.C.) came to the conclusion that movement of the soul was transmitted to the body by the movement of atoms. This opinion is not far from the current understanding of how movements come about, if one substitutes *atoms* with *ions* and *soul* with *intention*.

According to Plato (428–347 B.C.), self-motion was a sign of an immortal soul, which was supposed to possess a unique ability to be moved by itself (similar to Pythagoras). Plato compared human voluntary movements to a chariot moved by horses controlled by the soul (Figure 2.1). Movements of parts of the body were prescribed by the soul like those of marionettes. In our day, one could say that the soul (the unknown structures within the brain) produces *motor programs* to be implemented by the body parts (see Section 5.3).

Aristotle (384–322 B.C.) argued that for any movement there had to be a mover and a moved body. Only moving bodies are observable, while the mover (the soul) is not. Aristotle was arguably the first to pay particular attention to *coordination* of biological movement, which was for him synonymous to harmony. This harmony occurred naturally, by the design of the Creation. Despite some differences in philosophical views, all the mentioned philosophers would probably agree that only movements produced by living beings are purposeful. It took a few hundred years to make the next step.

In the second century A.D., the great Roman physician Galen (129–201) realized that voluntary movements of body segments were produced by pairs of muscles with opposing actions (Figure 2.2; now we call them *agonist–antagonist pairs*, for example flexors–extensors, adductors–abductors, etc. see Section 6.2). The muscles were supposed to produce force with the help of "animal spirits" delivered by nerves.

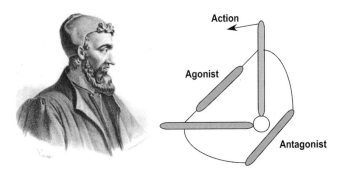

Figure 2.2 The great Roman physician Galen (left, lithograph by Pierre Roche Vigneron, Paris: Lith de Gregoire et Deneux, ca. 1865; Wikimedia Commons) was the first to realize that joints were controlled by pairs of muscles, agonist–antagonist pairs.

The Renaissance, dualism, and early biomechanics

Several great philosophers of the Renaissance contributed to the progress in understanding how voluntary movements were produced. Leonardo da Vinci (1452–1519) studied the functional anatomy of muscles; so he can be viewed as the first scientist to make movement in humans and animals the focus of his research. A century later, René Descartes (1596–1650) formulated the main ideas of *dualism*, a dominant branch of philosophy for many years. According to Descartes, every human being was composed of two independent entities, the soul and the body. The soul was responsible for thinking and decision-making, while the body obeyed the soul and the laws of nature. Following the traditions of Galen, Descartes thought that body movements were produced by the soul via animal spirits. Descartes realized that some movements were independent of the soul, for example, the beating of the heart. Other movements were induced by senses and mediated by the central nervous system, for example, protective arm movements during a fall. Descartes and the British anatomist Thomas Willis (1628–1678) viewed motor reactions to sensory stimuli as building blocks for voluntary movements and tried to link them to different brain structures. The term "reflex" for such actions was, however, introduced later by a French scientist, Jean Astruc (1684–1766).

Giovanni Alfonso Borelli (1608–1679) was a disciple of Galileo Galilei (1564–1642), one of the founders of classical physics. Borelli is now viewed as the father of biomechanics. He tried to integrate physiology and physics and performed numerous studies of muscles and their actions in a variety of static and dynamic tasks. In particular, Borelli estimated the maximal forces of major muscle groups using static tasks. He described muscles as being composed of thin elastic fibers. His analysis of the mechanics of jumping allowed him to conclude that release of the accumulated energy was important in such actions. According to Borelli, movements were produced by the soul, which vibrated nerves leading to the secretion of droplets of nerve juice. This was arguably the first theory on the importance of chemical processes in the production of active muscle force (see Section 3.1).

A Dutch scientist, Jan Swammerman (1637–1680), is credited for being the first to perform experiments on an isolated nerve–muscle preparation of a frog, a classical object of muscle physiology and biomechanics research. He stimulated the nerve of the preparation, observed the muscle contractions, and concluded that, during the contraction, muscle volume stays nearly unchanged. This observation contradicted the then dominant theory that muscle activation was induced by influx of "animal spirits" that were thought to be similar in properties to liquids or air.

Biological electricity and early motion analysis

The importance of electricity for intrinsic processes in animals was discovered only at the end of the eighteenth century. In 1791, a great Italian scientist Luigi Galvani (1737–1798) wrote that there was a link between neural tissue and electricity. In the following century, new instruments were invented to record electrical phenomena associated with neural and muscular activity, in particular *galvanometers*, named after Galvani. Carlo Matteucci (1811–1868) in 1838 showed that electrical currents could originate in muscles. A great French scientist, Etienne DuBois-Reymond (1818–1896) was the first to detect an electrical signal of the muscle; in 1849, he published illustrations of electrical signals recorded in human muscles and by doing so introduced a very important method of movement studies, *electromyography* (see Section 13.3).

In the middle of the nineteenth century, a German scientist called Eduard Friedrich Wilhelm Pflüger (1829–1910) performed influential studies on the *wiping reflex* in decapitated (headless) frogs. In Pflüger's experiments, such a frog preparation was suspended from a frame, and a small piece of paper soaked in a weak acid solution was placed on its back (Figure 2.3). After a short delay, the frog produced a coordinated motion of the hindlimb on the same side of the body and wiped the piece of paper off its back. When that particular hindlimb was amputated and another piece of paper was placed on the same side of the back, a longer delay was followed by a wiping motion of the remaining, contralateral hindlimb. Obviously, these movements could be controlled only by the spinal cord. Pflüger made two very important conclusions. First, the spinal cord is able to control targeted movements. Second, spinal reflexes can lead to activation of different muscle groups. These experiments and conclusions were all but forgotten for about a century, until in the second half of the twentieth century interest in the wiping reflex in frogs was revived in several laboratories.

Brothers Emst Heinrich (1795–1878), Wilhelm Eduard (1804–1891), and Eduard Friedrich Wilhelm Weber (1806–1871) were among the first to realize the importance of accurate mechanical observation and analysis of biological movement. Wilhelm and Eduard published in 1894 a book *The Mechanics of Human Walking Apparatus* based on studies performed between 1825 and 1838. In that book, they emphasized the importance of the mechanical (pendulum-like) motion of the leg during locomotion and suggested that this motion occurred under the action of gravity, without active participation of the muscles. This concept was not confirmed in later studies.

Etienne-Jules Marey (1830–1904) and Eadweard J. Muybridge (1830–1904) developed photographic methods specifically for the analysis of natural movements. They made sequences of photographs at a high speed and analyzed changes in the

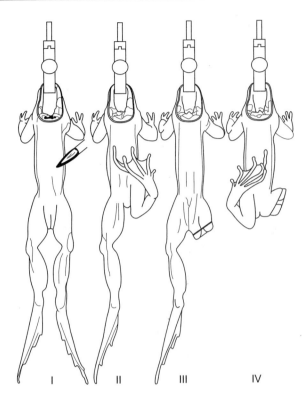

Figure 2.3 An illustration of Pflüger's experiments on decapitated frogs. Placing a stimulus on the frog's back (I) leads to a wiping motion by the ipsilateral (same side) hindlimb (II). If the hindlimb has been cut off (III), the wiping is produced by the contralateral (opposite side) hindlimb (IV). Reproduced from M. Verworn: *Die Mechanik des Geisteslebens*, 1907. Public domain.

configuration of the body and its segments in different phases of the movements. Ultimately, Marey achieved a speed of 60 frames per second in his recordings. He applied his inventions to the study of the gait of horses and humans as well as flying of birds and insects. Muybridge was famous for his photographs of locomoting humans and animals, particularly horses (Figure 2.4). These high-speed photographic methods allowed researchers to perform analysis of movement kinematics and to make inferences about the role of different forces in biological movements.

Action–perception, motor variability, and neuroanatomy

During the nineteenth century, the main question of how the soul controls the body was transformed into a different form better suited for research, namely, how the brain controls movement.

Hermann Ludwig Ferdinand von Helmholtz (1821–1894) contributed significantly to physics, biology, mathematics, engineering, medicine (he invented the ophthalmoscope—a device that allows us to look inside the eye), and philosophy. In

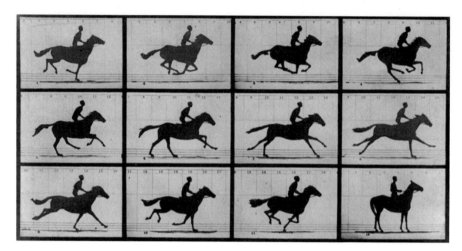

Figure 2.4 A sequence of photographs of the running horse made by Eadweard J. Muybridge in 1878. Images are from Wikimedia Commons. Library of Congress Prints and Photographs Division.

particular, von Helmholtz paid attention to the following observation. If you close one eye and move the other eye or the head in a natural way, changes in the image of external objects on the retina are correctly interpreted as your own motion while the environment is perceived as motionless. However, if you close one eye and press on the other eyeball with a finger, motion of the eyeball is associated with a feeling that the external world moves. Note that pressing on an eyeball leads to displacement of the image of the environment over the retina. This observation suggests that human perception depends not only on sensory signals but also on accompanying motor action. Approximately at the same time, the Russian physiologist Ivan Sechenov (1829–1905) also emphasized the role of activity in perception. Sechenov wrote: "We do not hear but listen, we do not see but look."

At the very end of the nineteenth century researchers started to pay attention to the fact that even well practiced human movements are frequently inaccurate. In 1899, Robert Sessions Woodworth (1869–1962) wrote a PhD dissertation under the direction of James McKenn Cattell (1860–1944). In that dissertation, Woodworth focused on errors and variability in motor performance. Based on those studies, he came up with arguably one of the first inferences on motor control: he concluded that control of a fast movement consists of an initial pulse and later corrections, an idea that in our day is frequently formulated as a combination of feed-forward and feedback control processes. Woodworth also studied the dependence of motor errors on movement speed and discovered that the errors increased with speed (see Section 12.1) when movements were performed with the eyes open but they stayed unchanged when similar movements were performed with the eyes closed (Figure 2.5).

In the late nineteenth and early twentieth centuries, progress in methods of studying the functional anatomy of the nervous system stimulated further research into the neural mechanisms involved in the control of movements. Santiago Ramon Y Cajal (1852–1934) provided essential support for the idea of the nervous system consisting of

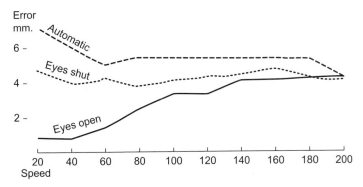

Figure 2.5 The dependences of motor error (in mm) on movement speed (in mm/s). Note the increase in the error with speed for movements performed with the eyes open, but not for movements performed with the eyes closed. Reproduced from R. S. Woodworth: *The accuracy of voluntary movement*, 1899. Public domain.

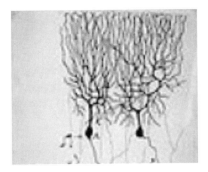

Figure 2.6 A drawing of the large Purkinje cells and small granule cells from the pigeon cerebellum by Santiago Ramón y Cajal, 1899. Instituto Santiago Ramón y Cajal, Madrid, Spain. The image is from Wikimedia Commons.

independent interacting neurons. Figure 2.6 shows drawings by Ramon Y Cajal of two types of neurons in the cerebellum—the tiny granule cells and the huge Purkinje cells famous for their dendritic trees (see Section 10.6). About the same time, Sir Michael Foster (1826–1907) and Sir Charles Sherrington (1852–1952) coined the term "synapsis" (later changed into "synapse") for hypothetical sites of interaction between pairs of neurons.

2.2   Classical biomechanics and neurophysiology of the twentieth century

Synergies, reflexes, and central pattern generators

Two great neurologists laid the foundation for many of the current approaches to the problem of control of multi-muscle systems. The notion of muscle synergies was introduced by the French scientist Joseph Felix Francois Babinski (1857–1932). Babinski compared the coordinated activity of muscles in patients with neurological disorders with that in healthy persons. In 1899, he linked impaired muscle coordination to pathology in the cerebellum and called such poorly coordinated movements "cerebellar asynergias." About the same time, the British neurologist J. Hughlings Jackson (1835–1911) introduced a theory of a three-level representation of movements in the central nervous system. He wrote about cortical representations of individual muscles and muscle groups in numerous combinations, which take part in most complex and highly specialized movements.

Sir Charles Sherrington was one of the founding fathers of contemporary neurophysiology. His contributions to the field are too many to be enumerated. In particular, Sherrington introduced the idea of *active inhibition* within the central nervous system as a method of movement coordination. He also described and emphasized the importance of reflex connections from peripheral receptors to motoneurons in the spinal cord producing muscle contractions. He was arguably the first to view muscle reflexes not as hardwired stereotypical responses to stimuli but rather as flexible mechanisms that formed the basis of motor behavior. Figure 2.7 illustrates the classical experiments by Sherrington on the reciprocal patterns of reflex activation in flexor and extensor muscles of the cat knee produced by the stimulation of peripheral nerves. The right-hand drawing illustrates a scheme including excitatory connections from *receptors* within a muscle on *motoneurons* that produce contraction of this muscle and inhibitory projections on motoneurons innervating the antagonist muscle. Sherrington thought of voluntary movements as combinations of reflexes with tunable parameters. As we will see later,

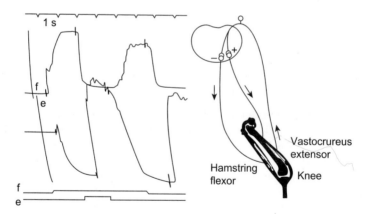

Figure 2.7 Sherrington's experiments on the reciprocal patterns of reflex activation. The left drawing shows flexor (f) and extensor (e) responses to the stimulation of the ipsilateral peroneal nerve (f—below) and contralateral peroneal nerve (e—below). The right drawing illustrates a scheme with excitatory connections from receptors within a muscle on motoneurons that produce contraction of that muscle and inhibitory projections on motoneurons innervating the antagonist muscle. Reproduced from Sherrington, C. S. (1913). Reflex inhibition as a factor in the co-ordination of movements and postures. *Quarterly Journal of Experimental Psychology, 6*, 251–310. Public domain.

these views were very important for the foundation of the equilibrium-point hypothesis, one of the most influential motor control hypotheses (see Section 8.3).

One of Sherrington's students, Thomas Graham Brown (1882–1965), focused on the ability of the spinal cord to produce coordinated movements in the absence of input from peripheral receptors, that is, in animals without reflexes. His studies of locomotion led him to conclude that the spinal cord contained neural structures able to produce rhythmic patterns without a sensory input. Later, such structures were termed *central pattern generators* (see Section 10.2). The argument on the role of reflexes mediated by sensory feedback signals and pattern generation by structures within the central nervous system continued for many years. Most recently, similar discussions took place between the competing ideas of motor programming vs. perception–action coupling and between internal models vs. equilibrium-point control (covered in Sections 5.1, 5.3, 8.3, 9.3, and 9.6).

Problems with mechanical analysis, progress in biomechanics

Contemporary motor control is based on the solid basis of the mechanical analysis of movements developed over the twentieth century. This analysis was built on classical Newtonian mechanics, which is one of the best developed fields of physics. Nevertheless, analysis of biological movement progressed slowly for a number of reasons. In particular, the mechanical properties of the elements in the human body cannot be measured with high accuracy, except in cadavers (see Sections 13.1 and 13.2). However, these properties in living organisms differ from those in cadaver specimens. For example, during active muscle contractions, the shape of the muscles and the blood flow through the muscles change, leading to changes in such basic characteristics as moment of inertia of the moving segments. Other properties of muscles that define the dependence of their force on muscle length and velocity (see Section 3.1) also change during active movements. One of the most common methods of identifying mechanical properties of inanimate objects is application of controlled force perturbations and measuring the object's response. In live muscles, however, the presence of reflex connections (see Section 3.4) leads to changes in the properties of the muscles after a very short time delay. As a result, two measurements of a system—before a perturbation and after a perturbation—cannot be directly compared because they reflect a system with two different sets of mechanical characteristics.

Several brilliant scientists contributed to our current understanding of the physiological and mechanical properties of the muscle. Sir Archibald Vivian Hill (1886–1977) studied both muscle mechanics and thermodynamics. Among his numerous contributions to muscle physiology and mechanics are the discovery of the mechanisms of heat production in the muscle, the introduction of the notions of *active state* and *series elastic element*, which are commonly used in modern models of muscle behavior, and the introduction of the famous *Hill equation* describing the relation between muscle force and rate of change of the muscle length (see Section 3.1). Hill focused on quantifying mechanical muscle properties using ingenious methods and ended up concluding that the classical physical notions of stiffness and viscosity were inapplicable to muscles.

A contemporary of Hill, Wallace Osgood Fenn (1893–1971) performed classical studies of heat production during muscle action and showed that muscles did not behave as pre-stretched passive springs. The increase of the total energy (mechanical work + heat) liberated during muscle contraction with the increase of mechanical work was later named the *Fenn effect*. Fenn also performed classical studies on the storage and release of energy in tendons and muscles and energy transfer among body parts.

Warren Plimpton Lombard (1855–1939) explored many issues related to motor activity, such as the knee jerk, muscular fatigue, and metabolism. He formulated the famous *Lombard paradox* after observing the coactivation of quadriceps and hamstring muscles during the transition from sitting to standing, despite the fact that these muscles have been traditionally viewed as antagonists to each other. The bi-articular rectus femoris has a smaller hip moment arm than the hamstrings. However, the rectus femoris moment arm is greater over the knee. This means that contraction from both rectus femoris and hamstrings will result in hip and knee extension. Hip extension also adds a passive stretch component to rectus femoris, which results in a knee extension force. The seeming paradox is due to the bi-articular muscle action and fits well the classical mechanics. One of the consequences of the Lombard paradox is that a bi-articular muscle can accelerate a segment in a direction opposite to the direction of the moment of force the muscle produces with respect to the axis of rotation of that segment.

Early electromyography

Studies of patterns of electrical muscle signals during voluntary movements became common in the middle of the twentieth century (see Section 13.3). One of the pioneers of these studies was Kurt Wachholder (1893–1961), who was the first to describe the triphasic electromyographic (EMG) pattern during fast single-joint movements performed by a human subject (see Sections 6.2 and 13.3). Wachholder and his colleague Hans Altenburger published a series of 11 papers between 1923 and 1928, in which they analyzed changes in the triphasic EMG pattern with changes in movement characteristics. They were particularly interested in interactions between a pair of muscles crossing a joint—an *agonist* and an *antagonist*.

In one of those studies, Wachholder and Altenburger asked a very simple question: How can muscles be relaxed at different joint positions in the absence of an external load? Indeed, if two muscles acting at a joint are relaxed at a certain position, motion of the joint would lead to stretching one muscle and shortening the other one. Muscle elastic properties should produce forces that have to move the joint back to the initial position. So, if a joint is to stay at the new position, muscle activation levels must change to counteract those elastic forces. This logic led Wachholder and Altenburger to perform meticulous studies of muscle activation levels at different joint positions. As a result, they concluded that muscles could indeed be relaxed at different joint positions, and that, consequently, elastic muscle properties were regulated by the central nervous system—an amazing insight for the 1920s!

The discovery of the system of *gamma-motoneurons*—small neurons in the spinal cord that send signals to muscle spindles, structures that contain receptors sensitive to muscle length and velocity—resulted in arguably the first motor control hypothesis, introduced by the British physiologist Patrick Anthony Merton (1920–2000). This hypothesis is discussed in detail in Section 7.2.

2.3 Nikolai Bernstein and the levels of movement construction

Bernstein—the father of motor control

The numerous contributions of Nikolai Alexandrovich Bernstein (1896–1966) to movement science lead us to consider him as the father of contemporary motor control. Bernstein was trained as a physician and worked for several years, during World War I and the Civil War in Russia, in a military hospital. Later, he joined the newly formed Institute of Labor, and developed there a number of methods for quantitative movement analysis and performed his now classical studies of the kinematics and kinetics of a variety of movements.

One of his novel methods for mechanical analysis of movements, *kimocyclography*, was based on the mentioned earlier works by Marey and Muybridge and also on the mechanical analysis of movements by Christian Wilhelm Braune (1831–1892) and his student Otto Fisher (1861–1917). Bernstein used a camera with a film that moved slowly at a constant speed. A rotating shutter opened the lens for a short time every revolution and made a shot of a set of light bulbs placed on the subject. This resulted in a sequence of stick-figure images spaced by time intervals reflecting the speed of the shutter rotation. Bernstein had absolute pitch and used it to measure the frequency of shutter rotation by the pitch of the accompanying buzz. For example, in his analysis of the mechanics of arm motion during piano playing by professional pianists, Bernstein achieved the amazing frequency of about 500 images per second. In those studies, he performed mechanical analysis of motion of the multi-joint chain (the arm), estimated the contribution of *interaction torques* (see Section 5.2), and concluded that motion of the proximal segments had minimal impact on the interaction of the fingers with the keys.

In the 1920s, Bernstein recorded professional blacksmiths hitting a chisel with a hammer. Figure 2.8 illustrates one of those studies with the consecutive positions of the arm segments and the hammer. Obviously, his subjects were perfectly trained, they had performed the same movement many times a day for years. Using kimocyclography, Bernstein noticed that the variability of the trajectory of the tip of the hammer across a series of strikes was smaller than the variability of the trajectories of individual joints of the subject's arm holding the hammer. Obviously, the brain could not send signals directly to the hammer, only to muscles that moved the joints. Rotations of individual joints produced motion of the hammer. How could noisy movements of the joints lead to accurate trajectories of the hammer? Bernstein concluded that the joints were not acting independently but correcting each other's errors. This observation suggested that, even in the best-trained subjects, the central nervous system did not produce a unique, optimal solution for the motor task but

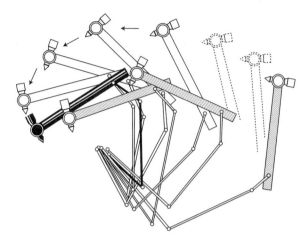

Figure 2.8 Consecutive positions of the arm segments and the hammer during a striking move-ment. Reproduced from Bernstein, N. A. (1923). Studies on the biomechanics of hitting using optical recording. *Annals of the Central Institute of Labor, 1*, 19–79. (in Russian). Public domain.

rather used a whole variety of joint trajectories to ensure a more accurate (less variable) trajectory of the hammer over repetitive strikes.

The name of Bernstein is associated with recognition of the importance of the problem of *motor redundancy* (see Section 3.5). This problem seems to emerge at any level of description of the neuromotor system. Any such level is characterized by more elements than the number of typical constraints associated with motor tasks. Bernstein formulated this problem as the *elimination of redundant degrees-of-freedom*. Currently, the problem of motor redundancy is commonly known as the *Bernstein problem*.

Construction of Movements According to Bernstein

Over much of his lifetime, Bernstein was developing a theory of the construction of movements. It was published in most detail in his book *On the Construction of Movements* in 1947 (never translated in full into English), and in a slightly washed-down but more accessible form for less prepared readers in a book called *Dexterity and Its Development* published in English in 1996. This theory is still very far from being obsolete although some of its elements, in particular links between the levels of movement construction and specific neurophysiological structures, would probably be described differently by Bernstein today.

Bernstein suggested a *multi-level system* for the construction of movements. The levels were associated both with certain classes of motor tasks and task components and with different involvement of neurophysiological structures and pathways. The main levels identified by Bernstein were:

- Level A, the *paleokinetic level*, or the rubro-spinal level;
- Level B, the *level of synergies* and patterns, or the thalamo-pallidal level;

- Level C, the *level of the spatial field*, or the pyramido-striatal level had two parts:
  - C1—striatal, extrapyramidal; and
  - C2—pyramidal, related to cortical control;
- Level D, the *level of actions* (object actions, meaningful actions, etc.), or the parietal-premotor level; and
- Level E, the *level of symbolic, highly coordinated actions* such as speech, writing, etc., based on "highest cortical" control.

As follows from this nomenclature, Bernstein already realized the crucial importance of such structures as the *spinal cord*, the *red nucleus*, the *basal ganglia* (*pallidum* and *striatum*), the *thalamus*, and different areas of the *cortex* for the control of movements (see corresponding sections in Chapter 10). Although this list does not mention the *cerebellum* explicitly, Bernstein was well aware of its importance.

According to Bernstein, nearly all human movements are built on several levels. One of the levels plays a leading role, while other levels play subordinate roles providing necessary support, which is typically not perceived consciously.

Level A

This level typically plays a subordinate role during natural actions, in particular ensuring adequate postural components of actions. Its sensory support comes primarily from *proprioceptors*, that is receptors that inform the central nervous system on body configuration and forces between body parts (see Section 3.3). Bernstein presents a few examples of movements when this level may be leading. These examples involve very quick vibrating actions (such as vibrato during piano playing), quick jerky reactions to unexpected stimuli (for example, the well-known startle reaction to an unexpected loud sound), and specific body postures, for example in some gymnastic exercises. One of the main functions of level A is to provide reliable reflex function mediated by the spinal cord. One of the best-known examples of this function is *reciprocal inhibition* (see Section 3.4).

Level A is also the level at which *muscle tone* is defined and regulated. Muscle tone is one of the most commonly used misnomers in the field of movement studies. Most commonly, this expression is used without a clear definition, based on the subjective impression by a clinician of the resistance offered by muscles (and other structures) to passive motion of a body segment. Bernstein offers an explicit definition of muscle tone: "tone is a fluid state of preparedness of the neuromuscular periphery to selective acceptance of the effector process (in our day, we would call this 'efferent process') and its realization." This definition implies that muscle tone reflects preparation to action and, thus, it can hardly be measured by asking a person to relax completely and then moving his or her body segments passively.

The name *rubro-spinal level* emphasizes an important role of the red nucleus, a relatively small structure in the brain, which is the origin of one of the fast-conducting descending pathways, the rubro-spinal tract (see Section 10.6). Bernstein knew that the red nucleus produced its output based on many processes involving the basal ganglia and the cerebellum. He viewed the rubro-spinal tract as playing a particularly important role in regulating the reflex function of the spinal cord and the *tone*.

Since level A provides support for virtually all voluntary actions by ensuring proper reflex function and preparation of spinal structures to neural commands from the brain, dysfunctions at this level lead to major movement disorders, particularly those associated with pathological changes in tone. These include *hypotonic* (lower than normal tone) and *hypertonic* (higher than normal tone) states as well as a complex disorder called *dystonia*. Bernstein also considered one of the main clinical signs of *Parkinson's disease*, parkinsonian tremor, a dysfunction of level A, while other major signs of this disease were attributed to higher levels.

Level B

At this level, large muscle groups are united to produce coordinated movement patterns. Like level A, level B uses proprioception as its main source of sensory information. Bernstein viewed level B as the level where synergies were formed. He used the word *synergy* as meaning "many muscles working together"; a somewhat different definition will be suggested and developed later (see Section 9.4). A typical example of a coordinated movement pattern involving numerous muscles is *loco-motion*. Note that locomotion can be produced by the spinal cord without any input from the brain (see Section 11.2); this suggests an important role of the spinal cord in level B processes. Sensory support for actions at level B is mostly proprioceptive.

Level B has been assumed to play an important role in the control of kinematic chains (such as multi-joint human limbs), taking into consideration reactive and *motion-dependent forces* (see Sections 5.1 and 5.2). These forces are very different for movements along the same trajectory performed at different speeds. So, level B is involved in movement construction in time and in correct switching of synergies in different movement phases.

Relatively few movements are controlled at level B. Examples involve locomotion (without a specific target), dance, and some gymnastic exercises. These movements are mostly body-centered and have no goal in the environment. There is a tendency towards repeatability of patterns in actions controlled at level B. While rarely leading in voluntary actions, level B provides very important background for most actions. In particular, it supports the natural tendency towards dynamically stable movements, that is movements that return to about the same trajectory after a small transient perturbation (see Section 9.3) without any smart corrective action from the neural controller.

Disorders at level B may lead to both hypokinetic and hyperkinetic syndromes, that is conditions characterized by poverty of movements and by excessive move-ments. A typical example of the former is the abovementioned Parkinson's disease. Examples of the latter involve dystonias and a few other disorders, including *Huntington's chorea*. Bernstein mentioned hyperkinetic asynergias (lack of coordi-nation within large muscle groups) as possible consequences of level B dysfunctions.

Level C

Actions at this level are performed in a *spatial field*. Spatial field is a portion of external space accessible for specific actions with all the associated forces, obstacles, and all the sensory signals relevant to the surrounding space and its objective perception (such as proprioception, touch, vision, and vestibular system). Today, psychologists would likely associate the notion of spatial field with the notion of *affordances* developed somewhat later by the famous American psychologist James Gibson (1904–1979). A typical action organized at level C is transporting an object from one point in space to another. Movements at this level are always leading from somewhere to somewhere, usually for a purpose. The spatial field and actions in this field are characterized by *geometry* and *metrics*: One can move an object along a straight or curved trajectory, over a larger or a smaller distance. Control of these movements is always associated with taking into account the action of external forces such as gravity and forces of interaction with external objects.

Bernstein identified two sublevels at level C. Simply put, level C2 cares primarily about achieving a desired ultimate result, while level C1 specifies a way of getting to that result. For example, the task of transporting a cup of hot tea from one place to another is formulated at level C2. Depending on a person's posture with respect to the cup and other factors, the task can be performed with the right hand or with the left hand, with or without standing up from the chair etc. A specific way of transporting the cup of tea is specified at level C1.

Since movements at level C involve targets, they may be characterized by *accuracy* and *variability*. Bernstein emphasized adaptive variability in such actions, that is variability in the way of executing a task that does not affect success of the task (later, we will address it as *good variability*, Section 9.4). He emphasized the phenomena of *error compensation* among the groups of involved joints or limbs and the *equifinality* of actions, which may even involve using different effectors in different trials. One of the most famous Bernstein's examples is writing a phrase with an implement held by different effectors, by the right hand, by the left hand, gripped by the teeth, and attached to one of the elbows or to one of the feet. With respect to actions at level C, Bernstein coined one of his most famous phrases: "Repetition without repetition." He implied that repeating an attempt to solve a task is associated with variable patterns of movements. The variability of movement patterns that could solve similar tasks led Bernstein to an assumption on the importance of *plasticity* within the central nervous system for changes in movement patterns with practice and in cases of motor disorders.

Pathologies at level C were supposed to be associated with such movement disorders as *ataxias* (discoordinated involvement of elements, such as joints) and *dysmetrias* (movements over incorrect distances). While Bernstein linked level C to the cortical structures and the basal ganglia, today ataxias and dysmetrias are viewed as linked to cerebellar disorders (see Section 10.6).

Level D

Actions controlled at the next level, level D, are performed nearly exclusively by humans. Bernstein mentioned possible involvement of this level in the control of some actions in elephants, dogs, and apes. This level deals with meaningful actions, not simply moving a cup of tea from one place to another but serving a guest with the cup of tea neatly placed on the plate. Level D actions can use any sensory system, the most important aspect is that the sensory signals should deliver relevant information. Bernstein emphasized the importance of shape and geometrical features such as *topology*, less so metrics. For example, if the task is to write the letter "a," there are many ways to perform the task, with different implements, on different surfaces, with letters of different size and style of writing. However, the final product should be ultimately recognizable as letter "a," not another letter or a non-letter. Distinguishing all objects that are recognized as letter "a" from all objects that are not is a complex issue, which is beyond the scope of this book.

Actions at level D involve *automatisms* and *motor skills*. Sometimes, these actions are counterintuitive. For example, to extract a screw from a wooden board, you do not try to pull it in the direction orthogonal to the board, but use a screwdriver to rotate it. In this example, the direction of action does not coincide with the direction of the desired outcome. Actions at this level demonstrate strong hand (foot) preference. For example, the non-dominant hand is better suited for steady-state tasks such as holding the nail, while the dominant hand is better at controlling fast actions such as hitting the nail with the hammer (see also Section 11.3).

Motor disorders at level D are mainly manifested by *apraxias*. This term implies problems with achieving a meaningful final result without obvious problems with motor coordination. A person may be perfectly able to use a screwdriver, but turns it in a wrong direction or tries to use it to pull the screw directly from the board.

Level E

This is a purely human level. It deals with actions that are associated with information transmission, for example using writing or speech to transmit a message to another person. Other examples of movements led by level E are those involved in musical performance, painting, and similar actions. Obviously, all the relevant sources of sensory information are used to construct and guide such movements.

Let me illustrate the described scheme with a reasonably common action, for example writing a brief letter to a friend on a piece of paper. The specific message one wants to transmit will lead the action at level E (Figure 2.9, top). At this level, the message will be converted into a sequence of words (one of many possible sequences that can be used to transmit the message). The next step is to ensure that all the characters are written legibly, spaced correctly, there are breaks between the words, the lines are parallel to each other, etc. Level D will take care of the proper arrangement of all the elements of the handwriting to ensure that they produce the desired sequence of words (Figure 2.9, bottom).

The writing movements will depend on many factors characterizing the spatial field where the movement takes place. For example, different grips may be used to write with a pen or a pencil; the grip may also depend on the friction of the surface of the pen/pencil. The piece of paper may be oriented differently with respect to the body. The paper may rest on a horizontal surface or on a slightly tilted surface. You may decide to write with smaller or larger letters. And so on. Level C2 will ensure that all the characters are written legibly and correctly (Figure 2.10, top). Level C1 will try to avoid clumsy postures of the arm and hand during the writing (Figure 2.10, bottom).

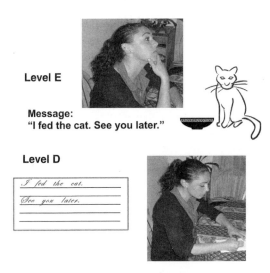

Figure 2.9 This figure and also Figures 2.10 and 2.11 illustrate the five (six) levels of movement construction using the action of writing a simple message to a friend. The specific message one wants to transmit will lead the action (level E, top). Level D (bottom) takes care of the arrangement of all the elements of the handwriting.

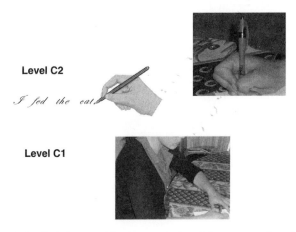

Figure 2.10 Level C will define specific characteristics of the motor action given the external conditions of its execution. Level C2 will ensure that all the characters are written legibly and correctly (top). Level C1 will try to avoid clumsy postures of the arm and hand during the writing (bottom).

Assume that the pen is held with the dominant hand. Its trajectory will depend on coordinated rotations of the many joints of the human hand and arm. These rotations will be produced by dozens of muscles and will also depend on the external forces such as those between the pen and the paper and the force of gravity. If you try to write faster, velocity-dependent forces and moments of force will change, and the muscle involvement will have to adjust correspondingly. There will also be reactive forces acting on the trunk, which will have to be counteracted by changes in the activation of postural muscles. All these adjustments are organized at level B (Figure 2.11, top).

Finally, level A will take care of proper functioning of the spinal reflexes (see Section 3.4) and ensure sufficient steady activation of postural muscles of the trunk and legs so that the body does not collapse on the floor in the process of writing (Figure 2.11, bottom). It will also be responsible for maintaining a proper background of activation of proximal muscles of the arm to make sure that the arm posture is adequate for the task.

Although Bernstein developed this scheme over 50 years ago, it is still far from obsolete. This was the first scheme that offered an explicit decomposition of a meaningful motor act into a set of hierarchically organized steps spanning all the levels of the central nervous system and incorporating notions from psychology to physiology to physics. Despite the recent progress in different subfields of motor control, there is still no other scheme that addresses all the main steps of action production and is as specific as the scheme offered by Bernstein.

Level B

Level A

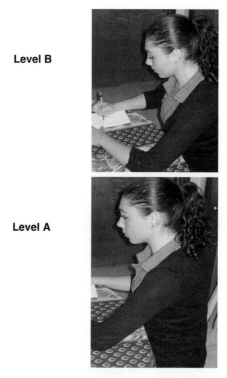

Figure 2.11 Adjustments of muscle activation necessary to perform the action given its speed, reactive forces among segments of the arm, and other factors will be performed at level B (top). Level A (bottom) will take care of providing adequate, steady activation of postural muscles of the proximal arm muscles, legs, and trunk.

Self-test questions

1. What makes the soul command the body to move according to Pythagoras and Aristotle?
2. How are the muscles made to produce force according to Galen?
3. Present examples of biological movements dependent on and independent of the soul (according to Descartes).
4. When was the idea that voluntary movements are based on combinations of automatic responses to sensory stimuli proposed?
5. How are movements produced according to Borelli?
6. When were the electrical processes in muscles discovered?
7. Describe the "wiping reflex" in the frog. What parts of the central nervous system are involved in this reflex?
8. When did photography start being used for movement analysis?
9. Present examples of motor action dependence on sensory stimuli and perception dependence on motor action.
10. When did movement errors become objects of scientific research?
11. When was the idea of synapse suggested? What is a synapse?
12. What are synergies and asynergias according to Hughlings Jackson, Babinski, and Bernstein?
13. Mention a few major contributions of Sir Charles Sherrington to neurophysiology.
14. What was the major discrepancy between the views on locomotion of Sherrington and Graham Brown?
15. Why is it hard to use Newtonian mechanics to study human movements?
16. What was the view of Sir Archibald Vivian Hill on the applicability of the classical notions of stiffness and viscosity to human muscles?
17. What is the Fenn effect?
18. What is the Lombard paradox?
19. Who were the first to describe the triphasic pattern of muscle activation during fast movements?
20. What discovery formed the foundation for the motor control hypothesis by Merton?
21. What method did Bernstein use to reach the very high time resolution in movement analysis?
22. What was the main observation made by Bernstein in his classical study of blacksmiths?
23. What is the Bernstein problem?
24. Name the main levels in the Bernstein scheme of movement construction.
25. What is muscle tone according to Bernstein?
26. What neurophysiological structures are associated with level A within the Bernstein scheme?
27. What movements are led by processes at level B?
28. At what level are synergies formed according to Bernstein?
29. Define spatial field.
30. What kind of movement pathologies may be expected when processes at level C malfunction?
31. Present examples of actions organized at level D.
32. Use a meaningful movement (not the example in the book) to illustrate the levels of movement construction according to Bernstein.

Essential references and recommended further readings

Bernstein, N. A. (1967). *The co-ordination and regulation of movements.* Oxford: Pergamon Press.
Bernstein, N. A. (1996). On dexterity and its development. In M. L. Latash, & M. T. Turvey (Eds.), *Dexterity and its development* (pp. 1–244). Mahwah, NJ: Erlbaum Publishers.

Cappozzo, A., Marchetti, M., & Tosi, V. (Eds.). (1992). *Biolocomotion: a century of research using moving pictures.* Roma: Italy. Promograph.

Gelfand, I. M. (1991). Two archetypes in the psychology of man. *Nonlinear Science Today, 1,* 11–16.

Gelfand, I. M., & Latash, M. L. (1998). On the problem of adequate language in movement science. *Motor Control, 2,* 306–313.

Gelfand, I. M., & Tsetlin, M. L. (1966). On mathematical modeling of the mechanisms of the central nervous system. In I. M. Gelfand, V. S. Gurfinkel, S. V. Fomin, & M. L. Tsetlin (Eds.), *Models of the structural-functional organization of certain biological systems* (pp. 9–26). Moscow: Nauka, (in Russian, a translation is available in 1971 edition by MIT Press, Cambridge, MA).

Hill, A. V. (1938). The heat of shortening and the dynamic constants of muscle. *Proceedings of the Royal Society of London, Series B, 126,* 136–195.

Hill, A. V. (1953). The mechanics of active muscle. *Proceedings of the Royal Society of London, Series B, 141,* 104–117.

Latash, M. L. (2006). A new book by Nikolai Bernstein: Contemporary studies in the physiology of the neural process. *Motor Control, 10,* 1–6.

Latash, M. L. (2008). *Synergy.* New York: Oxford University Press.

Latash, M. L., & Zatsiorsky, V. M. (Eds.). (2001). *Classics in movement science.* Urbana, IL: Human Kinetics.

Liddell, E. G. T., & Sherrington, C. S. (1924). Reflexes in response to stretch (myotatic reflexes). *Proceedings of the Royal Society of London, Series B, 96,* 212–242.

Meijer, O. (2002). Bernstein versus Pavlovianism: an interpretation. In M. L. Latash (Ed.), *Progress in motor control, Vol. 2. Structure-function relations in voluntary movement* (pp. 229–250). Urbana, IL: Human Kinetics.

Sherrington, C. S. (1906). *The integrative action of the nervous system.* London.

Sherrington, C. S. (1910). Flexion reflex of the limb, crossed extension reflex, and reflex stepping and standing. *Journal of Physiology, 40,* 28–121.

Smith, A. M. (1993). Babinski and movement synergism. *Revue Neurologique (Paris), 149,* 764–770.

Whiting, H. T. A. (1984). *Human motor actions: Bernstein reassessed.* Amsterdam: Elsevier.

3 Features of the system for movement production

Chapter Outline

3.1 The muscle

Excitability. The action potential

Neural and muscle cells belong to the class of excitable cells. This means that in certain conditions they can produce an electrical signal, a short-lasting change in the potential across the membrane that separates the cell from the environment. These are called *action potentials*. Typical responses of a membrane to external stimuli of different amplitude are illustrated in Figure 3.1. When the membrane is in a state of equilibrium, its transmembrane potential (*equilibrium potential*, V_{EQ} in Figure 3.1) is negative. If an external small stimulus is applied that changes the potential towards

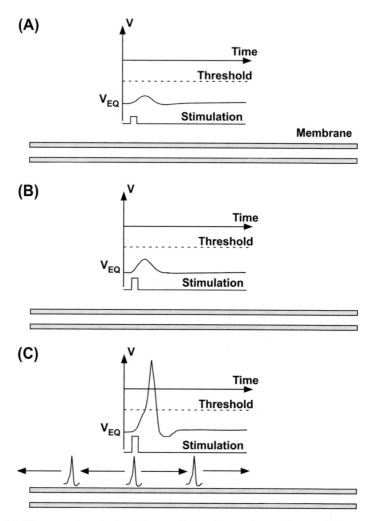

Figure 3.1 When an external stimulation applied to the membrane of an excitable cell leads to its depolarization, the effects of the stimulation depend on its magnitude. (A and B) When the stimulation amplitude is small, an increase in its magnitude leads to an increase in transient changes in the membrane potential, which quickly returns to its equilibrium value (V_{EQ}). (C) When the stimulation reaches a certain threshold, an action potential is generated representing a large-amplitude quick change in the membrane potential. If a membrane is stimulated at a certain site, an action potential will emerge and will travel in both directions from the site of stimulation (bottom drawing).

less negative values (*depolarization*), the effects of the stimulus depend on whether the membrane potential reaches a certain threshold value. Note that small stimuli, as in panels A and B of Figure 3.1, lead to relatively small-amplitude transient changes in the membrane potential that do not have effects over large distances. A larger stimulus (like the one in Figure 3.1C) produces a large-amplitude action potential. The shape and amplitude of the action potential do not depend on the amplitude of the stimulus. So, applying a stronger stimulus results in the same membrane response. An action potential is produced only if the membrane depolarization reaches a specific threshold value. Action potentials can travel over the membrane over large distances.

The characteristics of an action potential, such as its time profile and peak amplitude, are highly standardized for a given tissue and external conditions (in particular, temperature). As a result, all action potentials generated by a cell are identical to each other (there are important exceptions, for example action potentials generated by the large output cells of the cerebellum, the Purkinje cells, see Section 10.6). This is referred to as the *all-or-none law*. According to this law, a neuron or a muscle cell can generate either a standard action potential or nothing. As a result of this law, a neuron can send information to other cells by modulating the frequency of action potentials, not their amplitude.

Muscle contraction

Muscle contraction starts with a neural signal, an action potential arriving along a long neural fiber (the *axon*) from a neuron in the spinal cord (or in the brainstem, for neck and facial muscles), called an alpha-*motoneuron*, to a target muscle fiber (Figure 3.2A). When an action potential arrives at the junction between the neural fiber and a muscle cell, it triggers a sequence of physico-chemical effects that ultimately lead to changes in the membrane potential in the muscle cell. Such junctions are called *neuro-muscular synapses* (Figure 3.2B). Neuro-muscular synapses are obligatory: This means that an action potential arriving along a neural fiber always leads to the generation of an action potential in the muscle cell the fiber innervates.

An action potential running along the membrane of a muscle fiber triggers another sequence of physico-chemical events, ultimately leading to a brief episode of force production by molecular elastic links called *cross-bridges*. Muscles are unidirectional force generators, they can only pull but not push. That is why one has to have at least two muscles to control movement of a joint; these two muscles are commonly called *agonist* (a muscle that produces joint moment of force in a desired direction) and *antagonist* (a muscle that produces moment of force against the desired direction). Typical examples of agonist–antagonist pairs are flexor–extensor, adductor–abductor, etc.

If only one stimulus arrives at a muscle fiber, the cross-bridges disengage quickly and the muscle fiber relaxes. A typical time profile of force produced during such a single contraction (it is called *twitch contraction*) is shown in Figure 3.3A. Typical times of force rise and fall during a twitch contraction vary depending on muscle fiber properties; typical twitch contractions take about 50–100 ms to reach peak force. The phase of force decline is typically longer. This means that it is even harder to stop a muscle contraction abruptly than to initiate it quickly.

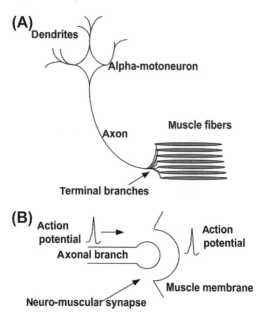

Figure 3.2 (A) A motoneuron is a neural cell which innervates a set of muscle fibers. It consists of a body, a tree of relatively short dendrites, and a long axon with terminal branches at its end. Each branch makes a synapse with a target muscle fiber. (B) The neuromuscular synapse is a complex anatomical structure consisting of a presynaptic neural fiber, the synaptic cleft, and a postsynaptic muscle fiber. An incoming action potential along the neural fiber always produces an action potential on the muscle fiber: This action is called obligatory.

If two stimuli come to a muscle fiber within a small time interval, the second stimulus may arrive while the first twitch contraction still continues. In this case, the second twitch contraction starts from an already elevated force level and reaches a higher peak force. If a sequence of stimuli comes to a muscle fiber at a high enough frequency, it may reach the state of *smooth tetanus* (Figure 3.3B), that is a state of high constant force production. Both twitch contractions and smooth tetanus are rare during everyday muscle function. More typically, muscle fibers receive action potentials that come at frequencies below those that could have produced smooth tetanus. Each muscle fiber produces a contraction consisting of peaks and valleys that neither reach the smooth tetanus force nor drop to zero; such contractions are called *saw-tooth tetanus* (as in the early portion of the contraction shown in Figure 3.3B). Whole-muscle contractions are typically smooth because the individual fibers produce twitch or saw-tooth tetanus contractions at different times.

Length and velocity dependence of muscle force

The magnitude of force produced by a muscle fiber in both twitch and tetanic contractions depends on that fiber's length and its rate of change (velocity). The dependences of muscle force on length and velocity depend partly on the properties of

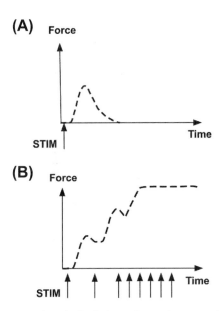

Figure 3.3 (A) Twitch contraction. A single incoming action potential along a neural finger produces a twitch contraction of the innervated muscle fiber. The twitch contraction is short-lasting (a few hundred milliseconds) and relatively low-amplitude. (B) Tetanic contraction. Here a sequence of action potentials comes at a high enough frequency to lead to overlapping twitches, ultimately resulting in a continuing muscle contraction—tetanus.

cross-bridges and partly on the properties of passive connective tissue, including those of tendons. In static conditions, longer muscle fibers produce larger forces in response to a standard stimulus up to a certain length, after which their force shows a drop (Figure 3.4). Note, however, that this drop is typically observed at fiber length values that are beyond the typical anatomical range. Sometimes, muscle behavior is described using the analogy of a non-linear spring with a damping element. This is a questionable analogy because some of the features of muscle contractions (see, for example, the

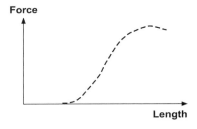

Figure 3.4 Force–length muscle characteristic. A typical dependence of the actively developed muscle force on muscle length (assuming constant level of muscle activation). In such studies, typically, muscle length is fixed at a certain value and a standard stimulation is applied. Then the muscle length is changed, and the procedure is repeated.

description of the studies of Fenn and Hill in Chapter 2) make them quite unlike those expected from damped springs. The simplest models of muscle contraction involve a force-producing element (cross-bridges), a parallel elastic element, a damping element in parallel with the contractile element, and another elastic element in series with the first three, reflecting the elastic properties of the tendons and other serially connected elements (Figure 3.5). Muscle action also depends on the external load.

When muscle fiber length changes, the force produced by the fiber shows a dependence on the fiber length velocity. When a muscle moves through a certain length while being stretched, its force is higher than that produced in static conditions (F_0) at the same length; when a muscle moves through the same length while it is shortening, the force is lower. This general relation is illustrated in Figure 3.6, which uses a more conventional way of plotting this relation, with positive velocity values corresponding to muscle stretch (traditionally, this illustration is drawn with positive velocity corresponding to muscle shortening). It was formalized by Sir Archibald Vivian Hill in the form of the famous Hill equation:

$$(F + a)V = b(F - F_0) \tag{3.1}$$

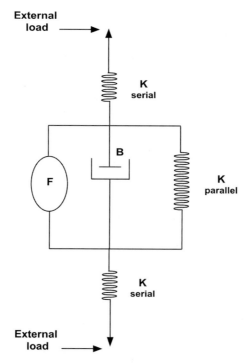

Figure 3.5 A typical Hill-type model of muscle action. Muscle fibers are represented as force generators (F) acting in parallel to a damping element (B) and a spring-like element (K parallel). Tendons can be modeled as spring-like elements (K serial) connected in series to the muscle fibers.

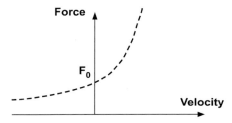

Figure 3.6 Force–velocity muscle characteristic. A typical dependence of active muscle force on velocity; F_0 corresponds to force produced by the muscle in static conditions.

where a and b are constants, F stands for muscle force, V is muscle fiber velocity, and F_0 is the force generated by the muscle at zero velocity, that is in static conditions.

Although muscles are unidirectional active force generators, both shortening and lengthening contractions happen all the time during natural movements. They are sometimes called *concentric* and *eccentric* contractions, respectively. This is because all joints are crossed by at least one pair of muscles acting in opposite directions. As a result, during any joint movements, one muscle stretches while the other one shortens. Commonly, both muscles show non-zero levels of activation during movements. This means that one of them performs a concentric contraction while the other one contracts eccentrically.

Motor units. Size principle

Human muscles are composed of large groups of muscle fibers innervated by neural cells (neurons) in the spinal cord or in the brainstem (for the muscles of the neck and head). The neurons that send action potentials to power-producing muscle fibers are called alpha-motoneurons. Each alpha-motoneuron sends its long branch (the axon) to a target muscle, the axon ends with a brush of relatively short branches, and each of these terminal branches makes a connection (innervates) a muscle fiber (Figure 3.7). In healthy

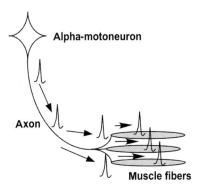

Figure 3.7 A motor unit consists of an alpha-motoneuron and muscle fibers innervated by its axon. These muscle fibers always contract together.

muscles, each muscle fiber is innervated by only one terminal branch. As a result, muscle fibers form groups that belong to a particular alpha-motoneuron innervating all the fibers from a group. When an alpha-motoneuron generates an action potential, all muscle fibers innervated by this alpha-motoneuron receive excitatory signals virtually simultaneously. Hence, an alpha-motoneuron and all the muscle fibers it innervates always work together and may be viewed as a unit of muscle action called a *motor unit*.

There are small and large motor units, fast and slow, fatiguable and fatigue-resistant. Motor unit size refers to the size of the alpha-motoneuron, the diameter of its axon, and the number of muscle fibers it innervates—all three typically correlate closely. Smaller alpha-motoneurons have thinner axons and innervate fewer muscle fibers (Figure 3.8A). They produce less force in twitch contractions (Figure 3.8B). In long-lasting, tetanic contractions, these motor units produce lower forces, they reach peak forces slowly, and they do not show a drop in force with time; in other words, they are fatigue-resistant (the left-hand plot in Figure 3.8C). In contrast, the largest motoneurons have thicker axons, innervate larger groups of muscle fibers, and produce more force. These motor units are typically faster and fatigue quickly (the right-hand plots in Figure 3.8). Note the different time scales in panels B and C of Figure 3.8.

During natural contractions with increasing force production, motor units are typically recruited in an orderly manner, starting from the smallest (slow) motor units,

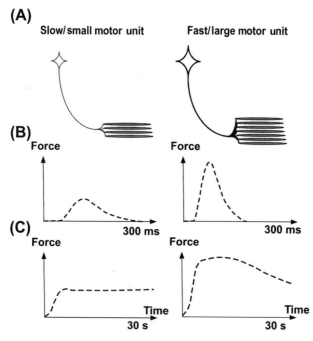

Figure 3.8 (A) An illustration of two motor units, slow/small and fast/large. (B) The fast/large motor unit shows quicker force production and higher peak force levels during a twitch contraction. (C) The fast/large motor unit shows a drop in force during a prolonged tetanic contraction (fatigue).

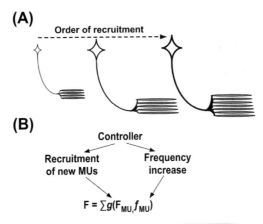

(A)

Order of recruitment

(B)

Controller

Recruitment
of new MUs

Frequency
increase

$$F = \sum g(F_{MU}, f_{MU})$$

Figure 3.9 (A) According to the size principle (Henneman principle), during natural contractions motor units are recruited in an orderly fashion, from small to large motor units. (B) The central nervous system has two mechanisms of increasing muscle activation level: recruiting new motor units (MUs) and increasing the firing frequency of already recruited motor units.

and then, with increased force requirements, gradually involving larger and larger (faster) motor units (Figure 3.9A). This rule is known as the *size principle* or the *Henneman principle*. Total muscle force represents a superposition of the forces produced by all the motor units within the muscle. Each motor unit can change its contribution to muscle force by changing the frequency of the action potentials generated by the respective alpha-motoneurons. In addition, muscle force can be modulated by changes in the number of recruited motor units. This gives the controller two methods of force modulation: (a) recruitment of motor units; and (b) changes in the frequency of action potentials of the recruited motor units (Figure 3.9B).

To summarize, human muscles are slow in force generation and in relaxation. The force they produce cannot be predicted in advance unless one knows all the details of movement kinematics, that is, changes in muscle length during the movement. Not surprisingly, Bernstein wrote in one of his early papers (in 1935) that the central nervous system could not in principle predict forces that would be produced as a result of its own central commands. These forces emerge as a result of an interaction of several factors, including the signals a muscle receives from the central nervous system and its actual state, length, and velocity.

3.2   Neurons and neural pathways

Neurons and action potential conduction

As mentioned earlier, neurons are threshold structures. This feature of neurons may be viewed either as a major complicating factor or a feature that is advantageous for the organism. The latter view has been developed in theories of motor control (to be described later, see Section 8.2) based on modification of neuronal activation thresholds. For example, such a method of control allows changing an input into a neuron or a group of neurons without producing any obvious output while preparing the system to produce an output when another input into the same neuron changes. It allows the system to behave in an adaptive way to changes in external variables that produce changes in inputs into neuronal pools.

Although the unit of information transmission (the action potential) is electrical, its speed of conduction within the human body is relatively slow, very far from the speed of the electric current. This is because action potentials do not truly travel along the membrane of excitable cells but rather emerge and disappear, giving rise to new action potentials on adjacent membrane segments. The process of action potential generation involves ion diffusion, which happens over short distances and, as a result, is fast, but not as fast as electric current. It takes just under 1 ms for the action potential to be generated after the membrane receives adequate excitation. This may not seem like a lot of time. However, consider that typical distances within the human body are on the order of 1 m, for example, the distance from the brain cortex to the lumbar enlargement of the spinal cord (which contains a number of neurons that control the lower part of the body) or the distance from the spinal cord, where the bodies of the alpha-motoneurons reside, to a muscle in a foot. Conducting an action potential generated over the membrane in the body of a neuron along its axon over a distance of about 1 m may take tens or hundreds of episodes of action potential generation along the axon. This may be expected to sum up to several tens or several hundred of milliseconds of time delay.

Myelinated fibers. Conduction delays

There are two types of neural fibers in the human body. Some of the fibers are covered with a sheath made of a fat-like substance, *myelin* (Figure 3.10). This sheath allows the action potentials to jump over relatively large distances between adjacent pairs of breaks in the *myelin sheath* (*Ranvier nodes*) and leads to a substantial increase in the conduction speed. For example, action potentials travel along the

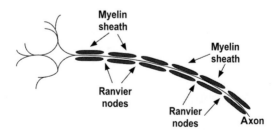

Figure 3.10 Myelinated axons are covered with a substance (myelin sheath) that increases the effective distance of local currents. Myelinated segments of the axon are interrupted with Ranvier nodes, where action potentials are generated. Under myelin, there are few ion channels, and action potential generation is impossible.

fastest conducting myelinated axons at a speed of up to 120 m/s. In contrast, axons that are not covered with myelin conduct action potentials at speeds of about 1 m/s or even slower.

However, even the fast-conducting myelinated fibers lead to time delays on the order of several tens of milliseconds over typical distances in the human body. For very fast actions and reactions such delays are not insignificant. For example, a tennis ball served at 150 km/h takes 25 ms to travel 1 m.

Loss of myelin can lead not only to slowing the conduction speed but even to total interruption of transmission of action potentials along the affected fibers. *Multiple sclerosis*, a progressive disease associated with loss of myelin, can lead to various functional consequences depending on the neural pathways affected, from loss of vision and other sensory functions to muscle weakness, poor coordination, uncontrolled contractions, and to cognitive dysfunction.

3.3 Sensory receptors

Types of receptors. Proprioceptors

The human body is equipped with a variety of sensors that allow adequate knowledge about one's own body and the external world. This information is vital for planning human actions and their correction in cases of unexpected changes in external forces, motor goals, etc. Human sensors represent cells or subcellular structures (*receptors*) that convert physical variables of different nature into changes of the membrane potential. These changes may lead to the generation of action potentials transmitted to other neural structures. Different receptors are specialized to respond to changes in such physical variables as temperature, light, and mechanical deformation.

Some sensors inform the central nervous system about the functioning of internal organs; this information (*interoceptive information*) is typically not consciously perceived. Other sensors, such as those located in the human eye, deliver information on such important aspects of the world as the location of external objects and visible parts of one's own body (*exteroception*). Still other receptors inform the brain on properties of objects that are in direct contact with the body (*haptic perception*) as well as on the relative position of body parts with respect to each other (*proprioception*). Proprioceptive information has been viewed as particularly important for the control of voluntary movements.

Proprioceptive information about the state of the limbs and the trunk is provided by specialized neural cells that reside in *ganglia* (many cells united by an anatomical and sometimes physiological principle) located close to the spinal cord (Figure 3.11). These cells have axons with two very long branches. One of the branches reaches a point somewhere in the body and ends with a sensory ending, a receptor that can generate action potentials in response to a particular physical stimulus. The other branch of the axon enters the spinal cord, where it can make connections with neurons at the level of the entry point; these connections can lead to quick responses to peripheral stimuli, commonly called *reflexes*. The central branch of the axon can also

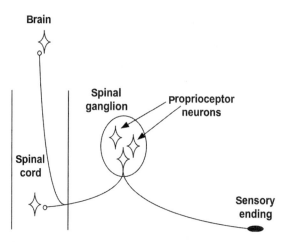

Figure 3.11 Proprioceptor neurons are located in spinal ganglia. They have no dendrites and long, T-shaped axons. The peripheral branch of the axon innervates a sensory ending, which generates action potential in response to appropriate physical stimuli. The central branch of the axon enters the spinal cord and makes projections to other neurons both at the same segment and at other spinal and supraspinal levels.

travel along the spinal cord to other neural structures, even all the way to the cortex of the large hemispheres of the brain.

Sensory endings of proprioceptors are typically sensitive to deformation, and their specific features depend on how they are located with respect to body tissues. Most endings can produce action potentials in response to other stimuli, for example electrical stimulation. There are several groups of proprioceptors that are of particular importance for motor control. They are sensitive to all the potentially important physical variables, such as joint position, muscle length and velocity, muscle force, etc. A more close analysis reveals, however, that signals from these receptors are commonly ambiguous and may require sophisticated analysis to extract the values of relevant physical variables with sufficient precision.

Muscle spindle

Arguably the most famous proprioceptor in the human body is the *muscle spindle*. Muscle spindles are sophisticated structures that house many sensory endings sensitive to muscle length and velocity. A cartoon illustration of a muscle spindle is shown in Figure 3.12. Spindles are scattered in skeletal muscles, oriented parallel to the power-producing muscle fibers and connected to those fibers with strands of connective tissue. There are also muscle fibers inside the spindle; these fibers have no connections to the muscle tendon, and their contraction has no visible external mechanical effect. To distinguish between the two types of muscle fibers, those that produce power are referred to as *extrafusal* in contrast to *intrafusal* fibers, which are muscle fibers located inside the spindles. The intrafusal fibers connect to the shell of

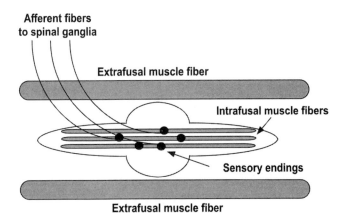

Figure 3.12 Muscle spindles are located in parallel to the power-producing (extrafusal) muscle fibers. Spindles contain intrafusal muscle fibers with sensory endings sensitive to mechanical deformation. The structure of the spindle makes some of the endings sensitive to muscle length while others are sensitive to both muscle length and velocity.

the spindle from the inside, while extrafusal fibers have elastic connections to the outside of the spindle shell. As a result, when extrafusal fibers change their length, the spindle and the intrafusal fibers are deformed in the direction of the length change.

There are two types of sensory endings on the intrafusal fibers, primary and secondary. The *primary endings* are innervated by afferent fibers that belong to group Ia, while the *secondary endings* are innervated by group II afferent fibers (Figure 3.12). The primary endings generate action potentials at a higher frequency when the muscle is longer and when the muscle is stretched (its velocity is positive). They may be completely silent when the muscle is shortened. The secondary endings are sensitive only to muscle length but not to its velocity. Typical dependences of the frequency of firing of a primary ending and a secondary ending to muscle stretch and shortening are shown in Figure 3.13 for a sequence of a quick ramp-like muscle stretch and a ramp-like muscle shortening. Note that the frequency of action potentials cannot drop below zero, so sometimes sensory endings show periods of silence, for example when the muscle shortens quickly.

The axons of the proprioceptive neurons that innervate primary spindle endings are some of the fastest conducting in the human body. They are thick, myelinated, and can transmit action potentials at a speed of up to 120 m/s, faster than the axons of cortical neurons that send signals to the spinal cord when a person wants to initiate a very quick action. This fact suggests that receiving adequate information on muscle length and its changes is crucially important for the central nervous system.

Gamma-motoneurons. Alpha–gamma coactivation

To add to the complexity of the design of muscle spindles, there is a specialized group of small neurons in the spinal cord called *gamma-motoneurons* (Figure 3.14), which

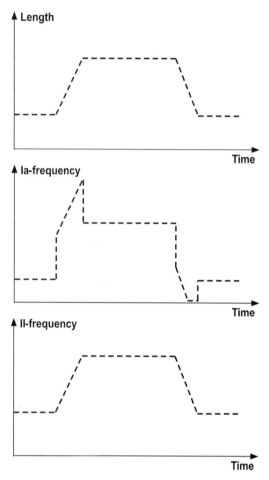

Figure 3.13 An example of responses of a primary spindle ending (middle panel) and secondary spindle ending (bottom panel) to a trapezoidal change in muscle length (top panel).

send signals to intrafusal muscle fibers. These motoneurons produce contractions of the intrafusal fibers, which, although they have no direct effect on the force the muscle produces, do change the sensitivity of the spindle endings to muscle length and velocity. In other words, this mechanism allows the sensors to be highly sensitive within the given range of muscle length and velocity values and to adjust this range of high sensitivity to changes in the muscle state. In particular, this mechanism allows the spindle endings to continue generating information for the central nervous system even when a muscle is being actively contracted. Gamma-motoneurons tend to be activated together with alpha-motoneurons (this phenomenon is called *alpha–gamma coactivation*). As a result, during active muscle contractions, muscle spindle endings do not show periods of silence and avoid a temporary interruption of information about muscle length and velocity.

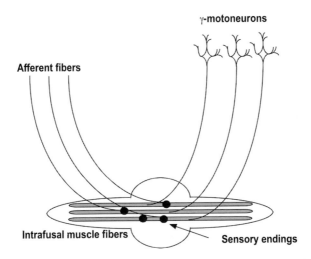

Figure 3.14 Gamma-motoneurons innervate intrafusal muscle fibers and lead to changes in sensitivity of spindle endings to muscle length and velocity.

Golgi tendon organs. Articular receptors

Proprioceptive sensory endings of another type are located at the junction between the extrafusal muscle fibers and tendons (Figure 3.15). They are sensitive to muscle force, which means that they generate action potentials at a frequency roughly proportional to the force produced by the muscle fibers on the tendon at that particular point. These endings are called *Golgi tendon organs*. They have no active mechanism of changing sensitivity that would be analogous to the system of gamma-motoneurons. Their action potentials are also transmitted along the very fast-conducting axons with a conduction speed only slightly slower than that of the axons innervating the primary spindle endings.

About 50 years ago, articular receptors were viewed as the primary source of information about joint position. These receptors are located inside the articular

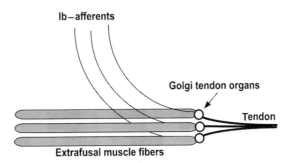

Figure 3.15 Golgi tendon organs are located at the junction between muscle fibers and tendons. They are sensitive to muscle force and are innervated by fast-conducting group Ib afferents.

capsule; their location seems to be optimal to signal joint angle and its changes. However, studies of the properties of these receptors produced disappointing results. First, most articular receptors are sensitive to joint position only when the joint is close to one of the limits of its anatomical rotation; relatively few receptors are able to signal joint position during natural movements in the mid-range of the accessible joint angles. Second, articular receptors change their activity when the joint capsule tension changes. For example, muscle co-contraction without joint motion leads to a substantial increase in the signals from the articular receptors, which are obviously not associated with joint angle change. Taken together, these results suggest that articular receptors are not reliable sources of joint position information. Rather, they may play the role of safety sensors informing the central nervous system that the joint may be in danger of being damaged. This hypothesis is supported by the fact that articular receptors show elevated response in cases of joint inflammation.

Complicating factors in proprioception

Even without help from articular receptors, muscle spindles and Golgi tendon organs seem adequate to supply the central nervous system with information on position and force. However, there are a few problems.

Natural limb movements are based on combinations of joint rotations. Muscles produce force vectors that generate moments of force in the joints. While forces are adequate variables to describe changes in linear velocity of material objects, rotations require different variables, which are moments of force. A *moment of force* is the product of a force vector and its moment arm. At different joint positions, moment arms of muscle action may differ (Figure 3.16) such that the same force can produce different moments of force while the same moment of force may require different forces to be produced. So, even if Golgi tendon organs were perfect force sensors, they would not be perfect sensors for moment of force, which is a much more adequate variable to describe mechanical consequences of muscle action.

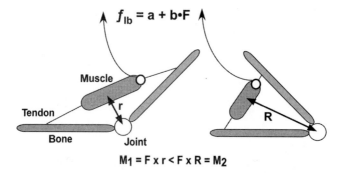

Figure 3.16 Signals from Golgi tendon organs are proportional to muscle force but not to joint movement of force because of possible changes in the lever arm of the muscle force. The two drawings show that the same muscle force can produce different movement of force values at two joint positions.

The location of muscle spindles parallel to the extrafusal fibers allows them to measure the length of the muscle fibers and its velocity. What matters for joint movements, however, is length of the "muscle + tendon" complex, which does not have a simple relation to muscle fiber length. When a muscle is relaxed, it is typically rather compliant, more compliant than the tendon. When the same muscle is activated, its fibers are typically stiffer than the tendon. So, under activation, muscle bellies can bulge and shorten causing tendon stretch even if there is no joint motion. How can the controller decide whether a drop in signals from a spindle corresponds to a joint motion, causing shortening of the muscle fibers, or to force production against a stop (a so-called *isometric contraction*) without any joint motion? Figure 3.17 shows two conditions where the length of the muscle fibers is different due to different forces produced against a stop, while joint positions are the same.

To complicate matters, the system of gamma-motoneurons can lead to changes in the activity of muscle spindle endings unrelated to joint motion. There are also bi-articular and multi-articular muscles crossing two joints or more each. Signals related to the muscle fiber length in those muscles cannot be easily deciphered in terms of individual joint rotations.

Efferent copy and its role in perception

A way to solve this problem dates back to a classical observation by von Helmholtz: If a person closes one eye and moves the other one in a natural way, he or she has an adequate perception that the eye moves, while the external world does not. If the same person moves the eye in an unusual way, for example by pressing slightly on the eyeball with a finger, there is a strong illusion that the external world moves. In both cases, an image of the external world moves over the retina, but this motion is interpreted differently depending on how it came about. Von Helmholtz interpreted this observation as pointing at an important role played by motor command in sensory perception. A term *efferent copy* (sometimes *efference copy*) was introduced by von Holst in 1954 to address hypothetical motor command signals that take part in

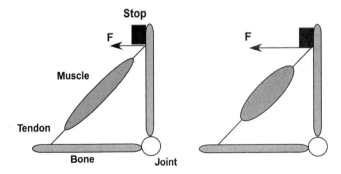

Figure 3.17 In isometric conditions, an increase of force produced against a stop leads to changes in the muscle fiber length (they shorten, while tendon length increases). As a result, signals from length-sensitive spindle endings change their level of firing while no joint motion occurs.

perception. Obviously, to use this idea one has to assume what these motor command signals are. At this point, let me make a general imprecise statement that motor command plays the role of a reference frame within which sensory signals are measured. This statement will be reconsidered later, after addressing some of the controversies in the area of motor control.

3.4   Reflexes

Classifications of reflexes

Historically, the term *reflex* was introduced to mean a motor action in response to a stimulus. Some researchers view reflex as an established useful notion, reflecting important physiological mechanisms within the body. Others, however, question the usefulness of this notion and suggest that the apparent dichotomy between reflexes and voluntary actions is artificial. All movements are actions, irrespective of the complexity of the involved neural pathways, typical time delays, methods of their initiation, and involved muscle groups. The two views were very nicely summarized in a collective paper written by several prominent researchers (Prochazka *et al.*, 2000).

It is indeed very hard to define the term "reflex" unambiguously, in such a way that all researchers would agree with this definition. There are motor reactions to sensory stimuli that come at relatively short time delays, shorter than the fastest voluntary (instructed) motor reaction. These reactions commonly involve muscle contractions in limited muscle groups. Patterns of these reactions are relatively immune to instructions to the person. It is hard to change them by "pure thinking." For some of these reactions, neural pathways that bring them about have been defined. It seems reasonable to keep a special term for these reactions, and reflex sounds quite appropriate. This is certainly not a reliable definition because it hinges on such imprecise words as "relatively," "commonly," etc. In addition, voluntary movements are always associated with changes in reflexes (assuming that this term is defined in a useful way) and, according to one of the main motor control theories, the equilibrium-point hypothesis (see Section 8.3), voluntary movements are produced by modulation of parameters of certain reflexes.

There are several classifications of reflexes based on their characteristics. For example, the great physiologist Ivan Pavlov classified reflexes into *inborn* and *conditioned* and tried to build a theory of all actions based on combinations of those reflexes. Another classification of reflexes into *phasic* and *tonic* is based on their typical time course: Phasic reflexes are transient, short-lasting, while tonic reflexes are steady-state. It is also possible to say that phasic reflexes are produced by a change in the magnitude of a stimulus while tonic reflexes are produced by the magnitude of the stimulus itself. Reflexes can lead to muscle contractions in the area of stimulus application; then, they are commonly called *homonymous* or *autogenic*. Alternatively, they can be seen in remote muscles; in such cases, they are referred to as *heteronymous* or *heterogenic*.

One of the classifications of muscle reflexes is based on the number of synaptic connections between neural cells in the loop that brings the reflex about. Figure 3.18

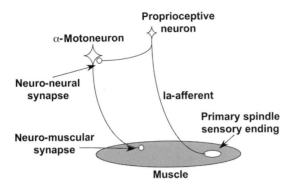

Figure 3.18 An illustration of the most common monosynapic reflex in the human body. Signals from primary spindle endings are delivered by Ia-afferents directly to alpha-moto-neurons innervating the same muscle. If a sufficient number of such signals come to an alpha-motoneuron, it can generate an action potential leading to a muscle twitch contraction.

illustrates the simplest reflex produced by stimulation of a primary spindle sensory ending, which leads to excitation of alpha-motoneurons innervating a muscle that houses the sensory ending. Such a reflex is called monosynaptic. This is a misleading term, because obviously the reflex chain involves two synapses, one between the sensory neuron and the alpha-motoneuron and the other between the axonal terminals of the motoneuron and the muscle fibers. However, since all muscle responses to a stimulus involve the neuromuscular synapse, this synapse is not counted.

Monosynaptic reflexes. H-reflex

There is only one well-studied monosynaptic reflex in adult humans, as illustrated in Figure 3.18. This reflex originates from the primary sensory endings in the muscle spindles. The axons of the proprioceptive neurons innervating these endings (afferent fibers, group Ia) make direct projections on alpha-motoneurons that send their axons to the same muscle. The spindle endings can be stimulated naturally, for example by a very quick muscle stretch (for example, produced by a tendon tap). Their afferent fibers can also be stimulated artificially by an electrical stimulator. The two versions of this reflex are called the *tendon tap reflex* (or *T-reflex*) and the *H-reflex* (after a German scientist, Johann Hoffmann (1857–1919), who described this reflex about 100 years ago). Muscle contractions produced by the monosynaptic reflex come after the shortest possible delay, which is mostly due to the conduction time along the afferent (sensory) and efferent (motor) axons. Typical delays (latencies) of mono-synaptic reflexes in the human arm and leg muscles are in the range 20–40 ms.

Monosynaptic reflexes are phasic, which means that they produce quick, transient twitch muscle contractions. They are inborn and can be seen in newborn babies. Typically, they are homonymous, although heteronymous monosynaptic reflexes (in particular, in antagonist muscles) have been described in babies and in some pathological states.

Oligosynaptic reflexes. Reciprocal inhibition

There are only a few more reflexes for which the neural pathways have been described with sufficient confidence. They all represent *oligosynaptic* reflexes. This group unites reflexes with two or three central synapses. Among the best-known reflexes in this group are those originating from the primary endings of the muscle spindles (Figure 3.19) and from the Golgi tendon organs (Figure 3.20).

The Ia afferents from muscle spindles make projections on a group of small neurons (Ia-interneurons) in the spinal cord, which in turn make inhibitory projections on alpha-motoneurons innervating a muscle with action opposing that of the parent muscle of the spindles, the *antagonist muscle*. This disynaptic reflex is called *reciprocal inhibition*. Golgi tendon organs have oligosynaptic reflex projections on alpha-motoneurons that innervate both the parent muscle (agonist muscle) and its antagonist muscle(s). The homonymous projections are inhibitory; they involve one interneuron (Ib-interneuron). The projections to the antagonist muscle are facilitatory; they involve two interneurons, including the Ib-interneuron. Muscle responses produced by oligosynaptic reflexes are also typically phasic. Their latencies are just a bit longer than those of monosynaptic reflexes. The difference is because of the longer time spent on synaptic transmission (on average, about 1 ms is lost at each synapse) and possible differences in the speed of conduction along Ia and Ib afferent fibers.

Polysynaptic reflexes. Flexor reflex

All other reflexes have undefined neural pathways. They are assumed to involve more than 2–3 central synapses and are called *polysynaptic*. These reflexes typically show longer delays between the stimulus and the response, they can be both phasic and tonic. Examples of phasic polysynaptic reflexes are the flexor reflex and the crossed

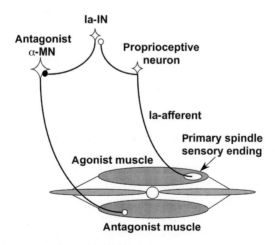

Figure 3.19 A scheme of reciprocal inhibition. Signals from primary spindle endings project on inhibitory interneurons (Ia-INs), which project on alpha-motoneurons (α-MN) innervating the antagonist muscle.

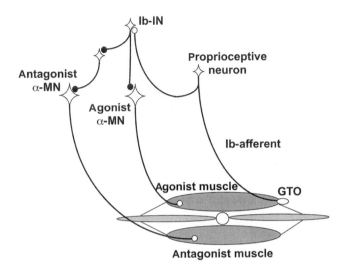

Figure 3.20 Signals from Golgi tendon organs (GTO) produce two kinds of oligosynaptic responses. First, they produce an inhibitory response in alpha-motoneurons (α-MN) innervating the muscle. These responses are mediated by inhibitory interneurons (Ib-IN). Second, they produce facilitation of antagonist alpha-motoneurons via Ib-INs and another pool of inhibitory interneurons.

extensor reflex. They originate from various peripheral receptors called *flexor reflex afferents*. Flexor reflex afferents respond to a variety of stimuli applied to the skin as well as to products of muscle metabolism, such as lactic acid. If these receptors or their afferent fibers are stimulated within an area of an extremity, a reflex response is seen in most flexor muscles of the extremity. This flexor reflex is commonly accompanied by a reflex response seen in extensor muscles of the contralateral extremity. Another polysynaptic reflex that we are going to consider in more detail a bit later is the tonic stretch reflex; as the name suggests, this reflex is tonic.

Pre-programmed reactions

One more group of semi-automatic actions can be produced by sensory stimuli at a delay shorter than the shortest delay before a voluntary (instructed) action to a comparable sensory stimulus (simple reaction time). These responses are sometimes viewed as reflexes and sometimes as voluntary actions. Imagine that a person holds a position in a joint against an external load by activating a muscle. The instruction is: "If a change in the external force happens, try to bring the joint to its original position as quickly as possible." Then, without any additional warning, a perturbation comes, for example a load increase stretching the activated muscle. Typical muscle responses are illustrated in Figure 3.21. If the perturbation is strong, it can lead to a mono-synaptic response in the muscle (M_1). This response is followed by two, not always well-differentiated, responses that come at the latencies of about 50–60 and 70–90 ms

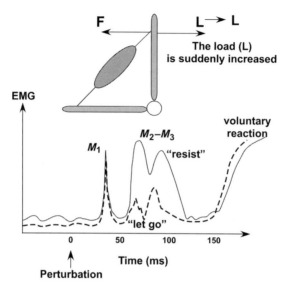

Figure 3.21 When a joint is suddenly loaded, the stretched muscles show a sequence of responses including a monosynaptic response (M_1), followed by two, sometimes not well differentiated, responses at a medium latency of 50–90 ms (M_2–M_3). If a person is instructed to resist the perturbation, M_2–M_3 are large. If the same person is asked to "let go," M_2–M_3 are reduced in size. No such instruction-dependent changes are seen in M_1.

respectively. They are referred to as M_2 and M_3. Later, a voluntary reaction can be seen, typically at a delay of about 150 ms.

Imagine now that the instruction has been changed into "let the joint move, do not react" ("let go" in Figure 3.21). A similar perturbation would produce a similar M_1 but much smaller M_{2-3}. Are M_{2-3} responses reflexes? On the one hand, they come with a rather short time delay. On the other hand, they are modulated by the instruction, making them similar to a voluntary action. These reactions have been described with a variety of terms, including the abovementioned M_{2-3}, long-loop reflexes, transcortical reflexes, functional stretch reflexes, triggered reactions, and pre-programmed reactions.

I would suggest viewing these reactions (let us call them pre-programmed reactions) as voluntary corrective actions to expected perturbations that are prepared by the controller (the central nervous system) in advance and triggered by adequate sensory stimuli. Such reactions have been described in association with a variety of functional motor actions, such as standing, walking, reaching, grasping, speaking, etc. Should they be called reflexes or not? This is a matter of convention, not science.

To summarize, actions can be more or less stereotypical, linked to a well-defined sensory signal or not, involve short or long delays. Highly stereotypical, short-latency actions linked to a specific sensory stimulus may be called reflexes. Very non-stereotypical actions that come at a much longer delay and have no obvious link to a sensory signal may be called voluntary actions. Any action that falls in-between these two extremes may be called simply an action.

3.5 Motor redundancy

Examples of motor redundancy

At any level of description on the system for movement production, there are always more elements than task constraints. For example, if you want to place the tip of an index finger on a particular point in space without moving the trunk (and nothing else matters!), you have to make sure that the three coordinates of the index finger describing its location in the external space coincide with those of the target point. The number of task constraints is three, corresponding to our three-dimensional space. The human arm has at least seven major axes of joint rotation, three in the shoulder, one in the elbow, two in the wrist, and one shared between the elbow and the wrist (pronation–supination). Actually, this number is higher because of the joints of the hand and the ability to move the scapula. But even with seven elemental variables (joint rotations), the task of finding a set of such variables to solve the task is equivalent to solving three equations (given by the three spatial coordinates of the endpoint) with seven unknowns. This is impossible to do. This means that the task can be solved (i.e. the target reached) in many (actually an infinite number of) different ways.

Figure 3.22 presents a two-dimensional illustration with three configurations of a three-joint system that are equally able to bring the endpoint of the arm into the target location. The number of such configurations is indeed infinite.

Consider the relatively simple elbow joint. It is crossed by at least three flexor muscles (biceps, brachialis, and brachioradialis) and three extensor muscles (the heads of the triceps). Imagine that you try to produce a certain moment of force in the elbow joint against a stop. What forces should be produced by each of the six

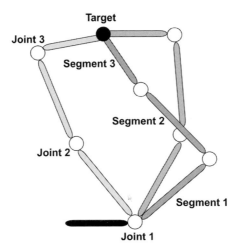

Figure 3.22 An illustration of kinematic redundancy. The three-joint system can reach a target endpoint location in two-dimensional space with an infinite number of joint configurations (three are illustrated).

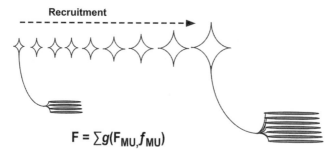

Recruitment

$$F = \sum g(F_{MU}, f_{MU})$$

Figure 3.23 For a given required level of static muscle force, there is no single combination of motor units and frequencies of their recruitment. The size principle guides the order of recruitment, but muscle force depends on both the number of recruited motor units and their frequency of firing.

muscles? Once again, we deal with a problem that cannot be solved. Now we have one equation with six unknowns:

$$M = \sum r_i \cdot F_i, \tag{3.2}$$

where M is joint moment of force, r stands for lever arm, and F is force. The index i refers to the muscles ($i = 1, 2 \ldots 6$).

Such examples can be continued. Imagine now that the task is to produce a certain level of activation of a muscle. The muscle consists of hundreds of motor units (Figure 3.23). What motor units have to be recruited and at what frequencies to satisfy the task? This single equation has hundreds of unknowns.

To bring the message home, let us make one more step. The process of generation of a single action potential involves motion of huge numbers of ions through the membrane. Which particular ions should move through the membrane from zillions of such ions that happen to be in a vicinity of the process? What do we have? One equation with zillions of unknowns!

This is ridiculous! Why should the system care which particular ions cross the membrane? It cares only about the overall characteristic of the process, that is the action potential, not about all the minor details of how the action potential comes about. So, let us agree that the last problem is patently ridiculous. But what about the previous few problems? Are they also ridiculous? The answer depends on whom you ask.

Most motor control researchers (not all of them!) would probably agree that the central nervous system does not care which particular motor units and at what particular frequencies contribute to a desired level of muscle activation. However, the opinions about the first two problems differ. Some researchers believe that the controller does solve such problems and selects certain (optimal) combinations of muscle forces and joint angles to satisfy task requirements. Others think that the controller cares only about overall task characteristics that are crucial for performing tasks properly.

Redundancy and abundance

The four problems we have just considered are examples of the *problem of redundancy*. During movement production, such problems are everywhere, at all levels of description and for all tasks. If one goes from action production to mechanisms of muscle activation, the problem becomes worse and worse. The great Russian physiologist Nikolai Bernstein (see Section 2.3) considered the problem of motor redundancy as the central problem of motor control. He formulated it as the problem of *elimination of redundant degrees-of-freedom*. A degree-of-freedom is an elemental variable at a selected level of analysis. Bernstein's formulation implies that the redundant degrees-of-freedom are indeed eliminated by the controller. In other words, the problem is somehow solved, and a unique solution is found.

There is, however, an alternative view. According to this view, the word "redundancy" misrepresents the design of the system for movement production. It is not redundant but abundant. Both words mean "something extra," but they have different connotations. *Redundancy* means something extra that one would like not to use, while *abundance* means something extra that one enjoys to have and to use. The *principle of abundance* states that the multi-element design of the system for movement production is not a source of unsolvable, ill-posed problems but a way to avoid solving them. This approach will be considered in more detail in Chapter 9.

3.6 Motor variability

Variability and redundancy

If you ask different people to solve the same motor task or even one person to solve the same task several times, all the variables you may wish to record will show different patterns in different persons and different trials. These phenomena are referred to as *motor variability*. Bernstein used a nice expression to describe motor variability, "repetition without repetition." This expression means that when a person repeats solving a task, no performance variable shows repeated patterns.

Motor variability is linked to motor redundancy, but they are not the same thing. Even if the best-trained person is asked to produce the same simple action twice, and the action involves using just one element (this is impossible, of course, but let us temporarily pretend that such tasks exist), the two trials will not be identical. One more time, let us turn to Bernstein. In one of his most famous studies (mentioned in Chapter 2), he recorded the repeated motions of the right arm of blacksmiths who performed the very standardized task of hitting a chisel with a hammer. These were trained blacksmiths who had performed thousands of such movements over the years, yet even in those subjects, the trajectories of the hammer differed across repetitive hitting movements (Figure 3.24). The trajectories of individual joints differed even more across trials, and we will discuss this unexpected result somewhat later (meanwhile, think why this result is unexpected; what could be expected if the brain sent noisy signals to muscles?).

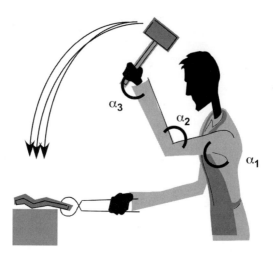

Figure 3.24 When a blacksmith hits an object with the tip of the hammer, trajectories of all arm joints show large variability. There is also variability in the trajectory of the tip of the hammer but it is smaller than what one could expect based on joint variability assuming that joint trajectories do not co-vary.

Noise vs. purposeful variability

There are two views on motor variability. The first considers it as a sign of imperfection of the system for movement production, "noise" within this system. Many researchers explore properties of this noise. For example, they are interested in whether the noise is "white" (with a flat spectrum over the widest possible bandwidth) or "colored" (having a structure), whether its magnitude depends or not on the level of the signal, etc.

The alternative view is that motor variability, or at least some of its components, is a reflection of a purposeful control strategy. In other words, the central nervous system could have produced more reproducible (less variable) patterns but, for some good reasons, it prefers to be more variable. We will return to this hypothesis in Sections 9.4 and 12.3.

Self-test questions

1. What is the difference between action potential and equilibrium potential?
2. Formulate the all-or-none law.
3. Give examples of obligatory and non-obligatory synapses in the human body.
4. Define twitch and tetanic contractions.
5. What muscle develops higher force in response to a standard stimulus—short or long, stretched or shortened?
6. Formulate the size principle.
7. What are the two methods of force modulation of a muscle available for the central nervous system?

8. What motor units fatigue quicker—fast or slow?
9. What motor units would you expect to find in large numbers in a slow muscle—small or large?
10. Why is the speed of conduction of the electrical action potential much slower than that of electric current?
11. What is the role of myelin?
12. Why are there Ranvier nodes in myelinated fibers?
13. Define haptic perception and proprioception.
14. Where are the bodies of proprioceptor neurons located?
15. What are the unusual features of proprioceptor neurons?
16. What is the role of muscle fibers inside the spindle?
17. What neurons innervate intrafusal fibers?
18. What mechanical variables are reflected in the activity levels of spindle sensory endings?
19. What is alpha–gamma coactivation?
20. Where are Golgi tendon organs located? What mechanical variables are they sensitive to?
21. What is the likely role of articular receptors?
22. What are the sensors of joint torque and the length of the "muscle + tendon" complex?
23. Define efferent copy.
24. What is a reflex? What classifications of reflexes do you know?
25. What monosynaptic reflexes do you know in the human body?
26. What oligosynaptic reflexes are produced by signals from the muscle spindle endings?
27. What reflexes do you know originating from activity of the Golgi tendon organs?
28. Give examples of polysynatic reflexes.
29. What is a pre-programmed reaction? What are its major differences from reflexes.
30. Formulate the problem of motor redundancy. Give examples of this problem at different levels of the neuromotor system.
31. What is the principle of abundance?
32. What did Bernstein mean by "repetition without repetition"?
33. Is motor variability a consequence of noise?

Essential references and recommended further readings

Bernstein, N. A. (1935). The problem of interrelation between coordination and localization. *Archives of Biological Sciences, 38*, 1–35, (in Russian; English translation in Bernstein 1967).

Bernstein, N. A. (1967). *The co-ordination and regulation of movements.* Oxford: Pergamon Press.

Chan, C. W. Y., & Kearney, R. E. (1982). Is the functional stretch reflex servo controlled or preprogrammed? *Electroencephalography and Clinical Neurophysiology, 53*, 310–324.

Craske, B. (1977). Perception of impossible limb positions induced by tendon vibration. *Science, 196*, 71–73.

Davids, K., Bennett, S., & Newell, K. M. (2005). *Movement system variability.* Urbana, IL: Human Kinetics.

DiZio, P., & Lackner, J. R. (1995). Motor adaptation to Coriolis force perturbations of reaching movements: endpoint but not trajectory adaptation transfers to the nonexposed arm. *Journal of Neurophysiology, 74*, 1787–1792.

Duysens, J., Loeb, G. E., & Weston, B. J. (1980). Crossed flexor reflex responses and their reversal in freely walking cats. *Brain Research, 197*, 538–542.

Enoka, R. M. (2002). *Neuromechanics of human movement* (3rd ed.). Urbana, IL: Human Kinetics.

Feldman, A. G., & Orlovsky, G. N. (1972). The influence of different descending systems on the tonic stretch reflex in the cat. *Experimental Neurology, 37*, 481–494.

Forssberg, H. (1979). Stumbling corrective reaction: A phase dependent compensatory reaction during locomotion. *Journal of Neurophysiology, 42*, 936–953.

Gelfand, I. M., & Latash, M. L. (1998). On the problem of adequate language in movement science. *Motor Control, 2*, 306–313.

Gielen, C. C. A. M., Ramaekers, L., & van Zuylen, E. J. (1988). Long-latency stretch reflexes as co-ordinated functional responses in man. *Journal of Physiology, 407*, 275–292.

Gottlieb, G. L., & Agarwal, G. C. (1979). Response to sudden torques about ankle in man: myotatic reflex. *Journal of Neurophysiology, 42*, 91–106.

Granit, R. (1970). *The basis of motor control*. London: Academic Press.

Henneman, E., Somjen, G., & Carpenter, D. O. (1965). Excitability and inhibitibility of motoneurones of different sizes. *Journal of Neurophysiology, 28*, 599–620.

Hill, A. V. (1938). The heat of shortening and the dynamic constants of muscle. *Proceedings of the Royal Society of London, Series B, 126*, 136–195.

Hill, A. V. (1953). The mechanics of active muscle. *Proceedings of the Royal Society of London, Series B, 141*, 104–117.

Latash, M. L. (2008). *Neurophysiological basis of movement* (2nd ed.). Urbana, IL: Human Kinetics.

Latash, M. L. (2010). Motor control: In search of physics of the living systems. *Journal of Human Kinetics, 24*, 7–18.

Latash, M. L., & Zatsiorsky, V. M. (1993). Joint stiffness: Myth or reality? *Human Movement Science, 12*, 653–692.

Liddell, E. G. T., & Sherrington, C. S. (1924). Reflexes in response to stretch (myotatic reflexes). *Proceedings of the Royal Society of London, Series B, 96*, 212–242.

Matthews, P. B. C. (1959). The dependence of tension upon extension in the stretch reflex of the soleus of the decerebrate cat. *Journal of Physiology, 47*, 521–546.

Matthews, P. B. C. (1970). The origin and functional significance of the stretch reflex. In P. Andersen, & J. K. S. Jansen (Eds.), *Excitatory synaptic mechanisms* (pp. 301–315). Oslo, Norway: Universitets forlaget.

Matthews, P. B. C. (1972). *Mammalian muscle receptors and their central actions*. Baltimore: Williams & Wilkins.

Merton, P. A. (1953). Speculations on the servo-control of movements. In J. L. Malcolm, J. A. B. Gray, & G. E. W. Wolstenholm (Eds.), *The spinal cord* (pp. 183–198). Boston, MA: Little, Brown.

Myklebust, B. M., & Gottlieb, G. L. (1993). Development of the stretch reflex in the newborn: reciprocal excitation and reflex irradiation. *Child Development, 64*, 1036–1045.

Newell, K. M., & Carlton, L. G. (1993). Force variability in isometric responses. *Journal of Experimental Psychology: Human Perception and Performance, 14*, 37–44.

Newell, K. M., & Corcos, D. M. (Eds.). (1993). *Variability in motor control*. Urbana, IL: Human Kinetics.

Nichols, T. R. (2002). Musculoskeletal mechanics: a foundation of motor physiology. *Advances in Experimental and Medical Biology, 508*, 473–479.

Nichols, T. R., & Houk, J. C. (1976). Improvement in linearity and regulation of stiffness that results from actions of stretch reflex. *Journal of Neurophysiology, 39*, 119–142.

Prochazka, A., Clarac, F., Loeb, G. E., Rothwell, J. C., & Wolpaw, J. R. (2000). What do reflex and voluntary mean? Modern views on an ancient debate. *Experimental Brain Research, 130*, 417–432.

Rothwell, J. C. (1994). *Control of human voluntary movement* (2nd ed.). London: Chapman & Hall.

Sainburg, R. L., Ghilardi, M. F., Poizner, H., & Ghez, C. (1995). Control of limb dynamics in normal subjects and patients without proprioception. *Journal of Neurophysiology, 73*, 820–835.

Sherrington, C. S. (1910). Flexion reflex of the limb, crossed extension reflex, and reflex stepping and standing. *Journal of Physiology, 40*, 28–121.

Turvey, M. T. (1990). Coordination. *American Psychologist, 45*, 938–953.

Von Holst, E. (1954). Relation between the central nervous system and the peripheral organs. *British Journal of Animal Behaviour, 2*, 89–94.

Von Holst, E., & Mittelstaedt, H. (1950/1973). Daz reafferezprincip. Wechselwirkungen zwischen Zentralnerven-system und Peripherie. *Naturwissenschaften, 37*, 467–476, 1950. The reafference principle. In The behavioral physiology of animals and man. The collected papers of Erich von Holst, R. Martin (translator) (Vol. 1, pp. 139–173). Coral Gables, FL: University of Miami Press.

4 Instructive examples

In this chapter a few examples are considered that emphasize important (from the point of view of the author) features of human motor actions. Most of these examples will be revisited in future chapters that address in more detail relevant aspects of motor control. So, the purpose of these examples is to illustrate a certain view on biological movements, a physicist's view. The first example is taken from the field of classical physics; it should be familiar to all readers.

4.1 Do stars and planets measure the distances to each other?

This sounds like a crazy question. And indeed it is. However, let us assume for the moment that we are unaware of the classical law of gravity and have no idea about the physical notion of field, in particular of gravity field. We only know that large bodies move in a way suggesting that they exert forces on each other. There are two possible approaches to the problem of understanding how these bodies interact with each other. One of them is the physical approach. It implies that there are natural laws that describe such interactions. These laws may be unknown, and the challenge is to discover them. The other approach is computational (it can also be called a "control theory" account). It assumes that forces are computed somewhere within the system

Fundamentals of Motor Control. DOI: 10.1016/B978-0-12-415956-3.00004-X and then signals are sent to force generating devices (actuators) to implement the results of such computations.

To illustrate the main difference between the physical approach and the computational approach, consider the law of gravity illustrated in Figure 4.1. Two objects with non-zero mass exert forces on each other proportional to the masses of the objects and inversely proportional to the distance between the objects squared. Figure 4.1A illustrates a physical account of the law of gravity. An object with mass M_1 creates a gravitational field with the strength of the field inversely proportional to the distance from the object squared (R^2). Another object with mass M_2 experiences the gravity force proportional to the strength of the field and to the mass of that second object. Figure 4.1B illustrates a computational account of the same law. There are two sensors located in the second object. They send signals to the first object related to the distance between the objects (R) and mass of the second object (M_2). The first object gets this information and computes a signal corresponding to the desired force value according to a formula that is stored in its memory (F_{COMP}). Then, the first object sends this signal to an actuator located at the second object, which transforms the symbolic value F_{COMP} into an actual force, F_{ACT}. This description can be repeated assuming sensors in object M_1 and computations performed by object M_2.

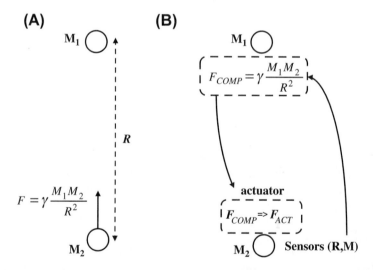

Figure 4.1 Physical and computational approaches to the gravity law. (A) The physical approach. An object with mass creates a gravitational field. Any other object with mass, placed in the field, experiences force proportional to the mass of the second object and inversely proportional to the distance between the two objects squared. (B) The computational (control theory) approach. The first object gets information from sensors located in the second object on its mass and distance between the objects. It computes a force (F_{COMP}) and sends a signal to an actuator located at the second object that converts this symbolic force into actual force F_{ACT}. Note that mathematically both illustrations lead to the same equation.

Mathematically, the schemes in the two panels lead to the same equation. I hope that all the readers would agree that Figure 4.1A illustrates the physical law of gravity, while Figure 4.1B illustrates how to model this law using non-gravitational (non-physical) means. So, if the purpose is to understand the physics of interactions between two material objects, Figure 4.1A is the only one to be used. If the purpose is to build a system that emulates the law of gravity, for example to illustrate it to high-school students, the scheme in Figure 4.1B may be preferred.

In situations when one deals with a known physical law, the difference between the two illustrations in Figure 4.1 is obvious. It becomes less obvious when the physics of the system under consideration is poorly known. It becomes very tempting to assume the existence of computations somewhere within the system (as in Figure 4.1B), which allows accounting for aspects of its behavior.

Our current knowledge on the physics of human movement production is very limited. The best developed field is mechanics of human movement, which is based on the classical apparatus of Newtonian mechanics. More biologically specific aspects, such as interactions within the central nervous system, are understood only superficially. When researchers perform specific studies, they commonly separate the object of their interest from the rest of the body (and, commonly, from the environment) and assume that this object receives an input from the rest of the body, and the input may be assigned intelligence. For example, the notions of *motor programs* and *control variables* (described in more detail in Chapters 5 and 7) are a poor-man way of describing a system, whose physics are unknown. These terms are temporary substitutes reflecting our current inadequate knowledge. All researchers who accept the physical approach sin in this way, but they hope that one day it will be possible to describe human behavior with a set of physical laws without resorting to such notions. In this context, "physical laws" include all natural laws that are commonly considered in courses of physics, chemistry, biology, physiology, etc.

4.2   Posture–movement paradox

By the middle of the twentieth century, a number of mechanisms that help stabilize the posture (of a joint, a limb, or the whole body) had been described. In particular, it was known that any mechanical perturbation of posture produces resistive forces due to a number of posture-stabilizing mechanisms. These involve both peripheral resistance of muscles generating force against changes in length as well as changes in muscle activation levels via involuntary (*reflex*) mechanisms.

A famous German scientist, Erich von Holst (1908–1962) asked a question: How is it that we can move from one posture to another without triggering resistance from all these posture-stabilizing mechanisms? Indeed, if a person stands quietly, and someone pushes him or her in the back (Figure 4.2A), many leg and trunk muscles show short-latency activation bursts that move the body back to the original posture. If the same person sways the body in the same direction and by the same magnitude voluntarily (Figure 4.2B), no such bursts of muscle activation are seen. How do all these involuntary mechanisms "know" when to resist a postural deviation and when not to interfere?

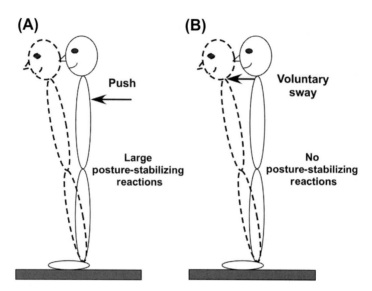

Figure 4.2 (A) If a standing person is pushed forward to a new posture by an external force, posture-stabilizing reactions will be seen in leg/trunk muscles trying to restore the initial posture. (B) If the same person sways forward voluntarily to the same new posture, no posture-stabilizing reactions are seen.

Principle of reafference

Von Holst formulated an answer to this problem in the form of the principle of reafference. He concluded that during voluntary movements the brain changed the coordinate with respect to which posture was stabilized, the referent coordinate. Posture-stabilizing mechanisms start to act when afferent signals report deviations from the referent coordinate, not from an absolute posture. Body deviations may result from an involuntary change of posture (as during an unexpected push, see Figure 4.2A) or from a purposeful central change in the referent coordinate. In the latter case, posture-stabilizing mechanisms turn into movement-producing ones (as in Figure 4.2B).

This conclusion is truly very important. According to it, postural control and voluntary movements are intimately linked to each other. Performing a voluntary movement involves a time change in the referent posture with respect to which posture-stabilizing mechanisms act. Any theory of motor control that ignores this basic feature of the system for the neural control of posture and movements is missing the point by a mile.

4.3   Opening a door with a mug of coffee in one's hand

Imagine that you walk down the hallway with a mug of hot coffee in your hand. As mentioned earlier, the human arm has quite a few kinematic degrees-of-freedom that,

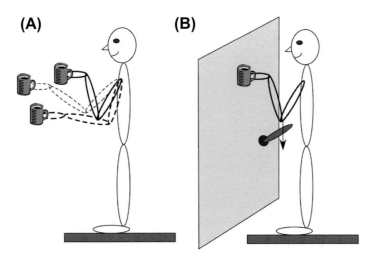

Figure 4.3 A person can carry a mug filled with coffee in the hand using variable joint configurations (three such configurations are shown in panel A). If the person comes to a closed door, he or
she can open the door by pressing on the handle with the elbow without spilling the coffee (B).

in this particular case, will be used to keep the mug vertical at all times (to avoid
spilling the coffee, Figure 4.3A). Now imagine that you are also carrying something
large and heavy in the other hand and that you come to a closed door with a handle
that you have to press down to open the door (Figure 4.3B). What will you do? One
commonly observed solution is to press down on the handle with the elbow of the arm
carrying the mug of coffee and push the door open. This action is typically done
smoothly and easily without any visible hesitation.

Now let us consider this situation as a task involving two problems of motor
redundancy. The first is to keep the mug vertical and the second is to move the elbow
downwards. Both share kinematic degrees-of-freedom of the same arm (and trunk).
The ease of performing this rather unusual task suggests that using a redundant set of
elements in one task does not interfere with using some of the same elements in
another task at the same time. This is not a trivial conclusion that speaks against the
idea of finding a single, optimal solution for the problem of motor redundancy
associated with the task of keeping the mug vertical (and, likely, for similar tasks
characterized by motor redundancy).

4.4   Tonic stretch reflex and voluntary movements

Tonic stretch reflex and its threshold

The tonic stretch reflex was first described by Charles Sherrington nearly one hundred
years ago. It represents an involuntary change in muscle activation and force with
a change in muscle length. The word "tonic" means that the changes in muscle

activation can be observed not only during the process of muscle length change (its stretch or shortening) but also at new steady states. Figure 4.4 illustrates a typical dependence of muscle force on muscle length recorded in an animal preparation where descending signals to the spinal cord coming from supraspinal structures were avoided, and hence, all muscle reactions could be safely viewed as involuntary.

When the muscle length is short, it shows no signs of activation. A very slow stretch of such a muscle leads to a relatively small increase in its force due to the elasticity of the peripheral tissues (not shown in the figure). At some value of muscle length, the muscle will start to show signs of activation. This value of muscle length is called the *threshold of the tonic stretch reflex* (λ in Figure 4.4A). Further stretch leads to a much quicker increase in muscle force (the solid curve) accompanied by an increase in the level of muscle activation. The involuntary mechanism leading to changes in muscle activation and force with its slow stretch is called the *tonic stretch reflex*, and the dependence of active muscle force on muscle length is called the *tonic stretch reflex characteristic*. The exact neurophysiological loop of this reflex is unknown. It likely reflects the action of numerous loops from the receptors activated by the stretch on the alpha-motoneurons innervating the muscle. Some of these loops are short-latency, including the monosynaptic reflexes from the primary spindle afferent; others are likely polysynaptic, with longer time delays.

A human muscle almost always acts against an external load, which may be produced by both external forces, and the action of other muscles. Given a certain load value, the combination of muscle force and length $\{F,L\}$, at which the system comes to an equilibrium, depends on the tonic stretch reflex characteristic. As illustrated in Figure 4.4B, a shift in the threshold of the tonic stretch reflex results in different $\{F,L\}$ combinations, when the system is at an equilibrium. The figure shows

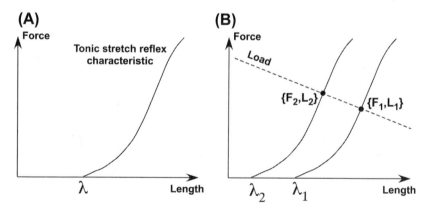

Figure 4.4 If a muscle is slowly stretched, at some length it will show active resistance to stretch (λ, the threshold of the tonic stretch reflex in A). Starting from that point, further stretch will lead to stronger resistance like in a non-linear spring (tonic stretch reflex characteristic). If a muscle acts against an external load (dashed line in B), the system "muscle + load" will reach an equilibrium at some combination of muscle length and force—the equilibrium point. A shift of λ (from λ_1 to λ_2 in B) leads to a shift of the equilibrium point resulting in changes in both muscle force and length.

a load characteristic that is position-dependent (has a non-zero slope), which is common in everyday life.

Descending control. Movements as shifts of equilibrium points

Several experimental studies on animals and humans have shown that a change in the descending signals from the brain shifts the tonic stretch reflex characteristic nearly parallel to itself along the x-axis. Figure 4.5 shows classical results of Anatol Feldman and Grigori Orlovsky (1972) of the shifts of the tonic stretch characteristics observed in a cat preparation in response to stimulation of various brain structures at different intensities. The plots in Figure 4.5 imply that the effects of changes in signals from the brain to a muscle can be described with only one parameter, the threshold of the tonic stretch reflex, λ. Note that actual muscle state is not defined by setting this parameter, only a dependence of active muscle force on muscle length is. Muscle state will equally depend on the current external force. If the external force (load) is fixed, a value of λ defines a unique equilibrium state when the system "muscle + tonic stretch reflex + load" is in a state of equilibrium. This state is referred to as the *equilibrium point* of the system. Movements are transitions between equilibrium points. They can be induced by a change in the load without a change in the descending command, by a change in the descending command without a change in the load, or by a change in both. These scenarios are illustrated in the three panels of Figure 4.6.

Based on the described experimental material and laws of physics, we can draw very important conclusions that descending commands cannot in principle specify such

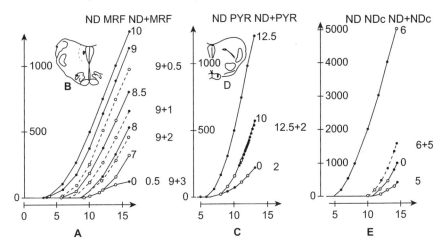

Figure 4.5 Stimulation of different brain areas results in nearly parallel shifts of the tonic stretch characteristic in the decerebrate cat. Stimulation was applied to ipsilater (ND) and contralateral (NDc) Deiters' nuclei, pyramidal tract (PYR), and mesencephalic reticular formation (MRF). Reproduced by permission from Feldman, A. G., & Orlovsky, G. N. (1972). The influence of different descending systems on the tonic stretch reflex in the cat. *Experimental Neurology, 37,* 481–494.

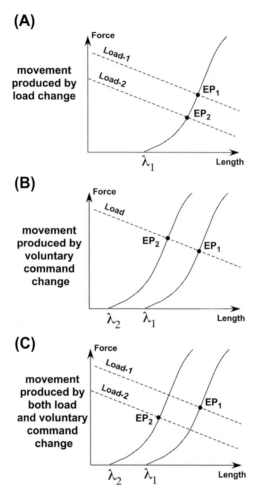

Figure 4.6 Changes in muscle length and/or force (a change in the equilibrium point, EP) can be produced by a change in the external load (Load-1 to Load-2 as in A), a change in the threshold of the tonic stretch reflex (λ_1 to λ_2 in B), or in both (as in C).

variables as muscle force, muscle length, and muscle activation level. A command can only specify the location of the tonic stretch reflex characteristic (force–length characteristic measured at steady-states) along the muscle length axis, while the three mentioned variables change along this characteristic and depend on the external load. Similar reasoning allows the claim that central commands cannot specify derivatives of these three variables, their ratios (for example, the slope of the characteristics, which is sometimes addressed as *apparent stiffness*), or any other variables that can be computed from the mentioned ones. Descending signals can only set a parameter λ that defines interactions between the muscle and the load (mediated by reflex loops), while all the variables typically measured in experiments emerge as results of this interaction.

4.5   Equifinality and its violations

Equifinality and equilibrium states

The term *equifinality* refers to a particular feature of voluntary movements, namely their ability to reach targets accurately in conditions when an unexpected transient external perturbation pushes the moving system off its trajectory. Imagine that you perform a very quick pointing movement into a target along a nearly straight trajectory (Figure 4.7). In one of the trials, early in the movement, unexpectedly, an external force acts for a very brief time on your moving arm and pushes it upwards (the dashed trajectory in Figure 4.7). Equifinality implies that if you do not try to correct the ongoing movement, the finger will land on the target accurately anyway (note the convergence of the original and perturbed trajectories). Phenomena of equifinality have been documented in many experiments using a variety of tasks, from single-joint action to whole-body motion, and a variety of subjects, from animals deprived of sensory information coming from the moving limb (deafferented animals) to healthy humans.

Equifinality is a natural consequence of the described method of control with setting thresholds of the tonic stretch reflex for the participating muscles. Indeed, if a set of λ values is used in each trial corresponding to accurate task performance and the external force field (loads for all muscles) is the same, there is a single

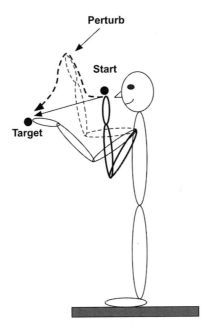

Figure 4.7 Example of equifinality. If a very fast reaching movement is perturbed in the middle of its trajectory by a transient force pulse (the dashed line), the final endpoint location in the perturbed trial will be about the same as in unperturbed trials (the solid line).

combination of muscle length values where the system will be in an equilibrium corresponding to a single joint configuration. Transient forces acting during the transition of the system from the initial equilibrium state to the final equilibrium state can change the trajectory along which the system moves, but not the final equilibrium state.

Violations of equifinality

Several studies reported violations of equifinality under specific experimental manipulations. Arguably, the most famous experiments of this kind were performed by two American researchers, James Lackner and Paul DiZio, on subjects who tried to produce accurate pointing movements while sitting in the center of a rotating centrifuge. The movements were well practiced without rotation of the centrifuge and then performed in total darkness to a light target. The subjects were unaware of the rotation because it started very slowly and the rotational acceleration was very low. In the absence of rotation, the subjects produced nearly straight trajectories into the target (Figure 4.8). During rotation, the trajectories became curved, deviated strongly from the straight line, and showed a compensation for the lateral deviation during the second half of the trajectory. However, this compensation was only partial, and the hand landed off the target (the dashed trajectory in Figure 4.8).

The deviations of the hand from the straight line were produced by the Coriolis force that perturbed the movement. To remind you, the Coriolis force acts on an object moving in a rotating reference system (see Section 5.1). For example, when you point quickly with a forward arm motion and simultaneously turn the trunk,

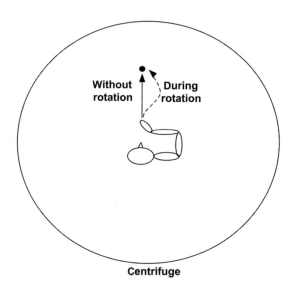

Centrifuge

Figure 4.8 During rotation in a centrifuge, the Coriolis force perturbs the reaching movement (compare the dashed—during rotation, and solid—without rotation trajectories). During rotation, the trajectory shows a tendency to come back to the same final position but there is a residual error.

Coriolis force acts on the hand. The magnitude of the Coriolis force is proportional to the linear velocity of the moving object. This means that its magnitude peaks at peak velocity and it is zero when the hand stops. So, Coriolis force acts only during the movement but not at the final steady-state. That is why, the residual errors in the final position were described as violations of equifinality.

These results may be interpreted in two ways. First, as a sign that the described hypothesis on the control of voluntary movements with parameters (λ) that produce shifts in equilibrium states is wrong. Second, as a sign that the controller adjusted the values of these parameters even when the subjects were unaware of such adjustments. The adjustments led to changes in the final equilibrium state of the system "hand + reflex loops + load," resulting in pointing errors. Since the method of control with shifts in equilibrium states is so well rooted in experimental material and laws of physics, I prefer the second interpretation.

4.6   Effects of deafferentation on voluntary movements

When the central nervous system stops receiving sensory (afferent) signals from a particular part of the body, this part is referred to as "deafferented." Deafferentation obviously has two major effects. First, the central nervous system receives no information on the state of the affected body part (unless it is substituted with another source of information, for example vision) and cannot use such information for movement planning or adjustment. Second, all the reflex loops originating from receptors in the affected body part stop functioning.

Deafferentation can be produced in experiments, for example by cutting all the dorsal roots that carry sensory information into the spinal cord from the targeted body part. In very rare cases, functional deafferentation happens in humans as a result of a state known as *large-fiber peripheral neuropathy*. In such cases, deafferentation is rarely complete, but sometimes patients report no sensation in the affected body part.

Motor deficits after deafferentation

The effects of depriving an animal of somatosensory information (*deafferentation*) on motor function are dramatic. Movements are still possible, but they are extremely inaccurate and discoordinated. In humans, it is virtually impossible to perform meaningful movements of affected body parts with closed eyes. In particular, a person with whole-body large-fiber peripheral neuropathy cannot stand with eyes closed. By the way, this last observation casts doubt on the crucial role of the vestibular system (which is unimpaired) in ensuring balance during standing (see Chapter 11).

Despite these dramatic impairments, animals and humans can learn how to produce reasonably accurate movements under visual control after deafferentation. Some features of natural movements are still present in movements of deafferented animals, for example equifinality under transient perturbations. Since the tonic stretch reflex is absent after deafferentation, such animals cannot use the "λ-control" and have to invent an alternative method of producing movements. The only available

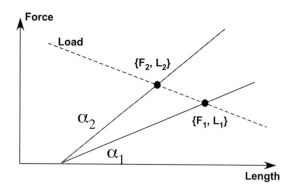

Figure 4.9 Force–length characteristics of a deafferented muscle. In a deafferented muscle, the tonic stretch reflex is absent. Such a muscle shows spring-like characteristics due to its peripheral properties. These characteristics change their slope with changes in the level of muscle activation (compare α_1 to α_2). When such a muscle acts against an external load, the system "muscle + load" reaches an equilibrium combination of force and length values.

method of control is to specify input into alpha-motoneuronal pools ("α-control"). This results in setting levels of muscle activation. Note, however, that a muscle under a fixed activation level produces length-dependent force with apparent stiffness (the slope of the dependence) depending on the α-signal (Figure 4.9). This means that muscle force and length values will depend on both the current value of the α-signal and the external load. So, despite the imposed change in the method of control, one of its major features, namely transitions between equilibrium points, remains unchanged, leading to equifinality under transient perturbations demonstrated in beautiful experiments on deafferented monkeys by the group of Emilio Bizzi in MIT.

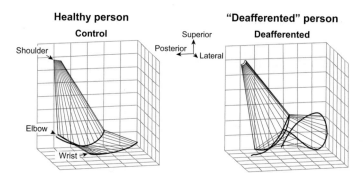

Figure 4.10 When a healthy person performs hand movements as if cutting a loaf of bread, the trajectories are slightly curved; the outward and inward portions of the trajectories are similar. When a person with large fiber neuropathy ("deafferented person") performs this task, the trajectories show major distortions with large differences between the outward and inward segments. Reproduced by permission from Sainburg, R. L., Ghilardi, M. F., Poizner, H., & Ghez, C. (1995) Control of limb dynamics in normal subjects and patients without proprioception. *Journal of Neurophysiology, 73,* 820–835.

Another documented difference in the movements of healthy humans and "deafferented" patients is the change in joint coordination during simple multi-joint movements such as slicing a loaf of bread—this study was performed by Robert Sainburg (currently at Penn State) and his colleagues. Healthy humans produce nearly straight, horizontal movements of the knife, with similar trajectories while moving from the body and towards the body. In contrast, "deafferented" patients produce highly curved knife trajectories (Figure 4.10) when they perform the movement without visual control, and the trajectories towards the body and from the body are rather different.

To summarize, voluntary movements are possible even when no sensory signals are coming from the moving body part to the central nervous system. However, these movements are profoundly impaired, showing the importance of sensory information for motor control.

Self-test questions

1. Define agonist and antagonist muscle.
2. Formulate the posture–movement paradox.
3. Formulate the principle of reafference.
4. Imagine a violin virtuoso performing a complicated passage while moving the violin around and turning the body. What can you conclude about the neural organization of the control of finger movements?
5. Suggest an example speaking against finding unique optimal solutions for tasks in conditions of motor redundancy.
6. Define tonic stretch reflex.
7. What is the threshold of the tonic stretch reflex?
8. Which of the following are specified by a value of the tonic stretch reflex: muscle length, muscle force, a combination of muscle length and force, and/or muscle activation level?
9. What studies provide evidence for the tonic stretch reflex threshold being specified by signals from different brain structures?
10. Which performance variables can be specified by a descending command from the brain independently of the external forces?
11. Define equifinality.
12. Present examples of equifinality during voluntary movements.
13. Present examples of violations of equifinality during voluntary movements.
14. Can spring-like muscle properties affect the movement of a deafferented animal?
15. Can reflexes change muscle activation in a deafferented animal?
16. What is the main difference between λ-control and α-control?
17. Present an example of disordered coordination in a person with large-fiber peripheral neuropathy.

Essential references and recommended further readings

Bernstein, N. A. (1967). *The co-ordination and regulation of movements*. Oxford: Pergamon Press.

Bizzi, E., Accornero, N., Chapple, W., & Hogan, N. (1982). Arm trajectory formation in monkeys. *Experimental Brain Research, 46*, 139–143.

DiZio, P., & Lackner, J. R. (1995). Motor adaptation to Coriolis force perturbations of reaching movements: endpoint but not trajectory adaptation transfers to the nonexposed arm. *Journal of Neurophysiology, 74*, 1787–1792.

Feldman, A. G. (1986). Once more on the equilibrium-point hypothesis (λ-model) for motor control. *Journal of Motor Behavior, 18*, 17–54.

Feldman, A. G., & Latash, M. L. (2005). Testing hypotheses and the advancement of science: Recent attempts to falsify the equilibrium-point hypothesis. *Experimental Brain Research, 161*, 91–103.

Feldman, A. G., & Orlovsky, G. N. (1972). The influence of different descending systems on the tonic stretch reflex in the cat. *Experimental Neurology, 37*, 481–494.

Lackner, J. R., & DiZio, P. (1994). Rapid adaptation to Coriolis force perturbations of arm trajectory. *Journal of Neurophysiology, 72*, 1–15.

Latash, M. L. (2008). *Synergy.* New York: Oxford University Press.

Liddell, E. G. T., & Sherrington, C. S. (1924). Reflexes in response to stretch (myotatic reflexes). *Proceedings of the Royal Society of London, Series B, 96*, 212–242.

Matthews, P. B. C. (1959). The dependence of tension upon extension in the stretch reflex of the soleus of the decerebrate cat. *Journal of Physiology, 47*, 521–546.

Merton, P. A. (1953). Speculations on the servo-control of movements. In J. L. Malcolm, J. A. B. Gray, & G. E. W. Wolstenholm (Eds.), *The spinal cord* (pp. 183–198). Boston: Little, Brown.

Newell, K. M., & Corcos, D. M. (Eds.). (1993). *Variability in motor control.* Urbana, IL: Human Kinetics.

Polit, A., & Bizzi, E. (1979). Characteristics of motor programs underlying arm movemnt in monkey. *Journal of Neurophysiology, 42*, 183–194.

Prochazka, A., Clarac, F., Loeb, G. E., Rothwell, J. C., & Wolpaw, J. R. (2000). What do reflex and voluntary mean? Modern views on an ancient debate. *Experimental Brain Research, 130*, 417–432.

Rothwell, J. C., Traub, M. M., & Marsden, C. D. (1982). Automatic and "voluntary" responses compensating for disturbances of human thumb movements. *Brain Research, 248*, 33–41.

Sainburg, R. L., Poizner, H., & Ghez, C. (1993). Loss of proprioception produces deficits in interjoint coordination. *Journal of Neurophysiology, 70*, 2136–2147.

Sainburg, R. L., Ghilardi, M. F., Poizner, H., & Ghez, C. (1995). Control of limb dynamics in normal subjects and patients without proprioception. *Journal of Neurophysiology, 73*, 820–835.

Schmidt, R. A., & McGown, C. (1980). Terminal accuracy of unexpected loaded rapid movements: Evidence for a mass-spring mechanism in programming. *Journal of Motor Behavior, 12*, 149–161.

Sternad, D. (2002). Wachholder and Altenberger 1927: foundational experiments for current hypotheses on equilibrium-point control in voluntary movements. *Motor Control, 6*, 299–302.

Von Holst, E. (1954). Relation between the central nervous system and the peripheral organs. *British Journal of Animal Behaviour, 2*, 89–94.

Von Holst, E., & Mittelstaedt, H. (1950/1973). Das reafferezprincip. Wechselwirkungen zwischen Zentralnerven-system und Peripherie. *Naturwissenschaften, 37*, 467–476, 1950. The reafference principle. In The behavioral physiology of animals and man. The collected papers of Erich von Holst, R. Martin (translator) (Vol. 1, pp. 139–173). Coral Gables, FL: University of Miami Press.

5 Control with forces and torques

Chapter Outline

The two major approaches to the problem of the neural control of movements are reviewed briefly in the first section. The first is based on the control theory and progress in engineering. It assumes that the central nervous system performs computations reflecting interactions between the body and the environment and among body parts. The second is based on neurophysiology and physics. This subdivision is certainly very crude, and there are approaches that are in the gray area, trying to incorporate ideas from both abovementioned approaches.

5.1 Force control

This approach is based on a seemingly natural postulate that, in order to produce movement of an effector from one point in space to another, the neural controller has to make sure that requisite time profiles of force (and moment of force) are applied to

Fundamentals of Motor Control. DOI: 10.1016/B978-0-12-415956-3.00005-1

the effector. This axiom, which is the foundation of the *motor programming approach*, looks so obvious that it takes an effort to realize that it may be questionable. Certainly, the only known way to produce a movement of a motionless material object is to apply force to that object. However, the formulation of the axiom implies that these forces are somehow pre-computed by the controller and then implemented by a sophisticated control system.

Newton's laws form the foundation of classical mechanics, a field of physics that describes how objects move under the action of forces (assuming that the velocities never approach the speed of light—a safe assumption for everyday human movements). Most people have learned in high school that in order to move a stationary object or to change the motion of an object that moves with a constant velocity vector it is necessary to apply a non-zero net force to that object. Biological objects do not violate this basic law of nature. However, does this mean that in order to move an object (for example, a limb) from one location to another, the neural controller has to pre-compute requisite forces and then generate neural signals resulting from this computation? To answer this question, let us consider a few common sources of force acting during human voluntary movements.

But first, let me remind you of a few basic definitions from classical physics. Physical variables can be classified into *scalars* and *vectors*. A scalar is characterized by magnitude but not by direction; in other words, a scalar is a physical quantity that does not change with changes in a coordinate system such as its rotations or translations. Examples of scalars are mass, distance, temperature, and speed. Vectors are characterized by both magnitude and direction. A change in coordinate system, in general, leads to a change in a vector. Examples of vectors are velocity, acceleration, force, and moment of force. Consider the two physical variables velocity and speed. The former is a vector, characterized by its magnitude (speed—a scalar) and direction. If velocity is measured in a coordinate system, and then the coordinate system is rotated, the direction of the velocity vector with respect to the axes of the new coordinate system will change while its magnitude (speed) will remain unchanged. Commonly, vectors are shown in bold fonts, while scalars are shown in non-bold fonts.

Gravity. Effects of joint rotations

One of the most common forces we experience in everyday life is gravitational force. This force obeys the law of gravity and can be described as $\boldsymbol{F}_G = m\boldsymbol{g}$, where $\boldsymbol{F}_G$ is the force due to gravity, $\boldsymbol{g}$ is the gravitational acceleration, and m is a coefficient called *mass*. For an object with constant mass on the surface of Earth, the force of gravity is also constant and is always directed downward, that is, towards the center of Earth. Humans learn the effects of gravity on motion of objects early in life and can predict the motion of objects induced by gravity with high accuracy. For example, if a standing person prepares to catch an object released from a certain height, and only the initial path of the object fall is visible, he or she can prepare for the impact by precisely timing the activation of postural muscles to the moment of impact (producing *anticipatory postural adjustments*, see Section 11.1). This requires predicting the fall time of the object under the action of gravity.

Human movements are produced by muscles that generate joint rotations. This makes *moments of force* in the joints (joint torques) adequate mechanical variables to analyze the mechanical interactions between the body segments and the environment. The effects of gravity on joint torques are position-dependent. Indeed, consider Figure 5.1. Although the mass (*m*) of the forelimb segment is the same and hence the force of gravity (*mg*) is the same, the moment this force creates in the elbow joint is different in the two joint configurations because of the difference in the lever arms ($R > r$).

Motion-dependent forces

Among motion-dependent forces (and torques) the most familiar one is *inertial force*. Inertial force is proportional to acceleration with the same coefficient *m* as in the equation for gravitational forces: $F_I = m\mathbf{a}$ (for rotations, the coefficient that links moment of force to angular acceleration is *moment of inertia*). Two more forces are motion-dependent, but they are typically less familiar to students. These are the *centripetal force* and the *Coriolis force* (Figure 5.2). The centripetal force (F_{CTR}, Figure 5.2A) acts at an object that performs a rotational movement. Its magnitude depends on the object mass *m*, tangential velocity *V*, and radius of the rotational movement *R*:

$$F_{CTR} = m\frac{V^2}{R}$$

This force is directed towards the axis of rotation. The Coriolis force (F_{COR}, Figure 5.2B) acts at an object that moves at a certain velocity in a rotating reference

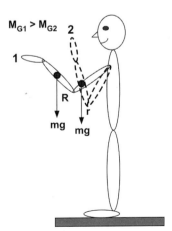

Figure 5.1 Torques produced by the gravity force are motion-dependent. In the presented example, the moment of force (*M*) produced by the weight of the forearm with respect to the elbow joint depends on the lever arm, which differs in the two illustrated configurations, $R > r$.

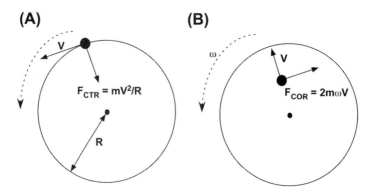

Figure 5.2 (A) Centripetal force acts on an object that performs a rotational motion. (B) When a linear motion happens in a rotating frame of reference, Coriolis force acts orthogonally to the velocity vector.

frame. For example, if you try to move a hand-held object in a horizontal plane while turning the whole body around the vertical body axis, the Coriolis force will act on the object. If the object moves in a plane orthogonal to the axis of rotation, $\mathbf{F_{COR}} = 2m\omega\mathbf{V}$, where ω is the angular velocity of rotation of the reference frame. This force acts orthogonally to the velocity vector $\mathbf{V}$.

Humans rarely act in a rotating environment, such as a centrifuge, although many arm movements are produced while rotating the trunk (consider, for example, the shot put). During limb movements that involve rotation of two joints, the distal link (e.g. the forearm) always moves in the rotating system of coordinates, due to the movement at the shoulder. When a person finds himself or herself in a rotating environment (usually, for experimental purposes), it is very hard to predict what the Coriolis force will do with motion of objects. The author once experienced being rotated in a large centrifuge where he tried to throw a tennis ball to another person (both stood close to the edge of the centrifuge). It was next to impossible to adapt the throwing movement to the very unexpected and very large effects of the Coriolis force that deflected the ball trajectory in a most unusual way.

We have to be grateful to *Newton's third law* and *friction forces* for the ability to stand, walk, and perform many other vital actions. These forces allow the body to counteract the force of gravity during standing and to produce horizontal forces that accelerate the body during walking and running. Figure 5.3 shows a cartoon of a person who tries to make a step forward. The vertical ground reaction force $(-Mg)$ supports the body weight, while friction ($\mathbf{F_{FR}}$) allows the application of a horizontal force acting on the center of mass (COM) and accelerating it in the required direction.

Sometimes we encounter unusual force fields. For example, if one tries to produce fast movements under water, the resistance of water generates a force directed against the velocity vector, with the magnitude that may be approximately considered proportional to the movement velocity squared. Such forces are also produced by air resistance, but they are commonly considered negligibly small, while they are not

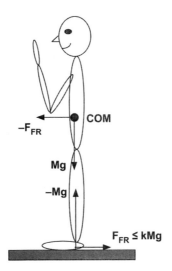

Figure 5.3 The ground reaction force supports the weight of the body, while friction allows moving the body with respect to the ground.

small during movements in more viscous media such as water. In laboratory studies, unusual force fields are frequently generated by programmable motors to study how the central nervous system adapts to such fields (see in more detail in Section 11.3).

To summarize, there is a plethora of forces acting on moving segments of the human body. So, let us get back to the main question: Does the brain solve equations of motion in order to generate neural signals that would lead to a desired movement? Note that the brain issues such signals before the movement is initiated and, given the time delays inherent to transmitting neural signals and converting them into forces by muscles, for fast movement, there may be no time for corrective actions. In other words, the neural command is generated in a *feed-forward* fashion (see Chapter 7).

Consider two examples. The first is playing billiards. The cue controlled by the player produces force only on the ball it touches. Further, that ball rolls and hits other balls that experience contact forces. So, the subject has no direct control over forces applied to the balls he or she wants to pocket. Does the player solve the equations of motion, keeping in mind the interaction between the balls and the surface of the table, mechanical laws of colliding balls, etc.? Intuition says that this is not the case. Indeed, the author (who plays pool poorly) was once given a piece of advice: Imagine a straight line from the center of the target ball to the hole and another ball, which touches the target ball and is located on that line (Figure 5.4). Now try to hit that imaginary ball straight in the center with the white ball. For a beginner, this is very good advice, which indirectly takes into consideration the basic mechanics of ball collision. Note that it is formulated not in terms of forces but in terms of positions and orientations. The author's game improved nearly instantaneously. Did this happen because his brain started to solve the equations of mechanics better? No. This happened because he learned a simple rule leading to success.

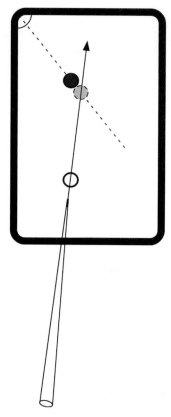

Figure 5.4 Knowledge of basic mechanics helps one to play billiards. Imagine a straight line from the center of the target ball to the hole and another ball, which touches the target ball and is located on that line. Try to hit that imaginary ball straight in the center with the white ball.

Motion in an elastic force field

Consider now playing pool on a billiard table covered not with a rigid surface but with an elastic one. A billiard ball would create with its weight a well on the surface and would be at equilibrium on the bottom of the well (Figure 5.5A). How could one move the object to a new location ("target" in Figure 5.5)? There are two approaches. First, to compute the requisite forces taking into account the mechanics of the task (in particular, the mass of the ball, the elasticity and friction of the surface, etc.) and then push the ball with the computed force (Figure 5.5B). Second, to press on the surface with a finger close to the ball. The ball will start falling down the slope (gradient of potential energy) towards the finger. Move the finger to the desired final location, and the ball will obediently follow (Figure 5.5C). No accurate knowledge of mechanical parameters and force computation is required, but adequate forces will emerge and act on the ball.

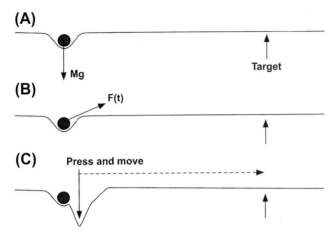

Figure 5.5 Two methods of moving a ball over an elastic surface. The ball creates a local potential well with its weight (A). To move it, one can either apply requisite (pre-computed) forces (as in B) or press on the elastic surface with a finger and move the finger to the target location (as in C).

Let us assume, for now, that the central nervous system uses the former approach, that is, that there are neural structures that model interactions within the different structures of the body and between the body and the environment and use these models to pre-compute requisite force–time profiles to fit specific motor tasks. This approach can be called "force control."

Force control. Inverse model

An important assumption of the force control approach is that the central nervous system has knowledge of the mechanical properties of the limbs and environment and uses this knowledge for the purposes of movement control. There is no physical or physiological explanation of how this knowledge is obtained, stored, and used. It is supposed to be essential in forming so-called *internal models*. This term has been used for a variety of meanings. The most general meaning is that an internal model is a neural process that allows us to predict the consequences of an action. There is no argument that the central nervous system can act in a predictive fashion; in earlier literature, this feature has been assigned to *neural representations* within the brain. A somewhat different definition implies that an internal model links realized changes in the body to expected perceptual consequences. It also seems similar in spirit to the notion of neural representation. The most specific definition states that internal models are processes within neural structures computing or predicting effects of the interactions among parts of the body and between the body and the environment. This definition is the most commonly used or implied in experimental studies in support of the idea of internal models. So this is the definition we are going to stick with here.

Two kinds of internal models within the central nervous system are typically considered within this approach. First, there should be models that pre-compute requisite forces based on the sensory information about the state of the body, the environment, and the task (Figure 5.6). A typical example would be a model that pre-computes descending neural signals necessary to produce muscle activations that move the index finger to a target. Since the model is supposed to be formed in the brain, the brain neural networks need to solve, explicitly or implicitly, a chain of problems.

First step

The initial and final positions of the fingertip can be characterized by three coordinates in the external space each. To place the endpoint of a multi-link chain into a certain point, one needs to define joint angles that satisfy the task (the *problem of inverse kinematics*). As mentioned earlier, the human arm is kinematically redundant: The number of major axes of joint rotation is more than three. Even if one does not count the joints within the hand, there are three axes of rotation in the shoulder (α_1, α_2, α_3 in Figure 5.7A), one in the elbow (α_4), two in the wrist (α_5, α_6), and one shared between the elbow and the wrist (pronation–supination, α_7). So, this step involves solving a problem of motor redundancy, that is, finding a solution for a system of equations where the number of unknowns (joint angle values) is larger than the number of equations (defined by endpoint coordinates). This problem has no single solution (two joint configurations are shown in Figure 5.7B for a cartoon arm with only three joints that performs a task of pointing in two dimensions). It can be formalized using the notion of a Jacobian, a matrix that links infinitesimal joint displacements to infinitesimal displacement vector of the endpoint in the external space:

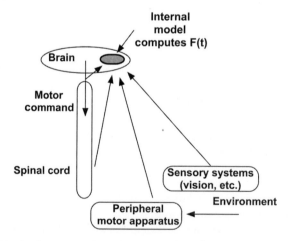

Figure 5.6 Within the force-control approach, there have to be models that pre-compute requisite forces based on the sensory information about the state of the body, the environment, and the task.

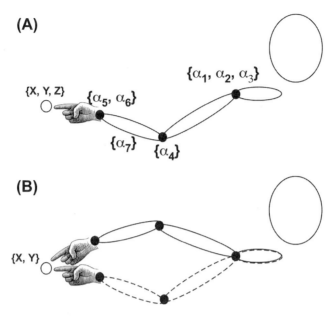

Figure 5.7 (A) There are more potentially independent axes of joint rotation in the three major arm joints, shoulder, elbow, and wrist, than the dimensionality of the space where we live (which is three). (B) This allows a target in space to be reached with different joint configurations even for a three-joint system moving in a two-dimensional space.

$$dX = Jd\alpha, \tag{5.1}$$

where J is the Jacobian matrix, X is the vector of the endpoint and α is the vector of joint angles. To solve the problem of inverse kinematics means finding $d\alpha$ that satisfy the equation:

$$d\alpha = J^{-1}dX. \tag{5.2}$$

Remember, a *matrix* is a rectangular arrangement of elements or entries (which are sometimes numbers). To specify the size of a matrix, a matrix with m rows and n columns is called an $m \times n$ matrix, while m and n are called its *dimensions*. A matrix with only one row is called a *row-vector*, and a matrix with one column is called a *column-vector*. Matrices are typically denoted using upper-case, bold letters. Two operations with matrices will be mentioned in this book, *transposition* and *inversion*. The transpose of a matrix A is another matrix A^T formed by turning rows into columns and vice versa. The inverse of a square matrix A (this means that the number of rows equals the number of columns, $n \times n$) is a matrix A^{-1} such that the product AA^{-1} equals an *identity matrix*, In, which is defined as an $n \times n$ matrix with diagonal elements that equal unity (1) and non-diagonal elements that equal zero.

Unfortunately, for a kinematically redundant system, the J matrix is not square and cannot be inverted. In engineering, commonly, additional constraints are used to invert the Jacobian matrix. One of the most common methods is the Moore–Penrose pseudo-inverse, which corresponds to the shortest distance in the joint angle space satisfying the abovementioned system of equation. There is no reason, however, to assume that the brain uses this strategy. Let us take it, however, that this problem has been somehow solved.

Second step

To implement the selected set of joint angles, the controller needs to define trajectories from an initial joint configuration to the final joint configuration. This problem also has many (an infinite number of) solutions. For example, the motion in all the joints may proceed simultaneously or in a staggered fashion (as illustrated in Figure 5.8 for a hypothetical system with only three joint angles). Assume that it is somehow solved, for example based on another criterion of optimality (to be discussed later).

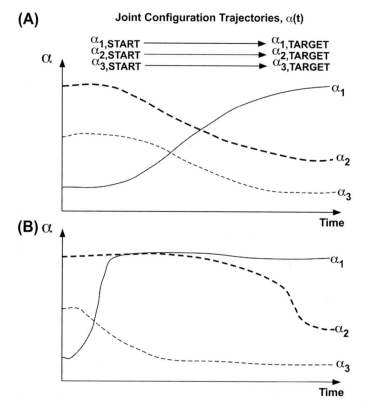

Figure 5.8 Even the same final joint configuration can be reached by an infinite number of joint angle (α) time profiles. For example, joints can move synchronously (as in A) or in a staggered fashion (as in B).

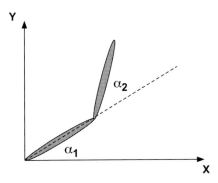

Figure 5.9 A simple two-joint system. Equations are in the text.

Third step

To move the joints, one has to apply appropriately timed joint torques. So the next step is to define a pattern of joint torques that would implement the required movement kinematics (the *problem of inverse dynamics*). This problem for a multi-segment effector involves solving rather complex equations of dynamics since forces acting on a segment depend not only on forces produced by muscles that attach to that segment and external forces such as gravity, but also on the so-called *interaction forces* that depend on the motion of adjacent segments. For a very simple, two-segment effector moving in a plane (Figure 5.9), the torques acting on the segments at the joints may be represented as:

$$
\begin{aligned}
\mathbf{T}_1 ={}& I_1(d^2\alpha_1/dt^2) + I_{1,2}(d^2\alpha_2/dt^2) - b_{cp1}(d\alpha_2/dt)^2 \\
& - b_{Cr}(d\alpha_1/dt)(d\alpha_2/dt) + \mathbf{G}_1 \\
\mathbf{T}_2 ={}& I_2(d^2\alpha_2/dt^2) + I_{2,1}(d^2\alpha_1/dt^2) + b_{cp2}(d\alpha_1/dt)^2 + \mathbf{G}_2
\end{aligned}
\tag{5.3}
$$

where subscripts 1 and 2 refer to the more proximal and more distal segment, $\mathbf{T}$ stands for torque (moment of force), I_1 and I_2 are inertial coefficients, $I_{1,2}$ and $I_{2,1}$ are inertial coupling coefficients (the inertial resistance of the first segment felt at the second joint and vice versa), b_{cp1} and b_{cp2} are centripetal coefficients, b_{Cr} is the Coriolis coefficient, and $\mathbf{G}$ stands for gravitational terms. For a movement in three-dimensional space performed by the human arm with seven major axes of joint rotation, the equations look much more unattractive.

Fourth step

All joints, even the simplest joints with only one axis of rotation, are crossed by several muscles (Figure 5.10). What forces should be produced by individual muscles to ensure the required pattern of joint torque? This is another problem of motor redundancy: One has to solve, for each rotational axis, one equation with the number of unknowns equal to the number of muscles crossing the joint and affecting that

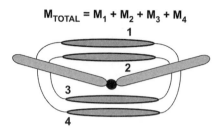

$$M_{TOTAL} = M_1 + M_2 + M_3 + M_4$$

Figure 5.10 Typically, joints are crossed by several muscles. This poses a problem of motor redundancy: How to share the required total joint torque among individual muscle torques.

rotation. This problem has been addressed using various *optimization* approaches that will be discussed later (see Section 9.2).

Fifth step

To produce active muscle force, action potentials have to be sent to the muscle by alpha-motoneurons of the appropriate pool. Muscle force depends on the level of excitation it receives from its motoneuronal pool and also on the actual muscle length and rate of its change (velocity). Therefore, to define signals that should be generated by alpha-motoneurons to a muscle to produce a required profile of muscle force, one has to take into account expected values of muscle length and velocity (Figure 5.11). There are many models of muscle force generation that, typically, involve at least two transformations, from muscle excitation to force production in the contractile elements (cross-bridges) and from force production by cross-bridges to tendon force acting at the points of tendon attachment. The first transformation may be approximated as an exponential function of excitation, which is low-pass filtered due to the properties of involved physico-chemical processes:

$$\begin{aligned}
\mathbf{F}_C &= a[\exp(bE) - 1]; \\
\mathbf{F}_C &= \tau^2(d^2\mathbf{F}_{CF}/dt^2) + 2\tau(d\mathbf{F}_{CF}/dt) + \mathbf{F}_{CF},
\end{aligned} \tag{5.4}$$

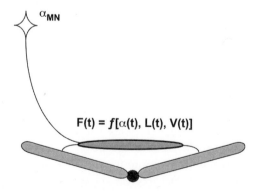

Figure 5.11 Muscle force is a function of its excitation level (defined by signals from alpha-motoneurons), length, and velocity.

where $\mathbf{F}_C$ is contractile force, $\mathbf{F}_{CF}$ is contractile filtered force, E is muscle excitation level, τ is a parameter of the filter, and a and b are coefficients. The second transformation takes into account the length and velocity dependence of muscle force:

$$\mathbf{F}_T = \mathbf{F}_{CF}[1 - f(\mathrm{d}L/\mathrm{d}t)/(\mathrm{d}L/\mathrm{d}t + d)] + k(L - L_0) \tag{5.5}$$

where $\mathbf{F}_T$ is tendon force, L is muscle length, L_0 is the resting length of the "muscle spring" due to the elastic properties, f is a term reflecting damping effects on the muscle force, and c and d are constants. An important point is that any error in estimating muscle length and/or velocity will necessarily lead to the production of erroneous force values.

Sixth step

Alpha-motoneurons produce sequences of action potential that depend on the total input to the motoneurons. These neurons receive signals from the brain ("the *controller*") and from peripheral sensory endings (*receptors*). The latter component is a complex function of signals related to muscle length, velocity, force, and may also depend on signals from skin receptors, joint receptors, and receptors located in other muscles. To ensure an adequate total input into a motoneuronal pool, the controller needs to take into account the predicted peripheral contribution and generate a central component that would make the total input into the motoneuronal pool adequate to produce the output computed at the previous step (Figure 5.12). There is a huge

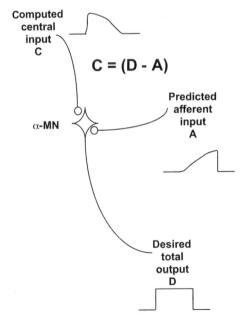

Figure 5.12 If a desired output of an alpha-motoneuronal (α-MN) pool is known (for example, a rectangular pulse), the controller has to predict contribution from reflex loops and send a command that, after being summed up with the reflex input, produces the required output.

problem, however: Since alpha-motoneurons are threshold elements, it is absolutely impossible to compute an input into an alpha-motoneuronal pool based on its output.

A formal model of this sequence of events (which involves more steps than those reviewed here) is sometimes termed the *inverse model* of the system. It is called "inverse" because it reverses the natural cause–consequence relationships at each of its steps as compared to what happens during natural movement production. Figure 5.13 summarizes the main steps involved in the inverse model for a pointing movement from a certain starting position to a certain final position.

Force control. Direct model

Since the signals from the controller have to be computed before movement initiation, most of the required information, such as time profiles of muscle length, velocity, and force, is unavailable and has to be predicted. Sensory signals inform the central nervous system on these variables but this information comes at a delay (afferent time delay, Δ_{AFF} in Figure 5.14). Signals from the controller also take time to reach alpha-motoneurons and muscles (efferent time delay, Δ_{EFF} in Figure 5.14). So the controller always deals with outdated information and sends commands that will be even more outdated when they reach the effectors.

To deal with this problem, one has to be able to predict (compute) what is likely to happen with the peripheral system after a certain time interval based on the recent history of both sensory information and commands sent to the system. An important

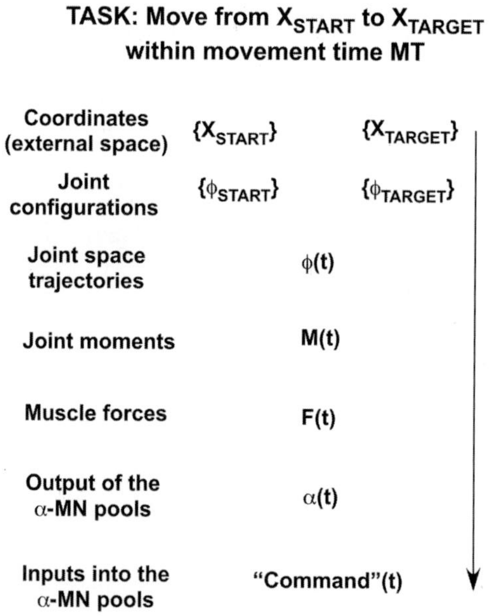

TASK: Move from X_{START} to X_{TARGET} within movement time MT

Coordinates (external space)	$\{X_{START}\}$	$\{X_{TARGET}\}$	I
Joint configurations	$\{\phi_{START}\}$	$\{\phi_{TARGET}\}$	N V
Joint space trajectories		$\phi(t)$	E R
Joint moments		$M(t)$	S E
Muscle forces		$F(t)$	M O
Output of the α-MN pools		$\alpha(t)$	D E L
Inputs into the α-MN pools		"Command"(t)	↓

Figure 5.13 A scheme illustrating the sequence of steps involved in an inverse model (grossly simplified).

Controller
Time delay
Δ EFF
Time delay
Δ AFF
Sensory
signals
Peripheral
Motor Apparatus
Environment

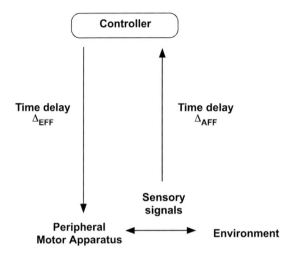

Figure 5.14 Time delays involved in delivering sensory information to the brain and execution of command signals from the brain.

component of any predictor is a *direct model* of the controlled system. It computes the effects of a particular command on the state of all the involved structures, such as the motoneurons, the muscles, the joints, and the endpoint. So these computations follow the natural course of events, justifying the term "direct." Figure 5.15 illustrates the

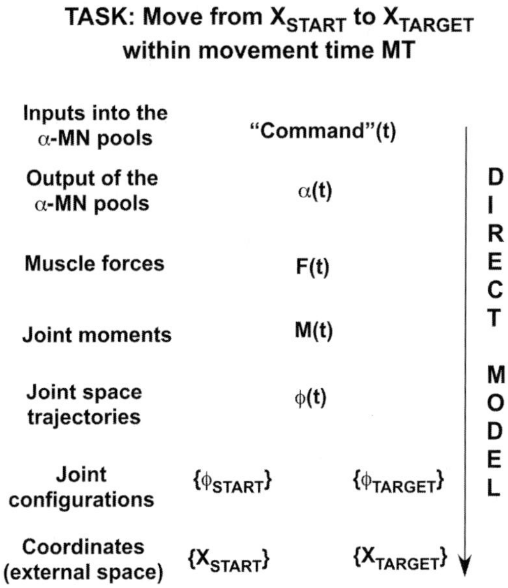

TASK: Move from X START to X TARGET
within movement time MT
Inputs into the
α-MN pools
"Command"(t)
Output of the
α-MN pools
α(t)
Muscle forces
F(t)
Joint moments
M(t)
Joint space
trajectories
ϕ(t)
Joint
configurations
{ϕ START}
{ϕ TARGET}
Coordinates
(external space)
{X START}
{X TARGET}
DIRECT MODEL

Figure 5.15 A scheme illustrating the sequence of steps involved in a direct model (grossly simplified).

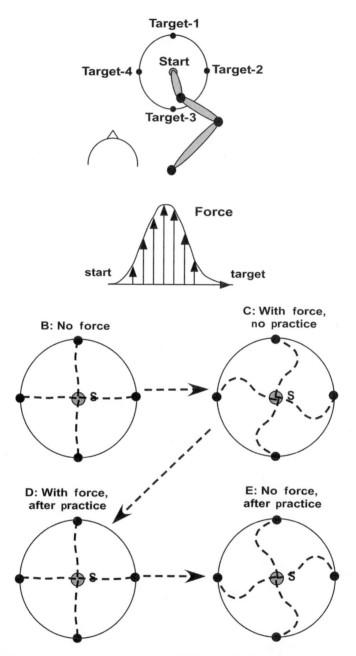

Figure 5.16 A person performs a center-out task illustrated in the top panel. An artificial force field can be produced by a programmable robot that generates force orthogonal to the vector of velocity and proportional to its magnitude. (B) Without the force field, the trajectories are nearly straight. (C) After the force field has been turned on, the trajectories become curved. (D) After some practice, the trajectories become straight again. (E) When the force field is turned off, the trajectories become curved in the opposite direction.

steps involved in the creation of the direct model. It involves similar steps to the inverse model (Figure 5.13), but in the opposite order.

Multiple direct and inverse models can be assembled into cascades to improve accuracy of their performance.

Much experimental support for the force-control approach comes from studies of *motor adaptation* in unusual force fields. A typical study of this kind would involve quick and accurate movement of a kinematically non-redundant effector into a target. Commonly, the experiments involved shoulder–elbow movements in a horizontal plane (Figure 5.16A). Subjects in such experiments demonstrate close to straight trajectories of the endpoint (Figure 5.16B). Then a force field is turned on, acting on the handle, for example the external force may be proportional to the absolute magnitude of the endpoint velocity and directed orthogonal to the velocity vector. In such conditions, movements become curved (Figure 5.16C). After some practice in the new conditions, the movement trajectory becomes straight again (Figure 5.16D). If the force field is unexpectedly turned off, the trajectories become curved in the opposite direction as compared to the trajectories observed when the force field was turned on for the first time (Figure 5.16E). These observations have been interpreted as suggesting that during the adaptation phase, the controller creates an internal model corresponding to inter-actions of the body with the artificial force field and learns to compute requisite muscle forces opposing the unusual motion-dependent forces produced by the force field. When the field was turned off, these self-generated forces were not opposed and produced deviations of the endpoint trajectory in the opposite direction.

The term "internal model" may be viewed as a metaphor for unknown processes within the body that allow it to show certain adaptive and predictive behaviors. Alternatively, it may be viewed as a reflection of computational processes within certain structures within the central nervous system. There is little argument that processes within the central nervous system allow the body to behave in adaptive and predictive ways; so, the former view on internal models is acceptable for many researchers (although, being a metaphor, it does not seem to be very useful for exact scientific research). The latter, more concrete meaning is much more debatable (see, for example, Section 4.1).

5.2 Are interaction torques special? The leading-joint hypothesis

Examples of interaction torques

Because of mechanical coupling, it is not easy to move just one joint of an extremity. The mechanical coupling is a result of two main peripheral factors. First, virtually all the major joints of the human body are spanned by at least one bi-articular muscle, that is a muscle that also crosses another, neighboring joint. Figure 5.17 illustrates a two-joint system with three segments (S1, S2, and S3)—two uni-articular muscles and one bi-articular muscle. Since muscles have elastic properties, motion of a joint, even a very slow motion, is accompanied by changes in the length of the bi-articular muscle, which

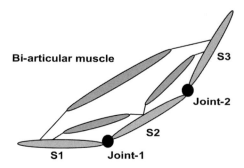

Figure 5.17 Bi-articular muscles provide coupling across adjacent joints. As a result, motion of one joint leads to a change in the torque applied to the other joint.

will produce torque at the other joint it spans. If no adjustments are made at the other joint, it will also move. Even in the absence of bi-articular muscles, motion of a joint within a multi-joint chain leads to torques in other joints, the so-called interaction torques (within a simple model, these are the sum of the contributions from inertial, centripetal, and Coriolis forces described earlier) (see Equation 5.3).

Consider a person sitting with the upper arm resting on a table with forearm and hand vertical (Figure 5.18). If this person tries to move the elbow joint without changing the wrist joint angle, muscles spanning the wrist joint will have to be activated in synchrony with and in proportion to activation of muscles that produce

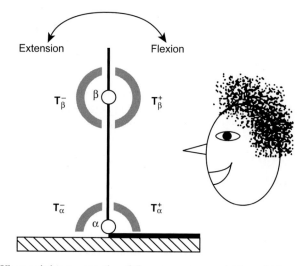

Figure 5.18 When a sitting person placed the upper arm on a table and tries to move one joint at a time, the elbow (α) or the wrist joint (β), the mechanical joint coupling requires simultaneous changes in the joint torques (T_α and T_β). Reproduced by permission from Latash, M. L., Aruin, A. S., & Shapiro, B. (1995). The relation between posture and movement: A study of a simple synergy in a two-joint task. *Human Movement Science, 14*, 79–107, © Elsevier.

the elbow movement. Otherwise, the hand will flap under the action of interaction torques. A fast movement in the wrist is also accompanied with interaction torques acting at the elbow (these are typically smaller than in the previous example because of typical differences in the characteristics of motion in the two joints). So, a fast wrist motion has to be accompanied by appropriately timed and scaled activation of muscles controlling the elbow if one wants to keep the elbow joint motionless.

The importance of interaction torques has been recognized in many approaches to motor control. In particular, the study of patients with peripheral large-fiber neuropathy ("deafferented patients") discussed earlier (see Section 4.6) showed movement trajectories compatible with the hypothesis that these patients lost the ability to predict and compensate for interaction torques. Within the force-control approach it is assumed that some kind of neural representation is used to directly compute and specify muscle forces and joint torques. In most such approaches, interaction torques are viewed as a nuisance, a factor that has to be predicted and taken care of by neural computations.

The leading-joint hypothesis

There is one exception. The *leading-joint hypothesis* offered by Natalia Dounskaia assumes that interaction torques play a central role in the movements performed by multi-joint limbs. The hypothesis also assumes that one joint of a moving limb plays a leading role and generates motion in all other joints with interaction torques. Other joints experience interaction torques produced by the leading joint motion and add muscle torques to the interaction torques to fit specific motor tasks. Because of such factors as larger accelerations and velocities (and larger muscles) typical of more proximal joints, more commonly, the most proximal joint is assumed to play the role of the leading joint. Muscles crossing the leading joint are assumed to be activated largely ignoring mechanical effects expected from motion of more distal joints. In some cases, rarely, another joint may play the role of the leading joint, and the most proximal joint becomes subordinate.

This principle of control is similar to moving a passive structure, a whip-like chain with several joints with force applied to its end (Figure 5.19). The joints in the passive chain will not be able to correct the interaction torques produced by the driving force. In contrast, in human limbs, muscles crossing the more distal joints can add to or subtract from the transmitted interaction torques.

The leading-joint hypothesis is not easily applicable to slow movements where interaction torques are low. It also sometimes views different joints as leading in different phases within a single action, which seems somewhat artificial.

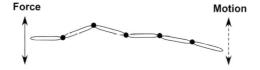

Figure 5.19 Applying force to one end of a chain of segments produces motion in all segments and in the endpoint.

5.3   Generalized motor programs

Essential and non-essential variables. Engrams

In the early 1960s the Russian mathematician Israel Gelfand (1913–2009) and physicist Michael Tsetlin (1924–1966) suggested that all variables describing biological systems, including those describing human movements, could be classified into *essential* or *non-essential*. Under essential variables they included those that defined salient features (patterns) of movements, while non-essential variables were supposed to define whether the movement was performed faster or slower, weaker or stronger. Note that this separation does not allow the identification of these groups of variables within such peripheral mechanical variables as forces or torques. For example, performing "the same" multi-joint arm movement faster or slower with a light object in the hand and with a heavy object in the hand is associated with non-linear scaling of the torque components in Equation 5.3.

The idea of essential and non-essential variables was close to the idea of *engrams* offered by Bernstein about 30 years earlier (see Section 2.3). Engrams were supposed to represent stored in memory patterns of neural variables that defined important features of movements (similarly to essential variables). These patterns could be scaled in magnitude and in time with parameters (similar to non-essential variables).

Generalized motor program

In the 1970s Richard Schmidt attempted to develop the idea of engrams for mechanical variables describing external movement patterns. His concept of a *generalized motor program* assumed that particular functions of control variables were stored in the central nervous system. These functions could be scaled in magnitude and also used at different time scales. For example, a classical study of professional typists by Carlo Terzuolo and Paolo Viviani showed that when professional typists typed the same phrase at different speeds, they preserved the relative timing of pressing individual keys. Other classical observations include the apparently preserved ability of a person to show individual features of handwriting when writing on a piece of paper and on a blackboard. Note that different joints and muscle groups are used during writing in these two conditions. Moreover, individual handwriting features were reported for writing with the non-dominant hand and even with the pen attached to the elbow or to a foot, or even gripped between the teeth. A classical set of handwriting samples by Bernstein is reproduced in Figure 5.20. All these observations suggest that learning a movement (a skill) is associated not with learning a set of commands to muscles but a pattern of a more abstract variable—an engram.

The idea of generalized motor program was developed further by trying to link the hypothetical neural variables to such peripheral variables as forces, torques, and patterns of muscle activation. So it is fair to say that the generalized motor program was the grandfather of the internal model; both ideas share a view that peripheral performance variables of the neuromotor system, such as forces and torques, are

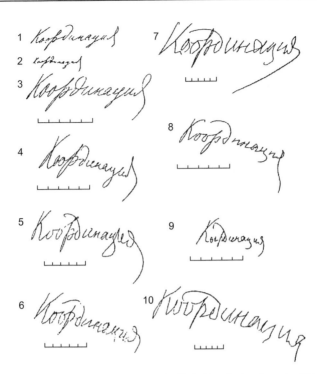

Figure 5.20 Examples of the word "Coordination" (in Russian) written by Nikolai Bernstein with the pencil grasped by the dominant hand, non-dominant hand, attached to the dominant and non-dominant elbows, to the right and left feet, and gripped with the teeth. Note the similarity of the writing samples. Reproduced from Bernstein, N. A. (1935). The problem of interrelation between coordination and localization. *Archives of Biological Science, 38,* 1–35. Public domain.

somehow pre-computed by neural structures before a movement starts. Note that engrams do not share these features since they refer to a topological pattern of the trajectory, not associated forces and torques.

Self-test questions

1. Are torques produced by gravity motion-dependent during multi-joint arm movements?
2. Write an equation for the centripetal force.
3. What is Coriolis force? How is it directed with respect to the linear motion of an object and rotation of the system where the object moves.
4. Present examples of Coriolis force affecting everyday movements.
5. What forces move the body when a person walks from one place to another?
6. Give examples of the problems of motor redundancy that the controller must solve to issue a neural command leading to requisite force profiles.
7. What are the main assumptions inherent in the force-control approach?

8. What is the inverse model?

9. What is the main problem in defining an input into an alpha-motoneuronal pool that would produce a desired output?

10. Why are direct models necessary?

11. What processes contribute most to time delays between issuing a neural command and observing its motor effect?

12. Why are the two groups of models called "inverse" and "direct"?

13. Why are endpoint trajectories nearly straight in a typical center-out task in the absence of any special force field?

14. After a person adapts to a force field and starts producing straight trajectories, turning the field off leads to curved trajectories. Why? In what direction will they be curved?

15. Present as many examples of interaction torques as you can.

16. Why do people activate wrist muscles when they try to perform a quick motion in a proximal joint, shoulder, or elbow?

17. Formulate the leading-joint hypothesis.

18. Which joint is leading in most arm movements?

19. Define essential and non-essential variables.

20. Define engram according to Bernstein.

21. What is a generalized motor program?

22. What is the main difference between the notions of engram and generalized motor program?

23. Present examples of studies that support the existence of generalized motor programs.

24. What is the major difference between the notion of generalized motor program and the notions of direct/inverse internal models?

Essential references and recommended further readings

Arbib, M. A. (1980). Interacting schemas for motor control. In G. E. Stelmach, & J. Requin (Eds.), *Tutorials in motor behavior* (pp. 71–81). Amsterdam: North Holland Publishing Company.

Bernstein, N. A. (1967). *The co-ordination and regulation of movements*. Oxford: Pergamon Press.

Dounskaia, N. (2005). The internal model and the leading joint hypothesis: implications for control of multi-joint movements. *Experimental Brain Research, 166*, 1–16.

Dounskaia, N. (2010). Control of human limb movements: the leading joint hypothesis and its practical applications. *Exercise and Sport Science Reviews, 38*, 201–208.

Dounskaia, N. V., Swinnen, S. P., Walter, C. B., Spaepen, A. J., & Verschueren, S. M. (1998). Hierarchical control of different elbow-wrist coordination patterns. *Experimental Brain Research, 121*, 239–254.

Enoka, R. M. (2002). *Neuromechanics of human movement* (3rd ed.). Urbana, IL: Human Kinetics.

Gelfand, I. M., & Tsetlin, M. L. (1966). On mathematical modeling of the mechanisms of the central nervous system. In I. M. Gelfand, V. S. Gurfinkel, S. V. Fomin, & M. L. Tsetlin (Eds.), *Models of the structural-functional organization of certain biological systems* (pp. 9–26). Moscow: Nauka, (in Russian, a translation is available in 1971 edition by MIT Press, Cambridge, MA).

Gribble, P. L., Ostry, D. J., Sanguineti, V., & Laboissiere, R. (1998). Are complex control signals required for human arm movements? *Journal of Neurophysiology, 79*, 1409–1424.

Hinder, M. R., & Milner, T. E. (2003). The case for an internal dynamics model versus equilibrium point control in human movement. *Journal of Physiology, 549*, 953–963.

Hollerbach, J. M., & Flash, T. (1982). Dynamic interaction between limb segments during planar arm movements. *Biological Cybernetics, 44*, 67–77.

Imamizu, H., Miyauchi, S., Tamada, T., Sasaki, Y., Takino, R., Putz, B., Yoshioka, T., & Kawato, M. (2000). Human cerebellar activity reflecting an acquired internal model of a new tool. *Nature, 403*, 192–195.

Kawato, M. (1999). Internal models for motor control and trajectory planning. *Current Opinions in Neurobiology, 9*, 718–727.

Kiemel, T., Oie, K. S., & Jeka, J. J. (2002). Multisensory fusion and the stochastic structure of postural sway. *Biological Cybernetics, 87*, 262–277.

Lackner, J. R., & DiZio, P. (1994). Rapid adaptation to Coriolis force perturbations of arm trajectory. *Journal of Neurophysiology, 72*, 1–15.

Latash, M. L. (1998). Control of multi-joint reaching movement. In M. L. Latash (Ed.), *Progress in motor control: Vol. 1. Bernstein's traditions in movement studies* (pp. 315–328). Urbana, IL: Human Kinetics, The elastic membrane metaphor.

Latash, M. L., & Zatsiorsky, V. M. (1993). Joint stiffness: Myth or reality? *Human Movement Science, 12*, 653–692.

Miall, R. C. (1998). The cerebellum, predictive control and motor coordination. *Novartis Foundation Symposium, 218*, 272–284.

Ostry, D. J., & Feldman, A. G. (2003). A critical evaluation of the force control hypothesis in motor control. *Experimental Brain Research, 153*, 275–288.

Schmidt, R. A. (1975). A schema theory of discrete motor skill learning. *Psychological Reviews, 82*, 225–260.

Schmidt, R. A. (1980). Past and future issues in motor programming. *Research Quarterly of Exercise and Sport, 51*, 122–140.

Shadmehr, R., & Mussa-Ivaldi, F. A. (1994). Adaptive representation of dynamics during learning of a motor task. *Journal of Neuroscience, 14*, 3208–3224.

Shadmehr, R., & Wise, S. P. (2005). *The computational neurobiology of reaching and pointing*. Cambridge, MA: MIT Press.

Viviani, P., & Terzuolo, C. (1980). Space-time invariance in learned motor skills. In G. E. Stelmach, & J. Requin (Eds.), *Tutorials in motor behavior* (pp. 525–533). Amsterdam: North Holland.

Winter, D. A., Prince, F., Frank, J. S., Powell, C., & Zabjek, K. F. (1996). Unified theory regarding A/P and M/L balance in quiet stance. *Journal of Neurophysiology, 75*, 2334–2343.

Wolpert, D. M., Miall, R. C., & Kawato, M. (1998). Internal models in the cerebellum. *Trends in Cognitive Science, 2*, 338–347.

Zatsiorsky, V. M. (1997). On muscle and joint viscosity. *Motor Control, 1*, 299–309.

Zatsiorsky, V. M. (1998). *Kinematics of human motion*. Champaign, IL: Human Kinetics.

Zatsiorsky, V. M. (2002). *Kinetics of human motion*. Champaign, IL: Human Kinetics.

6 Control with muscle activations

Chapter Outline

6.1 Introduction

A relatively large group of hypotheses assume that the central nervous system specifies certain patterns of total presynaptic input into appropriate alpha-motoneuronal pools, while mechanical characteristics of movement show time evolution reflecting these inputs, the input–output characteristics of the motoneuronal pools, the muscle properties, and the interactions among moving body parts and between the body and the environment. Since alpha-motoneurons receive projections from both descending pathways and reflex pathways (Figure 6.1), this group of hypotheses has to assume that the reflex inputs into the alpha-motoneuron are either very small (or even turned off temporarily) during movements, or accurately predicted by the controller and their predicted contribution is taken into account.

Reflexes during movements

The first assumption does not agree well with experiments. For example, imagine that a person is asked to press as strongly as possible against a stop. The muscles producing the action are activated close to their maximal level. Now, imagine that the stop is unexpectedly removed (Figure 6.2). The strongly activated muscles will show a period of complete or nearly complete silence after a short delay, about 40–50 ms, compatible with the action of reflexes from peripheral receptors. So, reflexes can turn off 100% of the strongest muscle activation; their effects are not small.

Fundamentals of Motor Control. DOI: 10.1016/B978-0-12-415956-3.00006-3

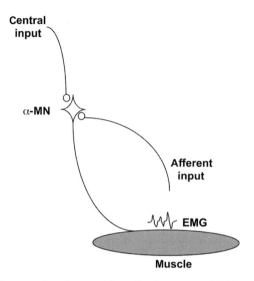

Figure 6.1 In a crude approximation, muscle activation pattern (EMG) may be viewed as reflecting an interaction of two signals converging on the alpha-motoneurons (α-MN)—a central input and an afferent input.

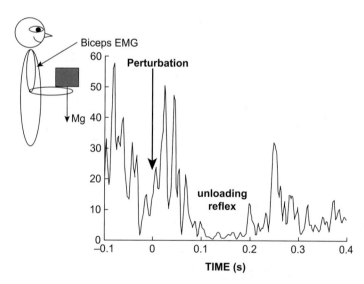

Figure 6.2 The unloading reflex. Initially, an elbow flexor (biceps brachii) showed a high level of activity to keep the elbow at 90° against the load. After the load has been suddenly removed (perturbation), the muscle shows a drop in its activation to nearly zero level at a delay of well under 100 ms. Reproduced by permission from Latash, M. L. (2008). *The neurophysiological basis of movement*, 2nd edn. Urbana, IL: Human Kinetics.

Strong reflex effects have been shown in a number of studies when a moving, rather than a stationary, effector was unexpectedly perturbed in the course of its trajectory by a change in the external force. These observations suggest that reflexes are not turned off during quick movements. A few recent studies have provided evidence for strong modulation of the amplitude of reflexes to muscle stretch during movements. However, typically, these studies do not consider that reflex effects can be modified using two parameters—gain and threshold. So, if a reflex is not observed or significantly reduced in response to a standard perturbation, this can mean that its gain has been reduced and/or that its threshold has been modified. Many earlier studies have suggested that there are large changes in the threshold of the tonic stretch reflex (see Chapter 4) during voluntary movements, while there has been no convincing evidence that the gain of this reflex is reduced during fast movements.

The other suggestion, that effects of reflex inputs into alpha-motoneurons are predicted by the controller, turns this hypothesis into another member of the *internal model* class (see Section 5.1). The main difference is that it starts not at the level of limb kinematics but at the level of the output of the alpha-motoneuronal pools recorded as the electromyographic signal (EMG, see Section 13.3). All the abovementioned problems inherent to the internal models approach remain inherent to this approach as well. In particular, consider that the threshold properties of alpha-motoneurons in principle do not allow inputs into these neurons to be pre-computed based on their desired output.

6.2   Dual-strategy hypothesis

Excitation pulse and tri-phasic activation pattern

The dual-strategy hypothesis was introduced by Gerald Gottlieb and his colleagues. It assumes that total presynaptic inputs into pools of alpha-motoneurons can be represented as rectangular pulses with modifiable height and duration (Figure 6.3). The height (H) and duration (D) of the excitation pulse are supposed to be selected based on the task requirements such as amplitude of movement, inertial load, and movement time. When an alpha-motoneuronal pool receives an excitation pulse, it is assumed to produce an output, which looks like a low-pass filtered version of the pulse (Figure 6.3). By itself, this is already a very strong assumption given that alpha-motoneurons are threshold elements.

The hypothesis was developed for single-joint movements controlled by a pair of muscles—an agonist and an antagonist. Later attempts at generalizing the hypothesis for multi-joint movements performed by kinematically redundant limbs were marginally successful. For single-joint movements, the parameters manipulated by the central nervous system included the height and duration of the excitation pulses to the two muscles and the delay of the antagonist excitation pulse. For movements performed in isotonic conditions (against an apparently constant external load), the hypothesis was able to account for patterns of agonist muscle activation that matched the experimental observations well. Such movements are typically accompanied by the so-called tri-phasic muscle activation patterns (Figure 6.4). Such a pattern consists

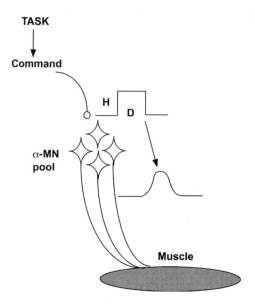

Figure 6.3 The dual-strategy hypothesis. The presynaptic input to an alpha-motoneuronal (α-MN) pool (command) represents a rectangular pulse with modifiable height (*H*) and duration (*D*). The processing of the pulse by the alpha-motoneurons leads to its low-pass filtering resulting in a smooth curve with characteristics that can be compared to those of observed EMG patterns.

of an initial activation burst in the agonist muscle (the muscle that produces torque in the direction required by the task), a delayed burst in the antagonist muscle (a muscle that produces torque in the opposite direction) during which the agonist is relatively quiescent, and a smaller second burst in the agonist muscle. During the first agonist

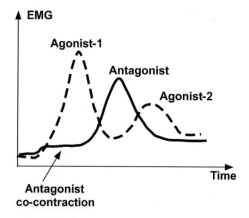

Figure 6.4 A typical tri-phasic electromyographic pattern consists of an initial agonist burst (Agonist-1), a delayed antagonist burst, and a second agonist burst (Agonist-2). During the first agonist burst, there is a low-level co-contraction of the antagonist muscle.

burst, there is a steady-state increase in the antagonist muscle activation, commonly known as *antagonist co-contraction*.

Speed-insensitive strategy

The term "dual-strategy hypothesis" is used because there are two hypothesized main patterns of modulation of the excitation pulses—those that involve changes only in the pulse duration while the height is kept constant and those involving pulse height modulation. In particular, for movements over different distances and/or against different inertial loads, when the subject is not trying to control movement time explicitly, the constant pulse height strategy has been assumed and termed *speed-insensitive strategy*. In particular, this strategy is used for movements performed under the instruction to move "as fast as possible." Figure 6.5 illustrates typical patterns of muscle activation during such movements performed over different distances against a constant inertial load, while Figure 6.6 shows such patterns when movements are performed over a fixed distance but against different inertial loads. Note the similar early rates of change of the first agonist EMG burst. There are other regularities in the patterns that are accounted for within the speed-sensitive strategy. These include the scaling of the peak of the first agonist EMG burst and of the delay before the initiation of the antagonist burst. Note also that the similarities in the EMG characteristics do not translate into similarities in the kinematic characteristics because the latter depend on the loading conditions. In particular, the early rates of velocity are similar across movements over different distances (Figure 6.5), while they differ across movements against different inertial loads (Figure 6.6).

Speed-insensitive strategy is not limited to movements performed "as fast as possible." For example, similar regular features of the EMG patterns can be seen if a subject is asked to move over different distances "at a comfortable speed" or "at the same speed." The last instruction is intuitively clear although it makes no physical sense. Indeed, speed is a time-varying variable during movements. For any of the movements illustrated in Figures 6.5 and 6.6, both average speed and peak speed change with changes in the movement distance and inertial load. So, no mechanical index related to velocity remains the same for such movements. The fact that human participants never ask for an explanation what "moving at the same speed" means tells us that there is likely an intrinsic neural variable that is kept constant for movements performed under such a vague instruction. Within the dual-strategy hypothesis, this variable is the height of the excitation pulse. Later in this chapter we will consider an alternative.

Speed-sensitive strategy

The other strategy implies modulation of the height of the excitation pulse with or without modulation of its duration. This *speed-sensitive strategy* is used, for example, when a person is asked to move over the same distance at various speeds, for example slowly, at a natural speed, fast, and as fast as possible. Figure 6.7 illustrates the EMG patterns for such movements. Another instruction to study movements performed under this strategy could be "move over different distances within the same movement time."

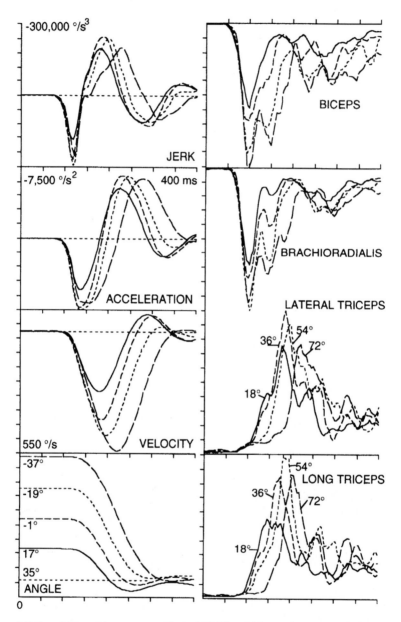

Figure 6.5 Speed-insensitive strategy: Typical EMG and kinematic patterns during movements performed "as fast as possible" over different distances. Note the similar rates of change of the agonist (biceps and brachioradialis) EMG over different times to different peak values. There is scaling of the antagonist (lateral and long heads of triceps) burst delay with movement amplitude without consistent changes in other characteristics of the triceps EMG burst. Reproduced by permission from Gottlieb, G. L., Latash, M. L., Corcos, D. M., Liubinskas, T. J., & Agarwal, G. C. (1992). Organizing principles for single joint movements. V. Agonist–antagonist interactions. *Journal of Neurophysiology, 67*, 1417–1427.

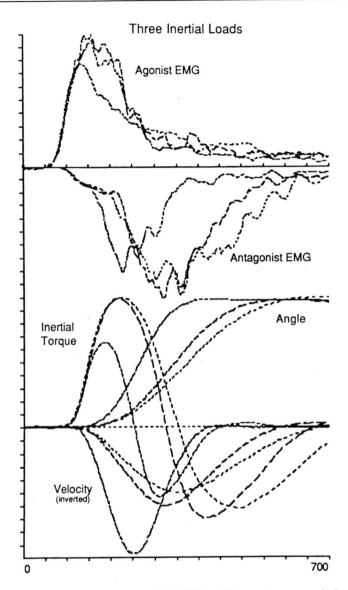

Figure 6.6 Speed-insensitive strategy: Typical EMG and kinematic patterns during movements performed "as fast as possible" over the same distances against different inertial loads. Note the similar rates of change of the agonist (biceps) EMG and different durations of the burst. There is scaling of the antagonist (triceps) burst delay with load magnitude without consistent changes in other characteristics of the triceps EMG burst. Reproduced by permission from Gottlieb, G. L., Corcos, D. M., & Agarwal, G. C. (1989). Strategies for the control of voluntary movements with one mechanical degree of freedom. *Behavioral and Brain Sciences,* *12*, 189–250.

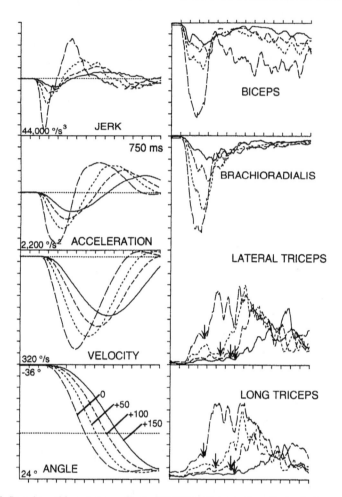

Figure 6.7 Speed-sensitive strategy: Typical EMG and kinematic patterns during movements performed at different speeds over the same distance. Note the different rate of change of the agonist (biceps and brachioradialis) EMG over about the same time interval to different peak values. There is scaling of the antagonist (lateral and long heads of triceps) burst delay and amplitude with movement speed. Reproduced by permission from Gottlieb, G. L., Latash, M. L., Corcos, D. M., Liubinskas, T. J., & Agarwal, G. C. (1992). Organizing principles for single joint movements. V. Agonist–antagonist interactions. *Journal of Neurophysiology, 67,* 1417–1427.

Note the following features of the EMG patterns performed under the speed-sensitive strategy. The rate of EMG rise differs from the very beginning of the first agonist burst, while the duration of the burst does not scale significantly. The antagonist burst is delayed for slower movements and its magnitude is smaller.

The dual-strategy hypothesis has been less successful in its attempts to account for the experimentally observed variations in the delayed muscle activation features of the tri-phasic pattern, such as the antagonist muscle burst and the second agonist muscle burst, and for muscle activation patterns in force production tasks (in isometric conditions). In particular, to account for the variety of experimentally observed EMG patterns, the hypothesis had to assume other patterns of excitation signals to alpha-motoneurons, such as excitation steps and excitation ramps.

The dual-strategy hypothesis ignored the contribution of reflex pathways to the muscle activation patterns. Its success in describing the behavior of the initial muscle activation was due to the fact that, during the first few tens of milliseconds, under constant loading conditions, muscle activation primarily reflects changes in descending signals to alpha-motoneurons. Reflex pathways require time (due to the transmission delays) to exert motion-specific effects on alpha-motoneurons. That is why the dual-strategy hypothesis struggled with delayed features of the tri-phasic pattern (in particular, characteristics of the antagonist burst) and with movements performed in substantially different conditions (for example, in isotonic and isometric conditions), when movement kinematics and kinetics were dramatically different. In such conditions, the reflex contribution of signals from the major proprioceptors, such as spindle endings and Golgi tendon organs, differed substantially, leading to EMG patterns that could not be accounted for by the assumption of a sequence of rectangular excitation pulses.

A natural development of the dual-strategy hypothesis is to reconsider the nature of the unknown central parameter that is kept constant under the instruction to move at "the same speed"; moving "as fast as possible" is a particular case of setting this hypothetical central parameter to its highest possible value. Within the original formulation of the hypothesis, this parameter was related to the height of the excitation pulse. An alternative is to relate this parameter to rate of change of a centrally defined neural variable, for example λ (threshold of the tonic stretch reflex) as introduced in Section 4.4. Shifting this parameter at a constant rate over different amplitudes produces movements assigned to the speed-insensitive strategy, while changing the rate of λ shift generates the speed-sensitive strategy (Figure 6.8). This is certainly a very crude scheme. It is more convenient to describe EMG patterns using a different pair of variables to the agonist–antagonist muscle pair, *reciprocal command* and *coactivation command* as described later, in Chapter 8. Several studies within the equilibrium-point hypothesis (see Section 8.3) have shown that these assumptions lead to predictions of EMG patterns that match experimental observations reasonably well.

6.3   Pulse–step model

Another model from this class, the pulse–step model developed by Claude Ghez and his colleagues, is also based on an assumption that the central nervous system controls movement and isometric force production by scaling patterns of muscle activation. This assumption makes the pulse–step model similar to the dual-strategy hypothesis. The model assumes that an input into an alpha-motoneuronal pool can be represented as a sequence of a short-lasting pulse and a longer lasting step (Figure 6.9). During movements in isotonic conditions, the amplitude of the pulse is assumed to control the rate of acceleration, while its duration would define movement amplitude. The step portion of the command would allow fixating the final position with a certain elevated

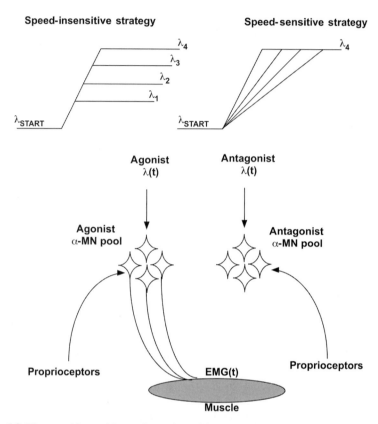

Figure 6.8 The speed-insensitive and speed-sensitive strategies may be associated with a shift of control variables to the muscles at the same rate over different amplitudes (top-left drawing) and over the same amplitude at different rates (top-right drawing). These variables, $\lambda(t)$ interact with the feedback from peripheral receptors and produce time-varying patterns of muscle activation, EMG(t). α-MN, alpha-motoneuron.

level of co-contraction of the opposing muscles. This last assumption is supported by a well-known phenomenon: Following a fast single-joint movement, the muscles crossing the joint show a substantial level of co-contraction that declines gradually with time after the movement termination.

In isometric conditions, the amplitude of the pulse would control the rate of rise of force and, indirectly, also the peak force, since quick force production is associated with relatively minor changes in the time to peak force. The step component would control the level of the terminal steady-state force. Figure 6.10A shows the torque and muscle activation patterns (EMGs) for a set of tasks involving the production of joint torque over a fixed torque magnitude with different rates of torque increase. Note the higher initial peaks of muscle activation for higher rates of torque rise and similar steady-state EMG levels at the final torque level. Note also the nearly symmetrical patterns in the agonist (biceps) and antagonist (lateral triceps) muscles. In terms of the dual-strategy hypothesis, these tasks belong to the speed-sensitive strategy.

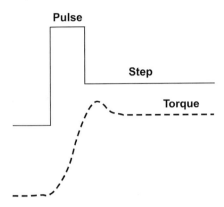

Figure 6.9 The pulse–step model assumes that excitation input into a motoneuronal pool consists of a short-lasting, high-amplitude pulse followed by a steady-state step. In isometric conditions, the pulse controls the rate of torque increase, while the step defines a new steady-state torque level.

Figure 6.10B shows the EMG and torque patterns for a set of tasks that required torque production "as quickly as possible" to different target levels. In terms of the dual-strategy hypothesis, these represent the speed-insensitive strategy. Note the similar initial segments of the agonist (biceps) EMG signals. Note, however, that the antagonist burst characteristics differ significantly from those typical of the speed-insensitive strategy during isotonic movements (compared with the patterns in Figure 6.5).

Recently, the pulse–step model has been revisited based on the more general idea that the central nervous system may implement separate plans for the control of trajectory (spatial trajectory or force/torque profile) of an effector and its final state (position or force). This development by Robert Scheidt and Claude Ghez is based on a computational model in the spirit of the ideas of force control. Indeed, a common feature of the force-control and muscle activation–control hypotheses is that the central nervous system is assumed to pre-compute some mechanical or muscle activation variables (or total inputs into the alpha-motoneuronal pools) based on the task and state of the neuromotor system. Getting back to Figures 5.13 and 5.15, which illustrate the main steps in the internal inverse and direct models, one either accepts that something of this kind takes place in the central nervous system or not. Which variables represent the ones that the controller pre-computes, forces, activation patterns, etc. is a relatively minor detail. The readers should form their own opinion after reading the whole book.

6.4   Control of multi-muscle systems: muscle synergies

The notion of multi-muscle synergies dates back to the end of the nineteenth century and early twentieth century. At that time, two great neurologists, J. Hughlings Jackson (1835–1911) and J. F. Babinski (1857–1932), introduced the idea that the brain controlled muscles not one by one but in groups. Such groups were supposed to be organized in a flexible, task-specific way, relatively similar across all healthy persons,

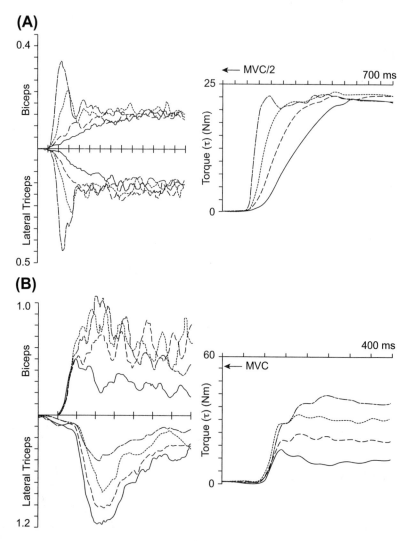

Figure 6.10 Electromyographic (left panels) and kinetic (right panels) patterns during isometric force production to the same torque target at different rates (A) and to different torque targets "as quickly as possible" (B). Averaged patterns over a series of trials are shown. The EMG signal for the antagonist muscle (lateral triceps) is inverted for better visualization. Reproduced by permission from Corcos, D. M., Gottlieb, G. L., Agarwal, G. C., & Flaherty, B. P. (1990). Organizing principles for single joint movements. IV. Implications for isometric contractions. *Journal of Neurophysiology, 64,* 1033–1042.

but changed in cases of motor pathologies. Babinski used the term *asynergia* for atypical patterns of activation of muscle groups, for example those seen in persons with cerebellar disorders. Later, N. A. Bernstein revisited the idea of synergies and defined them as large muscle groups working together in a coordinated, task-specific manner.

Recently, the notion of multi-muscle synergies has started to attract attention once again, encouraged by the development of methods of statistical analysis of large data sets. The basic assumption remains relatively unchanged since the times of Hughlings Jackson and Babinski: The brain is assumed to unite muscles into groups and then use one parameter per group to modify activation levels of all the muscles within the group in parallel. This definition implies that the brain is capable of defining muscle activations; in other words, it implies that reflex contributions to muscle activation levels are small or accurately predictable by the brain, or scale in proportion to the centrally defined activation levels.

Several methods have been used to identify muscle groups within which activation levels scale in parallel either in the course of performing an action or across actions with different parameters. There are certain common features across those methods. Most of them use surface electromyography to record muscle activation levels (see Section 13.2). The signals are typically rectified and then low-pass filtered or integrated over reasonable time intervals. These procedures result in a sequence of values reflecting activation of each of the muscles. Further, correlations among these values are computed over repetitive trials or time samples, and methods of analysis of large sets of correlation coefficients (referred to as *matrix factorization methods*) are used to identify muscle groups with close to parallel scaling of activation levels. A variety of such methods have been used, including *principal component analysis*, with and without factor extraction, *non-negative matrix factorization*, and *independent component analysis*. The main goal of each of these methods is to reduce the

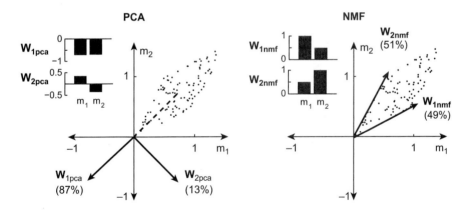

Figure 6.11 An example of a data set formed in the space of two variables, m_1 and m_2. Principal component analysis (PCA) applied to the set results in two orthogonal vectors, $\mathbf{W}_{1pca}$ and $\mathbf{W}_{2pca}$ that account for 87% and 13% of the original variance respectively. Non-negative matrix factorization (NNMF) applied to the same set produces two vectors, $\mathbf{W}_{1nmf}$ and $\mathbf{W}_{2nmf}$ that account for 51% and 49% of the original variance, respectively. Reproduced by permission from Ting, L. H., & Chvatal, S, A. (2010). Decomposing muscle activity in motor tasks: methods and interpretation. In F. Danion, & M. L. Latash (Eds.). *Motor control: theories, experiments, and applications* (pp. 102–138). New York: Oxford University Press.

high-dimensional original data set (many muscle activation indices) to a lower-dimensional set of variables (a few synergies).

As is frequently the case in studies of muscle activations, the choice of particular methods of analysis is based on the goals of specific studies. If magnitudes of muscle activation are used as the initial set of variables, non-negative matrix factorization has an obvious advantage because this method excludes negative values upfront (the lowest level of muscle activation is zero). On the other hand, if deviations of muscle activation from a certain baseline are analyzed, both positive and negative values have to be considered, and then principal component analysis (commonly it is used with factor extraction, turning it into *factor analysis*) may have an advantage.

Figure 6.11 illustrates principal component analysis (PCA) and non-negative matrix factorization (NNMF) applied to a data set that forms an ellipse (a two-dimensional

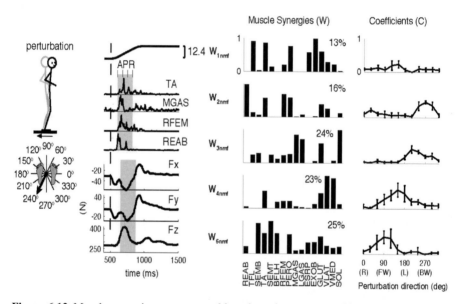

Figure 6.12 Muscle synergies reconstructed based on electromyographic data (EMGs) recorded in a standing person during perturbations in different directions using non-negative matrix factorization. The left panel shows the design of the study and typical EMG and mechanical time profiles. The right panel shows the weights of muscle activation indices (**W**) in individual synergies and the changes in their gains for perturbations in different directions. R, right; FW, forward; L, left; BW, backwards; REAB, rectus abdominis; TFL, tensor fascia latae; SEMB, semimembranosus; TA, tibialis anterior; SEMT, semitendinosus; BFLH, biceps femoris, long head; RFEM, rectus femoris; PERO, peroneus; MGAS, medial gastrocnemius; LGAS, lateral gastrocnemius; ERSP, erector spinae; EXOB, external oblique; GLUT, gluteus medius; VLAT, vastus lateralis; VMED, vastus medialis; SOL, soleus. Reproduced by permission of Oxford University Press from Ting, L. H., & Chvatal, S, A. (2010). Decomposing muscle activity in motor tasks: methods and interpretation. In F. Danion, & M. L. Latash (Eds.). *Motor control: theories, experiments, and applications* (pp. 102–138). New York: Oxford University Press.

surface) in the original space of three variables. Both methods belong to linear decomposition techniques. This means that they both allow the original data set to be represented as the sum of weighted base vectors, with some residual error of course. The fact that the data in the three-dimensional space form a two-dimensional ellipse allows them to be represented by just two new vectors (appropriately selected). PCA defines two vectors in the original three-dimensional space that are orthogonal to each other and coincide with the main axes of the data ellipse (dashed lines in Figure 6.11). NNMF defines two vectors that are not orthogonal to each other but are found through a search process that minimizes the deviation of the computed values from the observed ones (solid, thin lines in Figure 6.11).

More commonly, data do not form perfect ellipses; they have as many dimensions as there are original variables (muscle activations). However, most of the data variance may be confined to a relatively low-dimensional sub-space, an ellipsoid. Then, a few basic vectors (*eigenvectors*—vectors with length equal to one) may be sufficient to describe the data set within an acceptable error margin.

Such methods have been applied to a variety of tasks involving large muscles groups, such as postural tasks (standing, swaying, preparing for a perturbation, and

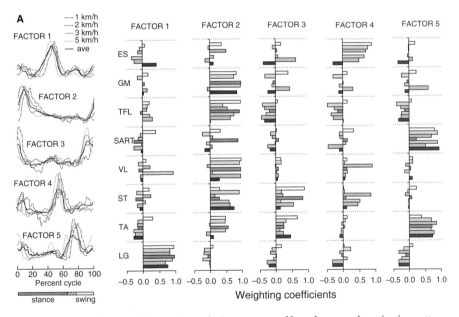

Figure 6.13 Sets of muscle factors (synergies) reconstructed based on muscle activation patterns recorded in humans during walking. The left panel shows the time profiles of the gains at individual synergies during the walking cycle at different speeds. The right panel shows the contribution of individual muscles to the factors. The data for individual subjects are shown. ES, erector spinae; GM, gluteus maximus; TFL, tensor fascia latae; SART, sartorius; VL, vastus lateralis; ST, semitendinosus; TA, tibialis anterior; LG, lateral gastrocnemius. Reproduced by permission from Ivanenko, Y. P., Poppele, R. E., & Lacquaniti, F. (2004). Five basic muscle activation patterns account for muscle activity during locomotion. *Journal of Physiology, 556*, 267–282.

reacting to a perturbation), locomotor tasks (with or without additional task components), multi-digit actions, and arm actions.

Two groups have applied the NNMF method to analysis of large muscle activation data sets in postural and walking tasks. One of them is led by an American researcher, Lena Ting, and the other one involves several prominent Italian researchers such as Francesco Lacquaniti and Yuri Ivanenko. An example of applying NNMF to a task of reacting to a postural perturbation is presented in Figure 6.12. The complex multi-muscle response pattern can be described with six vectors in the muscle activation space with time-varying coefficients. At each time, the activation level of each muscle is computed as the sum of the contributions of each of the five synergies taken with appropriate coefficients.

Another example is presented in Figure 6.13. In this case, the NNMF method was applied to multi-muscle activation patterns during locomotion. Five synergies were extracted. They were able to describe observed muscle activation patterns with high accuracy. When the same task (walking) was combined with another task of bending and picking up an object, the number of synergies increased.

Muscle groups with a somewhat different composition were found when PCA with factor extraction was applied to voluntary sway tasks. Typical groups (the

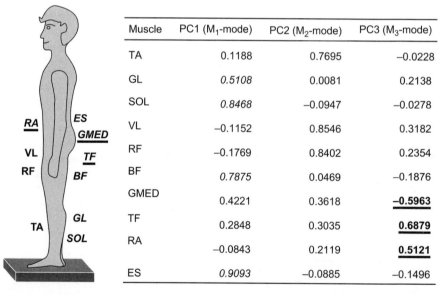

Muscle	PC1 (M₁-mode)	PC2 (M₂-mode)	PC3 (M₃-mode)
TA	0.1188	0.7695	−0.0228
GL	*0.5108*	0.0081	0.2138
SOL	*0.8468*	−0.0947	−0.0278
VL	−0.1152	0.8546	0.3182
RF	−0.1769	0.8402	0.2354
BF	*0.7875*	0.0469	−0.1876
GMED	0.4221	0.3618	**−0.5963**
TF	0.2848	0.3035	**0.6879**
RA	−0.0843	0.2119	**0.5121**
ES	*0.9093*	−0.0885	−0.1496

Figure 6.14 Muscle groups (M-modes) computed using principal component analysis with factor extraction for a standing person based on the muscle activation data. Three M-modes are shown with different fonts. The table presents the loading coefficients (significant ones are shown in bold) for a set of leg/trunk muscles. TA, tibialis anterior; GL, gastrocnemius lateralis; SOL, soleus; VL, vastus lateralis; RF, rectus femoris; BF, biceps femoris; GMED, gluteus medius; TF, tensor fascia latae; RA, rectus abdominis; ES, erector spinae.

authors called them *muscle modes* or *M-modes* rather than synergies) united muscles crossing different joints on the dorsal side of the body and on the ventral side of the body (see the M_1 and M_2 M-modes in Figure 6.14). Sometimes, muscles acting at the same joint could be found in the same M-mode with the same sign: Such cases were referred to as *co-contraction modes*. M-mode composition has been shown to be rather robust across similar tasks performed by a person and also across young, healthy persons.

Most studies view the linear scaling of activations levels across large muscle groups as multi-muscle synergies. An alternative approach is to view such variables as elements on which synergies are built. This approach is considered in more detail in Section 9.4.

Self-test questions

1. What are the assumptions of muscle activation control hypotheses with respect to reflex effects on activity of motoneurons?
2. Are reflex contributions to muscle activation weak or strong in a healthy person?
3. What are the main similarities and differences between muscle activation–control and force-control models?
4. Describe the tri-phasic EMG pattern.
5. What is the role of the antagonist burst?
6. What is the role of the second agonist burst?
7. Suggest a functional role of antagonist low-level coactivation during the first agonist burst.
8. What are the main parameters of the excitation pulse?
9. Define speed-sensitive and speed-insensitive strategies.
10. What are the typical features of EMG patterns for movements performed under the speed-sensitive strategy?
11. What are the typical features of EMG patterns for movements performed under the speed-insensitive strategy?
12. Can one decide whether movements are performed under the speed-sensitive or speed-insensitive strategy by looking at kinematic profiles? At kinetic profiles? At EMG profiles?
13. What variables are kept at the same values when a person performs movements over different distances "at the same speed"?
14. What were the main problems of the dual-strategy hypothesis with actions performed in isometric conditions and with late EMG events such as the antagonist burst?
15. How can the dual-strategy hypothesis be reformulated using the notion of shifts of the tonic stretch reflex?
16. What is the assumed purpose of the pulse in the pulse–step model?
17. What is the assumed purpose of the step in the pulse–step model?
18. Present arguments for and against the idea that control of a fast movement has two distinct components, control of the trajectory and control of the final position.
19. What is asynergia?
20. What methods are used commonly to identify multi-muscle synergies?
21. What are the main assumption underlying the methods of identification of muscle synergies?
22. Present arguments in favor of principal component analysis and non-negative matrix factorization as methods of synergy identification.

Essential references and recommended further readings

Brown, S. H., & Cooke, J. D. (1990). Movement-related phasic muscle activation. I. Relations with temporal profile of movement. *Journal of Neurophysiology, 63*, 455–464.

Cooke, J. D., & Brown, S. H. (1990). Movement-related phasic muscle activation. II. Generation and functional role of the triphasic pattern. *Journal of Neurophysiology, 63*, 465–472.

Corcos, D. M., Gottlieb, G. L., & Agarwal, G. C. (1989). Organizing principles for single joint movements. II. A speed-sensitive strategy. *Journal of Neurophysiology, 62*, 358–368.

Corcos, D. M., Gottlieb, G. L., Agarwal, G. C., & Flaherty, B. P. (1990). Organizing principles for single joint movements. IV. Implications for isometric contractions. *Journal of Neurophysiology, 64*, 1033–1042.

Danna-Dos-Santos, A., Slomka, K., Zatsiorsky, V. M., & Latash, M. L. (2007). Muscle modes and synergies during voluntary body sway. *Experimental Brain Research, 179*, 533–550.

d'Avella, A., Saltiel, P., & Bizzi, E. (2003). Combinations of muscle synergies in the construction of a natural motor behavior. *Nature Neuroscience, 6*, 300–308.

Feldman, A. G., Adamovitch, S. V., Ostry, D. J., & Flanagan, J. R. (1990). The origin of electromyograms—Explanations based on the equilibrium point hypothesis. In J. M. Winters, & S. L-Y. Woo (Eds.), *Multiple muscle systems. Biomechanics and movement organization* (pp. 195–213). New York: Springer-Verlag.

Ghez, C., & Gordon, J. (1987). Trajectory control in targeted force impulses. I. Role of opposing muscles. *Experimental Brain Research, 67*, 225–240.

Gielen, C. C. A. M., van der Oosten, K., & Pull ter Gunne, F. (1985). Relations between EMG activation patterns and kinematic properties of aimed movements. *Journal of Motor Behavior, 17*, 421–442.

Gordon, J., & Ghez, C. (1987). Trajectory control in targeted force impulses. II. Pulse height control. *Experimental Brain Research, 67*, 241–252.

Gottlieb, G. L., Corcos, D. M., & Agarwal, G. C. (1989a). Strategies for the control of voluntary movements with one mechanical degree of freedom. *Behavioral and Brain Sciences, 12*, 189–250.

Gottlieb, G. L., Corcos, D. M., & Agarwal, G. C. (1989b). Organizing principles for single joint movements. I: A speed-insensitive strategy. *Journal of Neurophysiology, 62*, 342–357.

Gottlieb, G. L., Corcos, D. M., Agarwal, G. C., & Latash, M. L. (1990). Organizing principles for single joint movements. III: Speed-insensitive strategy as a default. *Journal of Neurophysiology, 63*, 625–636.

Ivanenko, Y. P., Poppele, R. E., & Lacquaniti, F. (2004). Five basic muscle activation patterns account for muscle activity during human locomotion. *Journal of Physiology, 556*, 267–282.

Ivanenko, Y. P., Cappellini, G., Dominici, N., Poppele, R. E., & Lacquaniti, F. (2005). Coordination of locomotion with voluntary movements in humans. *Journal of Neuroscience, 25*, 7238–7253.

Krishnamoorthy, V., Latash, M. L., Scholz, J. P., & Zatsiorsky, V. M. (2003). Muscle synergies during shifts of the center of pressure by standing persons. *Experimental Brain Research, 152*, 281–292.

Latash, M. L. (1993). *Control of human movement*. Urbana, IL: Human Kinetics.

Latash, M. L. (2008). *Neurophysiological basis of movement* (2nd ed.). Urbana, IL: Human Kinetics.

Scheidt, R. A., & Ghez, C. (2007). Separate adaptive mechanisms for controlling trajectory and final position in reaching. *Journal of Neurophysiology, 98*, 3600–3613.

Shapiro, D. C., & Walter, C. B. (1986). An examination of rapid positioning movements with spatiotemporal constraints. *Journal of Motor Behavior, 18*, 373–395.

Shapiro, M. B., Prodoehl, J., Corcos, D. M., & Gottlieb, G. L. (2005). Muscle activation is different when the same muscle acts as an agonist or an antagonist during voluntary movement. *Journal of Motor Behavior, 37*, 135–145.

Ting, L. H., & Chvatal, S. A. (2010). Decomposing muscle activity in motor tasks: methods and interpretation. In F. Danion, & M. L. Latash (Eds.), *Motor control: theories, experiments, and applications* (pp. 102–138). New York: Oxford University Press.

Torres-Oviedo, G., & Ting, L. H. (2007). Muscle synergies characterizing human postural responses. *Journal of Neurophysiology, 98*, 2144–2156.

Torres-Oviedo, G., Macpherson, J. M., & Ting, L. H. (2006). Muscle synergy organization is robust across a variety of postural perturbations. *Journal of Neurophysiology, 96*, 1530–1546.

Tresch, M. C., & Jarc, A. (2009). The case for and against muscle synergies. *Current Opinions in Neurobiology, 19*, 601–607.

Wallace, S. A. (1981). An impulse-timing theory for reciprocal control of muscular activity in rapid, discrete movements. *Journal of Motor Behavior, 13*, 144–160.

7 Control theory approaches

The approaches discussed in this chapter are based on a few assumptions. The first is that the system for movement production can be divided into a controller and a controlled part. The neural controller is assumed to perform certain computational operations (see Section 4.1 and Chapter 5). This is a non-trivial assumption: Neurons are threshold elements with strongly non-linear characteristics when the membrane potential is above the threshold for action potential generation; hence, 2 plus 2 for a neuron may happen to be 4 or 7, while 6 multiplied by 0.5 may happen to be 3, 1, or even zero. Further, it is assumed that the results of those symbolic computations are somehow realized by the muscles as time-varying mechanical variables. Accepting or rejecting these assumptions form the core of the ongoing argument between skeptics and champions of the control theory approach to motor control.

7.1 The basic notions

State and control variables

Consider a simple system consisting of two components—a *controller* and a *controlled object* (Figure 7.1). The controller receives an input from a neural structure responsible for making decisions on what and when to do; this input may be referred to as the *Task*. At this point, we are not going to ask how decisions are made and accept their existence as an axiom. The Task specifies a desired state of the controlled object. Let us assume that state of the object can be described with a set of variables, $X_i(t)$,

Fundamentals of Motor Control. DOI: 10.1016/B978-0-12-415956-3.00007-5

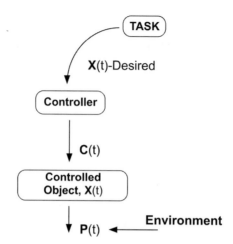

Figure 7.1 A simple system consisting of two components—a controller and a controlled object. The controller generates a control vector $C(t)$ based on a desired state of the object, $X(t)$-Desired. The actual state of the object, $X(t)$ will depend on its interaction with the environment, which produces performance variables, $P(t)$ that are typically measured in experiments.

which can be represented as a time-varying vector $X(t)$. At any time t_0, the object can be described with a set of values for each of the variables, that is, with a vector $X(t_0)$. The controller may also receive information on the current (initial) state of the controlled object, but this is not necessary. The controller communicates with the controlled object using another set of time-varying variables, $C_i(t)$, which we are going to call the vector of *control variables*, $C(t)$.

   Performance variables measured in experiments form yet another vector, $P(t)$, which reflects the interaction between the object and the environment. Performance variables can be measured at different levels of the neuromotor hierarchy using a variety of methods. For example, these may represent joint trajectories or joint torques or levels of activation of a set of muscles, and so on. Within the actual neuromotor system, the border between $C(t)$ and $P(t)$ is blurred. For example, the mentioned dual-strategy hypothesis and the pulse–step model consider the input into the alpha-motoneurons as $C(t)$, while movement kinematics and kinetics are considered as $P(t)$. Other hypotheses, however, may view patterns of activation of alpha-motoneuronal pools as $P(t)$. Some studies assume (usually implicitly) that anything that happens in the brain is control, $C(t)$, while anything in the spinal cord and in peripheral structures is performance, $P(t)$, but it is easy to present examples against such a simplistic view. For example, complex coordinated motor patterns, such as those during locomotion, can be produced by the spinal cord isolated from the brain (see Section 10.1).

Feed-forward and feedback control

The controller always receives an input, *Task*, corresponding to a desired state of the object or its desired change in time $X_{DES}(t)$. However, it may or may not receive information about the current state of the object $X(t)$. If the controller specifies a control vector $C(t)$ independently of information on the current state of the controlled object, this type of control is called *open-loop* or *feed-forward* control (Figure 7.2A). These two terms are not perfect synonyms but within this book we will not consider differences between them. During open-loop control, a motor command is issued for a whole motor act before the outcome of the earliest change in the command is taken into account by the controller. A typical example of open-loop control is hitting a flying ball in tennis or baseball. The central nervous system sends commands to the muscles involved in this motor act before the contact with the ball is made, and the brevity of this contact does not allow the controller to adjust the commands.

If the controller changes the control vector based on its effects on the state of the object, this type of control is called *closed-loop* or *feedback* control (Figures 7.2B). An important component of a feedback control system is an error-detection mechanism, which uses signals about the current actual state of the controlled object, $X_{ACT}(t)$. Signals related to $X_{ACT}(t)$ are compared to the desired progression of the state of the object $X_{DES}(t)$. A structure called the *comparator* computes an *error*, $\Delta X(t)$ between $X_{ACT}(t)$ and $X_{DES}(t)$ and uses it to adjust the vector of control variables $C(t)$: $dC(t)/dt = f[\Delta X(t)]$.

Two basic types of feedback control can be distinguished, negative and positive. The main purpose of the negative feedback control is to minimize deviations of $X_{ACT}(t)$ from $X_{DES}(t)$. Hence, feedback signals on an error $\Delta X(t)$ are used to adjust the control vector in such a way that the adjustment brings $\Delta X(t)$ down, closer to zero (Figure 7.3A). Negative feedback control systems tend to counteract any deviations of the state variables of the controlled object from their desired values or their desired time evolution. A typical example from the area of motor control is stabilization of posture, in particular vertical posture during standing (see Section 11.1).

Positive feedback acts to amplify errors in state variables of the controlled object. In other words, an error $\Delta X(t)$ leads to an adjustment of $C(t)$, which leads to further

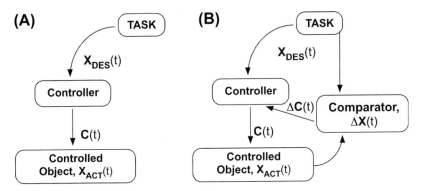

Figure 7.2 (A) Feed-forward control. The control vector $C(t)$ does not depend on the actual state of the object $X_{ACT}(t)$. (B) Feedback control. The control vector is modified by $\Delta C(t)$ based on the difference, $\Delta X(t)$, between a desired state of the object, $X_{DES}(t)$, and its actual state, $X_{ACT}(t)$, computed by the comparator.

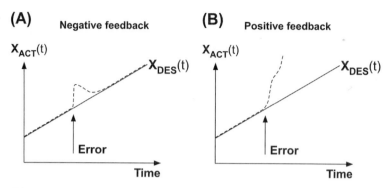

Figure 7.3 In cases of errors, that is, deviations of actual object state, $X_{ACT}(t)$, from its desired state, $X_{DES}(t)$, negative feedback (A) with small or zero time delay leads to a decrease of the error, while positive feedback (B) leads to an increase in the error.

increase in the magnitude of $\Delta X(t)$ (Figure 7.3B). Positive feedback systems tend to bring about qualitative changes in the behavior of the system. In the field of neuro-physiology, positive feedback underlies the generation of an action potential when the membrane potential reaches the threshold.

Gain and delay in feedback loops

Two important parameters characterize feedback loops—gain and delay (Figure 7.4). Gain (G) can be defined as the ratio between the magnitude of a corrective vector ΔX_{COR} and the magnitude of the original error vector ΔX that gave rise to the correction: $G = |\Delta X_{COR}|/|\Delta X|$. If $G = 1$ in a negative feedback system, a seemingly perfect correction mechanism issues a corrective signal that annihilates the error completely. However, the perfection of such a system may be only seeming because of the unavoidable time delays involved in any feedback control systems. The

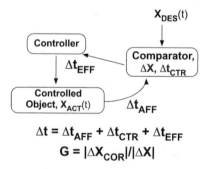

Figure 7.4 Two important characteristics of a feedback loop are its time delay, Δt, and gain G. The former is composed of the afferent conduction time (Δt_{AFF}), efferent conduction time (Δt_{EFF}), and central processing delay (Δt_{CTR}). The latter is the ratio between the magnitude of a correction (ΔX_{COR}) and the magnitude of an error (ΔX).

correction takes place after a delay from the time when the original error emerged. In artificial systems with electrical means of signal transmission, conduction delays may be negligible. In the human body, however, the speed of action potential transmission is not as high (see Section 3.2). This means that transmitting signals from sensory receptors that inform the central nervous system on $X_{ACT}(t)$ and transmitting signals from the comparator to the muscles that introduce corrections may take substantial time. In addition, the presumed computation of ΔX_{COR} may also take time. As a result, correction will take place some time after the signal was generated informing on a deviation between $X_{ACT}(t)$ and $X_{DES}(t)$. The controlled object is likely to change its state over this time interval. As a result, the correction may become suboptimal or detrimental, even if the gain of the negative feedback loop is unity.

Time delay may turn into an important drawback of feedback control, particularly if the magnitude of the delay is large and the motor process is fast. Therefore, if speed is vital, feed-forward control may be preferred, while if accuracy is important and speed is not, feedback control may have an advantage. One possibility to adjust the relative contribution of the feed-forward and feedback components of a control system is through regulation of the gain in the feedback loop.

7.2 Servo-control and Merton's servo-hypothesis

In motor control, much attention has been paid to a particular combination of feed-forward and feedback control loops called the *servo*. The purpose of a servo is to keep the vector of state variables, $X(t)$ at a desired value $X_0(t)$ specified by a feed-forward system. Keeping $X(t)$ close to $X_0(t)$ is achieved with the help of a feedback mechanism. A sensor is used to measure current values of $X(t)$ and to supply these measurements to the comparator. The comparator compares the measured value to the specified one and changes its output (ΔX) based on the error (i.e. the difference between $X(t)$ and $X_0(t)$). Good servos allow only very small errors to emerge and correct them promptly. In other words, they have high gains and small time delays.

In the early 1950s, P. A. Merton suggested arguably the first motor control hypothesis, called the *servo-hypothesis*. Merton suggested that the control of muscle spindles with the system of gamma-motoneurons was part of a servo mechanism controlling muscle length.

Sensors of muscle length and velocity located in muscle spindles receive signals from small motoneurons (gamma-motoneurons, Figure 7.5). These signals change the sensitivity of the spindle receptors to muscle length and velocity. The afferent signals from the primary spindle endings make excitatory projections on alpha-motoneurons innervating the same muscle.

Gamma-motoneurons and voluntary movements

Merton suggested that voluntary muscle activation started with a descending command to gamma-motoneurons that changed the sensitivity of the sensory endings in muscle spindles to muscle length. The effect of an increased gamma-activity is

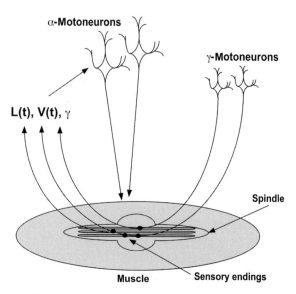

Figure 7.5 Reflex feedback from sensory endings in the muscle spindle depends on muscle length (*L*), velocity (*V*), and level of activation of gamma-motoneurons.

similar to the effect of an increase in muscle length since both lead to an increase in the spindle afferent activity level. So, the descending signal to gamma-motoneurons may be viewed as simulating a new value of muscle length.

The changed activity of the spindle endings leads to a change in the activation level of alpha-motoneurons innervating the muscle via the stretch reflex mechanism. This produces muscle contraction leading to a movement (i.e. to a change in muscle length, assuming that the movement is not blocked). In particular, an increase in the spindle activity will lead to an additional muscle contraction leading to muscle shortening, which will lead to a decrease in the spindle activity. So, the stretch reflex mechanism acts as a negative feedback system.

The movement will continue until muscle length comes to a new value at which the activity of muscle spindles leads to a muscle contraction exactly balancing the external load (i.e. to a new equilibrium state). Figure 7.6 illustrates the presumed sequence of events leading to voluntary movements within the servo-hypothesis.

If the descending command to gamma-motoneurons remains constant, the mechanism of the stretch reflex is assumed to ensure constant muscle length despite possible changes in external load (i.e. to work as a perfect servo). For example, if the load increases, it stretches the muscle, leading to an increase in the activity of muscle spindle endings. This leads to additional activation of alpha-motoneurons and an increase in muscle contraction force. According to Merton's hypothesis, the increase in muscle force will exactly balance the external load change so that muscle length will not change.

Figure 7.7 illustrates the servo-hypothesis with the help of force–length muscle characteristics. The central command specifies the location of a characteristic

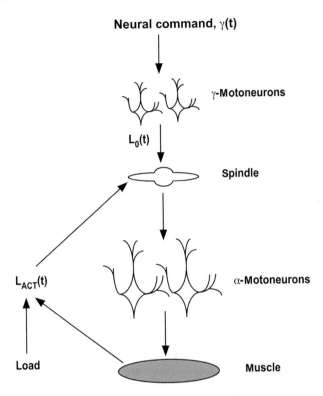

Neural command, $\gamma(t)$

γ-**Motoneurons**

$L_0(t)$

Spindle

$L_{ACT}(t)$ α-**Motoneurons**

Load   **Muscle**

Figure 7.6 Within Merton's gamma-model (servo-model), voluntary movements are initiated with a signal to gamma-motoneurons that specifies the muscle length (L_0) at which the muscle will be in an equilibrium state. Tonic stretch reflex will act to activate the muscle and produce muscle shortening until its actual length (L_{ACT}) becomes L_0.

corresponding to a certain value of muscle length. In order for the servo mechanism to ensure perfect compensation of possible changes in the external load, the characteristic must be nearly parallel to the y-axis; then, muscle length will not depend on muscle (and external) force. Voluntary movements are performed by shifting such force–length characteristics along the x-axis, so that the control variable may be associated with the signal to gamma-motoneurons (γ_1, γ_2, γ_3 in Figure 7.7).

Problems with the servo-hypothesis; alpha–gamma coactivation

Unfortunately for the servo-hypothesis, its main testable predictions were not supported in experiments. In particular, the servo-hypothesis predicts that voluntary movements are initiated by a change in the activity of gamma-motoneurons while changes in the activity of alpha-motoneurons follow at a delay, which allows signals to be transmitted from the gamma-motoneurons to the spindles and from the spindles to the alpha-motoneurons. Note that gamma-motoneurons have relatively thin myelinated axons that conduct at a modest velocity of about 20 m/s. So, a signal from

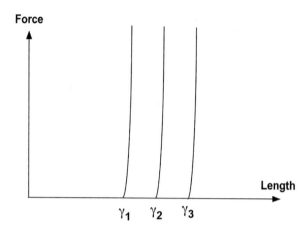

Figure 7.7 The servo-model may be illustrated as a family of nearly vertical muscle characteristics on the force–length plane. The location of each line is defined by the gamma-command. A distinctive feature of the model is that desired muscle length is achieved independently of the external load (which requires the force-length characteristics to be nearly parallel to the *y*-axis).

a gamma-motoneuron sent to a spindle in a foot muscle will take about 50 ms to reach its destination. This is longer than the typical quickest reflex delay, from changes in the state of a muscle spindle ending to muscle activation (about 30 ms). If one adds to this value the time it takes action potentials to travel from the brain to the lumbar portion of the spinal cord (where alpha-motoneurons controlling leg muscles are located), the total time will become comparable to, or even longer than, the shortest voluntary reactions time delays (about 100 ms).

The development of new methods, in particular direct recordings from human peripheral nerves pioneered by the Swedish scientist Ake Vallbo, allowed experimental assessment of the relative timing of changes in the activity of alpha- and gamma-motoneurons during voluntary muscle contractions. These observations showed that during virtually all voluntary movements, changes in the activity of alpha- and gamma-motoneurons happen simultaneously. This phenomenon has been termed *alpha–gamma coactivation*. So, movements are not initiated by a signal to gamma-motoneurons, although changes in their activation level take place and are likely to play an important role in the process of muscle activation.

To deal with the finding of alpha–gamma coactivation, a British scientist, Peter Matthews, suggested that the servo-mechanism worked as postulated by Merton, while voluntary movements were initiated by a combination of a feed-forward command signal (to alpha-motoneurons) and a signal to the length-controlling servo (to gamma-motoneurons) (Figure 7.8).

There was, however, another big problem. The servo-hypothesis implies a very high (close to an infinite) gain in the stretch reflex loop, such that any change in the external load is readily balanced by a change in muscle force without visible

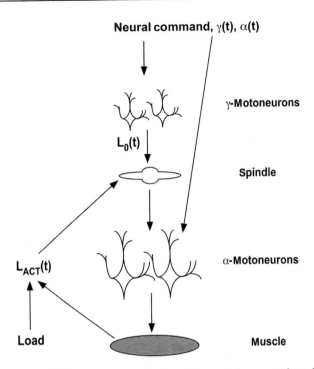

Figure 7.8 The idea of alpha–gamma coactivation. The central command sends signals simultaneously to alpha- and gamma-motoneurons. The former initiate the action, while the latter define the target muscle length value.

changes in the muscle length (corresponding to the nearly vertical force–length characteristics in Figure 7.7). However, the measurements of the gain in the stretch reflex loop demonstrated relatively low values, showing that the mechanism of this reflex cannot be considered a perfect servo. Thus, eventually, the servo-hypothesis was replaced by new theories including the *equilibrium-point hypothesis* described in the next chapter.

7.3   Optimal control

Optimal control is a branch of mathematics developed to find ways to control a system that changes in time, such that certain criteria of optimality are satisfied. Let us assume that instantaneous rate of change in the state variables of a system is defined by their initial values ($\mathbf{X}_0$ at time $t = 0$) and by the current values of the control variables:

$$\frac{d\mathbf{X}(t)}{dt} = f[\mathbf{X}(t), \mathbf{C}(t), t], \ \mathbf{X}(0) = \mathbf{X}_0. \tag{7.1}$$

If one knows the control function $\mathbf{C}(t)$ over a time interval from 0 to T, when the system is analyzed, the initial state of the system $\mathbf{X}_0$, and the form of the function f, Equation 7.1 can be integrated (solved) to find the trajectory of the state variables $\mathbf{X}(t)$. It is possible to choose a time profile $\mathbf{C}(t)$ such that the state and control variables optimize (minimize or maximize) an *objective function* (sometimes addressed as *cost function*) I over the same time interval:

$$I = \int_0^T F[\mathbf{X}(t), \mathbf{C}(t), t]\mathrm{d}t + S[\mathbf{X}(T), T] \qquad (7.2)$$

In this equation, F is a function reflecting the costs of the process associated with changes in both control and state variables. For example, this function may reflect a desire of the controller to minimize energy expenditure, fatigue, "effort" (a not very well-defined notion related to changes in control variables), and other characteristics of the action. The S-function in Equation 7.2 gives the so-called salvage value of the final state $\mathbf{X}(T)$. Its purpose is to make sure that the control is not only optimal (in a sense of minimizing I) during the process but it makes sense at the final state. For example, minimization of joint motion may be interpreted as making no motion at all, but the salvage function does not allow such a solution. Typically, there are constraints imposed on each component of I. For example, values of the control and state variables are usually limited to a certain range compatible with human anatomy and physiology, while the final state $\mathbf{X}(T)$ is expected to comply with certain task-specific criteria.

For example, consider the (unsolvable) problem of finding an optimal tennis serve. Obviously, $\mathbf{C}(t)$ will be constrained by the abilities of the player, there will be geometrical constraints on $\mathbf{X}(t)$ to make sure that the racket is always in contact with the hand, and $\mathbf{X}(T)$ will be constrained by the requirement to hit the ball. In this example, the cost of the process may be of a relatively little importance while the final outcome (mechanical characteristics of the hit) is. Because of the complexity of the human motor control system, it is very hard to formulate Equations 7.1 and 7.2 sensibly. As a result, there are only a few examples of application of the optimal control theory to problems of motor control.

Optimal feedback control of a redundant system

A method of *optimal feedback control* was applied by two researchers, Emo Todorov and Michael Jordan, to address the control of a redundant system. These researchers formulated a cost function, similar to function I in Equation 7.2, in such a way that it included a measure of internal effort spent on control and a measure of accuracy of performance of the whole system. Namely, the model minimized the weighted sum where the first summand was the squared difference between a function of effector outputs (equivalent to $\mathbf{P}(t)$ introduced earlier) and its required value, and the second summand was the effort defined as the variance of the control signals during task execution.

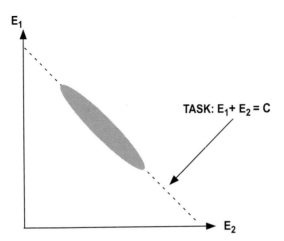

Figure 7.9 Optimal feedback control may result in a non-uniform distribution of data points within a redundant system. The figure illustrates the task of producing a constant sum of two elemental variables E_1 and E_2. The deviations from the required value of $(E_1 + E_2)$ are corrected while the compensated changes in the individual forces that do not affect the sum are not. The slanted line corresponds to perfect performance. The dotted ellipse shows a possible distribution of data points.

The controller re-computes a new desired trajectory at every moment in time, making no effort to correct deviations away from the previously planned behavior unless those deviations interfere with important performance characteristics and lead to an increase in the cost function. This idea suggests a particular method of producing flexible behaviors leading to a desired goal, which is one of the trademarks of voluntary movements (see Sections 3.5 and 9.4). Figure 7.9 illustrates a typical data distribution computed based on this type of control applied to the task of producing a constant output with two noisy effectors, which, on average, contribute equally to the output. Each point in this graph corresponds to a combination of effector forces in different attempts at performing this task starting from a relaxed state. Note that the controller allows relatively small deviations of the points from the slanted line corresponding to perfect performance of the task. In contrast, deviations along the line are much larger. We will return to such data point distributions and their interpretations in Section 9.4.

Self-test questions

1. Define state variables and control variables.
2. Select a level of analysis of a human movement and suggest examples of state variables and control variables.
3. What is the main difference between feed-forward and feedback control?
4. What are the main two parameters that describe functioning of a feedback loop?

5. Does a negative feedback loop with the gain of −1 always produce effective error correction?
6. What is the role of gamma-motoneurons in the servo-hypothesis?
7. What feedback loop forms the core of the servo-hypothesis?
8. What is the typical speed of action potentials along the axons of gamma-motoneurons?
9. What would be a typical time delay from activation of a gamma-motoneuron to muscle activation?
10. What is the slope of force–length muscle characteristics within the servo-hypothesis?
11. How can force be controlled in isometric conditions according to the servo-hypothesis?
12. What spinal neurons are expected to be activated first during the initiation of a muscle contraction according to the servo-hypothesis?
13. What is alpha–gamma coactivation?
14. Define optimal control.
15. What is the role of the salvage value of the final state of a system in optimal control?
16. How can optimal control produce multiple solutions for a typical redundant motor task?

Essential references and recommended further readings

Hasan, Z. (1986). Optimized movement trajectories and joint stiffness in unperturbed, inertially loaded movements. *Biological Cybernetics, 53*, 373–382.
Kiemel, T., Oie, K. S., & Jeka, J. J. (2002). Multisensory fusion and the stochastic structure of postural sway. *Biological Cybernetics, 87*, 262–277.
Kuo, A. D. (2005). An optimal state estimation model of sensory integration in human postural balance. *Journal of Neural Engineering, 2*, 235–249.
Marsden, C. D., Merton, R. A., & Morton, H. B. (1976). Stretch reflex and servo action in a variety of human muscles. *Journal of Physiology, 259*, 531–560.
Matthews, P. B. C. (1970). The origin and functional significance of the stretch reflex. In P. Andersen, & J. K. S. Jansen (Eds.), *Excitatory synaptic mechanisms* (pp. 301–315). Oslo: Universitets forlaget.
Mergner, T. (2010). A neurological view of reactive human stance control. *Annual Reviews in Control, 34*, 177–198.
Merton, P. A. (1953). Speculations on the servo-control of movements. In J. L. Malcolm, J. A. B. Gray, & G. E. W. Wolstenholm (Eds.), *The spinal cord* (pp. 183–198). Boston: Little, Brown.
Nelson, W. (1983). Physical principles for economies of skilled movements. *Biological Cybernetics, 46*, 135–147.
Peterka, R. J. (2000). Postural control model interpretation of stabilogram diffusion analysis. *Biological Cybernetics, 82*, 335–343.
Peterka, R. J. (2002). Sensorimotor integration in human postural control. *Journal of Neurophysiology, 88*, 1097–1118.
Todorov, E. (2004). Optimality principles in sensorimotor control. *Nature Neuroscience, 7*, 907–915.
Todorov, E., & Jordan, M. I. (2002). Optimal feedback control as a theory of motor coordination. *Nature Neuroscience, 5*, 1226–1235.
Vallbo, A. B. (1971). Human muscle spindle response at the onset of isometric voluntary contractions. Time difference between fusimotor and skeletomotor effects. *Journal of Physiology, 218*, 405–431.

8 Physical approaches

Chapter Outline

In contrast to control theory approaches, physical approaches do not assume that the central nervous system performs computations. They do not separate the body into two parts—a controller and a controlled object. Rather, they try to describe the interactions within the body and its sub-systems (including neuronal pools) and between the body and the environment using laws of physics (for a beautiful early review see the book by Peter Kugler and Michael Turvey 1987). The physics of inanimate nature is a highly developed science. However, it has major troubles dealing with typical problems of motor control. First, in contrast to movements in the inanimate world, movements of biological objects are intentional and purposeful. These two notions cannot be easily incorporated into contemporary physics. Another problem is that the body is a very complex system, which makes it hard to apply the currently available physical tools; many crucial variables are not directly measurable or even identifiable. So, motor control turns into "physics of unobservable objects."

When researchers perform specific studies, they commonly separate the object of their interest from the rest of the body (and the environment) and assume that this object receives an input from the rest of the body, reflecting the task. For example, the

Fundamentals of Motor Control. DOI: 10.1016/B978-0-12-415956-3.00008-7

notions of *motor programs* and *control variables* are a second-rate way of describing a system for which the knowledge of its physics is next to non-existent. These terms are temporary substitutes reflecting current inadequate knowledge. Researchers who accept the physical approach frequently use such terms with an understanding that they reflect not results of neural computations but the outcome of physical processes that are yet to be discovered.

8.1 Mass-spring models

Muscle, joint, and limb "stiffness"

Models of this group are based on well-established experimental facts that muscles without reflexes demonstrate dependences of force on length and velocity (Section 3.1), which are sometimes imprecisely called "viscoelastic properties." In addition, the *tonic stretch reflex* action also contributes to the dependence of muscle force on its length and velocity (Section 4.4). These models received strong support from experiments demonstrating *equifinality* of movements under transient perturbations (see Section 4.5). Indeed, they predict that, if parameters of the system remain unchanged, a transient perturbation should not affect its equilibrium state achieved after the perturbation is over.

One has to be careful applying established physical notions such as *stiffness* to complex objects such as muscles, joints, and limbs. Stiffness is a property of a particular group of objects (springs) that possess certain features. First, they deform under the action of an external force. Second, they generate force against deformation. Third, they accumulate potential energy under deformation, and this energy can be released if the deforming force is removed. If there is a linear relationship between the magnitude of external force and the magnitude of induced deformation, the behavior of such objects may be described with the well-known Hooke's law:

$$F = -k(L - L_0), \tag{8.1}$$

where L_0 is "zero length" of the spring (its length when there is no external force applied), L is its length, F is applied external force, and k is a coefficient called stiffness. The minus sign shows that the spring shortens under the action of compressive force. In our universe, there are no deformable objects that would elongate under the action of a compressive force; so, "negative stiffness" is a nonsensical expression. Similarly, to stretch an ideal linear spring, one has to apply force proportional to the desired magnitude of the stretch (F is negative in Equation 8.1, resulting in $L > L_0$; see also Figure 8.1).

The definition of stiffness makes this notion applicable to deformable objects. Applying this notion to objects that do not deform but move under the action of force is highly questionable. For example, if an external torque is applied to a joint, the joint will not deform but move to a new position (Figure 8.2). Formally, one can compute the ratio of torque magnitude to the joint displacement and call the result "joint

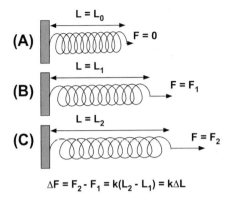

$$\Delta F = F_2 - F_1 = k(L_2 - L_1) = k\Delta L$$

Figure 8.1 A perfect linear spring can be characterized by zero length (L_0) and stiffness (k). At L_0, the spring produces no force (A), stretching a spring, for example from L_1 to L_2 (as in B and C), results in a force change (ΔF) proportional to the length change (ΔL).

stiffness," but the meaning of this procedure is not at all clear. When a joint is moved to a new steady-state by an external torque, muscles and tendons crossing the joint are either shortened or stretched (deformed). Passive structures such as tendons may be assigned stiffness values. Assigning stiffness values to a muscle is by itself questionable because of the complex muscle behavior under length changes. And it is very unlikely that the combined effects of torque changes on joint angular position could be described in a meaningful way with a single parameter such as stiffness.

Nevertheless, in quite a few studies, spring-like properties are assumed for complex systems, forces are applied, displacements are measured, and the ratio of the former to the latter is called *stiffness*. This may be very confusing and misleading because the apparent force–displacement relations may be due to physical properties of the object different from those of ideal springs. To distinguish between stiffness measured in a spring and a stiffness-like property measured in an arbitrary object, the notion of *apparent stiffness* has been introduced. It implies that the object behaves like a spring but may not be a spring at all.

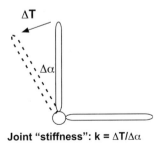

Joint "stiffness": $k = \Delta T/\Delta\alpha$

Figure 8.2 The notion of joint "stiffness" (more precisely, apparent stiffness) may be introduced as the ratio between the change in torque (ΔT) produced by a small joint displacement ($\Delta\alpha$) to the magnitude of this displacement.

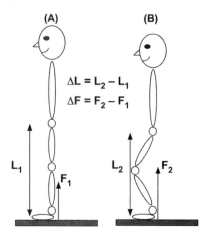

(A)   **(B)**

$\Delta L = L_2 - L_1$
$\Delta F = F_2 - F_1$

L_1 F_1 L_2 F_2

Limb "stiffness": k = −ΔF/ΔL

Figure 8.3 Formally, one can introduce the notion of limb "stiffness" (apparent stiffness) as the ratio between a change in the ground reaction force (ΔF) and a change in the distance between the most proximal and most distal segment (ΔL) compare the forces (F) and length (L) values at postures A and B.

The situation becomes even more complicated when the notion of stiffness is applied to a limb, such as a leg or an arm. Indeed, one can measure the distance between a proximal and a distal point on a limb and call this distance *limb length*. Now one can apply a force to the limb leading to a change in its configuration and compute the ratio of the force magnitude to the change in the limb length (Figure 8.3). Such computed values are sometimes called *limb stiffness*. Note that the limb is not deformed in such an experiment, but rather its configuration is changed. Imprecise applications of the notion of stiffness have led in some cases to claims of negative stiffness that make no sense within classical physics.

Simple linear oscillator

Consider a mass on a spring and assume that the spring has no mass of its own (Figure 8.4). The force produced by the spring will accelerate the mass: $F = md^2x/dt^2 = -kx$, where x is mass coordinate measured from zero length of the spring ($x = 0$, when $L = L_0$). The mass will oscillate with the frequency $f = 1/2\pi\sqrt{(k/m)}$. This system will continue to oscillate forever unless some kind of energy dissipation is introduced. Most commonly, a linear damping element is considered that leads to a decrease in the amplitude of the oscillation (Figure 8.5, top). Such an element produces force against the velocity vector: $F_D = -b(dx/dt)$, where b is a constant called *damping*. Sometimes b is imprecisely referred to as *viscosity* (which means resistance to motion in liquid or gas).

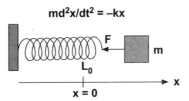

Figure 8.4 An illustration of a typical mass–spring system. Spring force ($-kx$) is equal in magnitude and directed against the inertial force ($m{\cdot}d^2x/dt^2$).

Motion of a damped mass–spring system without an external force acting on it can be described as:

$$m\frac{d^2x}{dt^2} + b\frac{dx}{dt} + kx = 0$$

Two useful parameters can be introduced, $\omega_0 = \sqrt{(k/m)}$ and $\sigma = b/2\sqrt{(mk)}$. The former is called *natural frequency* of the oscillator (expressed in radians per second) and the second one is called the *damping ratio* (dimensionless). If $\sigma < 1$, the system is called underdamped; it will oscillate with an exponential drop in the amplitude of the oscillation (Figure 8.5A). Systems with $\sigma > 1$ are called overdamped; they do not oscillate, but rather show a smooth transition to the resting length of the spring, $x = 0$ (Figure 8.5B). Available estimates of muscle damping (mostly unreliable, achieved under many simplifying assumptions) suggest that muscles are underdamped. Note, however, that these estimates typically did not consider damping produced by reflex

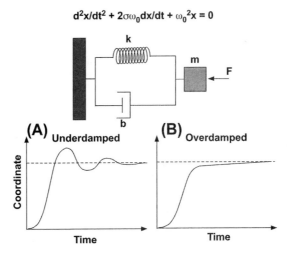

Figure 8.5 A mass–spring system with a damping element (top). The two bottom graphs show typical trajectories of the mass in an underdamped (A) and overdamped (B) system.

loops. Since spindle primary endings are sensitive to velocity, their reflex effects contribute to damping at a reflex time delay. This contribution can be substantial, affecting the σ parameter.

Human movements show some features of damped mass–spring systems, in particular fast movements are commonly accompanied by oscillations at the movement termination suggesting that, within this model, the system is underdamped or critically damped ($\sigma = 1$). Observations that humans can stop a quick movement efficiently led James Houk and his colleagues to a model that included non-linear damping. Within that model, the damping force was assumed to be proportional to a power function of velocity $F_D = b(dx/dt)^{\{1/5\}}$. This assumption allowed the movements to be performed at high velocities and to stop with minimal terminal oscillations because of the increased relative role of damping at low velocities.

Problems with simplified mass-spring models

Earlier models of motor control used mass–spring analogies to reflect only the properties of the peripheral structures (muscles and tendons) while muscle force was supposed to be generated independently of the parameters of the model. In other words, cross-bridges were assumed to generate the force driving the mass–spring system:

$$m\frac{d^2x}{dt^2} + b\frac{dx}{dt} + kx = F_{CB},$$

where F_{CB} stands for the force produced by cross-bridges.

Further, it was discovered, however, that voluntary muscle activation is associated with major changes in parameters of the mass–spring equation, and even the functional form of the equation may become suspect. In particular, such parameters as *stiffness* (k), *damping* (b), and *zero length* of the assumed spring (L_0), all change with changes in muscle activation. Strong non-linearities of the damping and stiffness terms have also been demonstrated. Although mass–spring models may still be useful for analysis of some problems, results of analysis using such models should be taken with a huge pinch of salt. The second-order linear equations of motion are too simplified to reflect important features of voluntary movements.

8.2   Threshold control

The elements of the central nervous system, neurons, are excitable cells that, at rest, are characterized by polarization of the cellular membrane such that the electric potential inside the membrane is negative as compared to the extracellular space. Neurons have *threshold properties*. This means that changes in the overall input into a neuron do not lead to changes in its output (Figure 8.6A,B) unless the input results in depolarization of the neuronal membrane (reduction in absolute magnitude of the negative potential) over a threshold value (Figure 8.6C). If this happens, the neuron generates a standard electric pulse called the *action potential*. Characteristics of the action potential (its amplitude and duration) do not depend on the magnitude of the

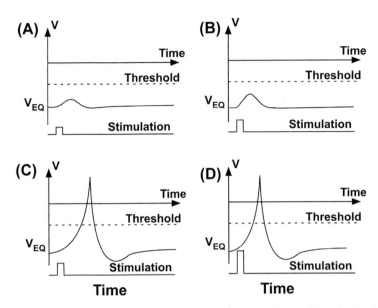

Figure 8.6 Neurons are threshold elements that respond to small stimuli applied to the membrane with proportional transient changes in the membrane potential (A and B). When the stimulus reaches a certain threshold, an action potential is generated (C). Increasing the stimulus further leads to no change in the membrane response (D, all-or-none law).

input; this feature is referred to as the *all-or-none law*. There are notable exceptions from this rule such as the simple and complex spikes produced by Purkinje cells in the cerebellum, but this material is outside the scope of the current discussion. The process of action potential generation involves ion current flow through specialized sites at the membrane called *ion channels*. After generating an action potential, the membrane cannot be excited over some time, even by very strong stimuli, due to inactivation of the channels for sodium ions. This time interval is known as the *refractory period*.

The threshold property of the neurons may be viewed as a complicating factor if one wants to build movement control on internal models pre-computing inputs into neuronal pools that would generate desired outputs. Indeed, the all-or-none law does not allow computation of an input even into a single neuron based on its output, for example a single action potential (see the two different inputs that produce the same action potential in Figure 8.6C,D). This property, on the other hand, may be viewed as an important feature of the design of the central nervous system that allows it to use certain modes of control that differ from typical control schemes in engineering.

Using activation threshold as a control variable

Consider a neuron that has two inputs, from a central structure (controller) and from another source, for example from receptors within an effector (Figure 8.7). The output

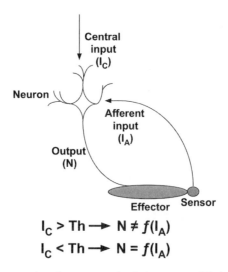

$$I_C > Th \longrightarrow N \neq f(I_A)$$
$$I_C < Th \longrightarrow N = f(I_A)$$

Figure 8.7 Threshold properties of neurons make their response (N) dependent on the afferent input (I_A) only when the central input (I_C) is below the threshold (Th).

of the neuron (N) changes the state of the effector, which is measured by the receptors that project back onto the neuron. The output of the neuron will depend on whether the combined signals from the two sources reach the threshold and how frequently this happens; the latter factor will define the frequency of action potentials generated by the neuron. If the controller sends to the neuron an excitatory signal that is very strong, such that the neuronal membrane potential is always above the threshold for action potential generation ($I_C > Th$), the neuron will generate action potentials at the highest possible frequency independently of the feedback it receives from the other source because of the all-or-none law. (Feedback signals that effectively decrease the descending excitation can modulate the output of such a neuron, but let us, for now, consider only reflex excitatory inputs.) In other words, the neuron will produce a standard output to the effector that will not depend on the interaction between the effector and the environment. This mode of control can be used by the central nervous system, for example, in cases of deafferentation, that is loss of sensory signals from an affected body part to the central nervous system.

In contrast, if the controller sends to the neuron a *subthreshold* excitatory stimulus that by itself does not lead to action potential generation ($I_C < Th$), the output of the neuron will depend on the amount of excitation it receives from the other, peripheral sources (or from another source within the central nervous system). When the state of the effector is such that it produces enough excitatory input via the sensory pathways that takes the neuronal membrane to its threshold, the neuron will generate action potentials that will lead to a change in the effector's state. This change will reduce the excitation the neuron receives from the periphery if the effector is free to move.

Figure 8.8 shows a graph of the dependence between the output of a neuron (frequency of action potentials it generates) and a state variable of the effector that

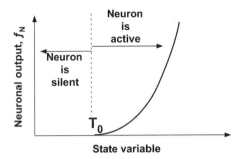

Figure 8.8 An illustration of a dependence between the output of the neuron (f_N) and a state variable of the effector that defines the sensory input into the neuron.

defines the sensory input into that neuron. For example, if the effector is a single muscle, this variable may be associated with muscle length (and also perhaps with its velocity and force). The signal from the controller defines a minimal value of excitation from the sensory signals that leads to action potential generation by the neuron, that is, it defines the threshold (T_0) for neuronal activation expressed in units of the relevant peripheral variable. Within a certain range of values of this variable, the neuron will not receive enough excitation and will remain silent (to the left of T_0). To the right of T_0, the output of the neuron (the frequency of action potential generation) will increase with an increase in the magnitude of the peripheral variable. A change in the signal from the controller changes the range within which the neuron responds to changes in the peripheral variable (Figure 8.9). Shifting the threshold to higher values decreases the range within which the neuron is active (T_1 in Figure 8.9), while shifting the threshold to lower values of the peripheral variable increases this range (T_2).

It is important to emphasize that subthreshold depolarization of the neuronal membrane does not change the absolute magnitude of the membrane threshold. It changes the difference between the current membrane potential and its threshold value, which we will refer to as the *activation threshold*.

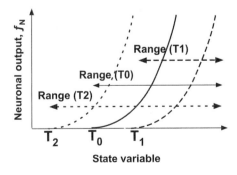

Figure 8.9 Shifting the threshold to higher values by the controller decreases the range of the state variable within which the neuron is active (T_1) while shifting the threshold to lower values of the variable increases this range (T_2).

Persistent inward currents

The mode of control with membrane potentials has recently attracted much attention in relation to the ability of the dendritic membrane to show steady depolarization. Dendrites have been shown, both theoretically and experimentally, to have long-lasting changes in the membrane potential induced by persistent inward currents. A *persistent inward current* is a depolarizing current produced by voltage-sensitive channels that do not show the phenomenon of inactivation (this is why they can be long-lasting or persistent). These channels are specialized for calcium ions. Significant recent progress in our understanding of the role of persistent inwards currents has come from studies by the group of the American neurophysiologist C. J. Heckman.

Figure 8.10 illustrates the dependence between voltage and current over a membrane in the absence of persistent inward currents (solid curve) and when these currents are present (dashed curves). Note that when the current is zero, the membrane is at the equilibrium potential. The solid line shows only one value of the membrane potential when the current is zero; it corresponds to the resting membrane potential (equilibrium potential, V_{EQ}). The thick dashed line shows three crossings of the abscissa axis. The first and third are stable while the intermediate one is not. The second stable resting potential (U_{EQ} in Figure 8.10) can be above the threshold for the generation of action potential (V_{TH}), shown by the vertical dashed line. If the dendritic membrane reaches a potential U_{EQ}, the dendrite would start generating action potentials and would continue doing so without any external stimuli as long as the membrane potential stays above the threshold value and the neuron does not run out of energy. Persistent inward currents (PIC) can potentially lead to muscle activation in the absence of a descending command to the corresponding alpha-motoneuronal pool. Potentially, this is an important mechanism of producing sustained, long-lasting muscle contractions, for example those of postural muscles.

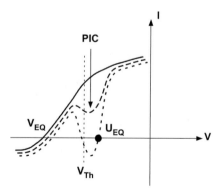

Figure 8.10 Dependence between the voltage (V) and current (I) over a membrane in the absence of persistent inward currents (PIC, solid curve) and when PIC are present (dashed curves). Note that strong PIC can lead to emergence of additional equilibrium voltages on the membrane—one unstable and the other stable (U_{EQ}).

8.3   The equilibrium-point hypothesis

The equilibrium-point hypothesis is based on three pillars. The first is the mentioned threshold property of neurons. The second is a physical principle stating that a system with negative feedback based on position and velocity will move towards an equilibrium state defined by parameters of the system and its interaction with the environment. The third is a body of experimental material suggesting that the neural control of a muscle can be adequately described with changes in the threshold of the tonic stretch reflex.

The experimental basis of the equilibrium-point hypothesis

About 50 years ago, Peter Matthews performed experimental studies on the dependence of muscle force on muscle length in decerebrated cat preparations. He stretched the soleus muscle at a constant slow velocity and measured the force and length of the muscle. Experimenting with the denervated (passive) and intact (active) muscle allowed Matthews to show that muscle force depended on muscle length due to the properties of peripheral tissues and that in an intact muscle the force–length dependence was dramatically different, with much higher forces produced at comparable length values. He placed an electrical stimulator at the site of the transection of the neural axis and used different stimulation levels to simulate different descending commands. Other important results included the dependence of the force–length relation on the speed of muscle length change and on its direction. The muscle showed hysteresis: Larger forces were generated during stretch than during shortening for similar length values. At a fixed stimulation frequency applied to the motor nerve, Matthews observed a dependence between muscle force and length, $F(L)$ similar to the curves shown in Figure 8.11. A change in the stimulation level led to translation of the $F(L)$ curve along the abscissa axis, which could be described as

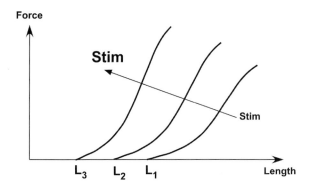

Figure 8.11 An illustration of Matthews' experiments on decerebrate cats. Increasing the frequency of the stimulation applied to the motor nerve led to a shift of the force–length muscle characteristics along the length axis with no major changes in their shape.

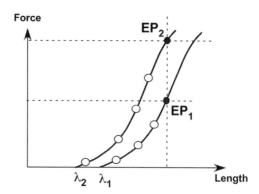

Figure 8.12 In Feldman's experiments, the subjects occupied a posture corresponding to a combination of load and muscle length (equilibrium point, EP_1). Unloading the muscle led to a sequence of combination of muscle force and length (open circles) that could be approximated by a smooth line—the tonic stretch reflex characteristic. If the same procedure started from a different force–length combination (EP_2), a different tonic stretch reflex characteristic was reconstructed.

a change in the threshold for active muscle force production (compare the thresholds L_1, L_2, and L_3 in Figure 8.11).

Later, Anatol Feldman and Grigory Orlovsky explored the force–length muscle characteristics, $F(L)$, in decerebrated cats during the stimulation of specific supraspinal structures such as the pyramidal tract, Deiters' nucleus, and mesencephalic reticular formation. This study also documented the nearly parallel translation of the $F(L)$ muscle characteristics with changes in the strength of the stimulation (see Section 4.4).

Qualitatively similar results were reported by Feldman in 1966 based on his pioneering human experiments. In those experiments, no surgical intervention was used; rather, the subjects were asked to hold a position against a load and "not to intervene" when the load changed. The results were interpreted under an assumption that "non-intervention" was equivalent to an unchanged supraspinal command. Under this instruction, a change in the load was accompanied by movement of the effector to a new *equilibrium state* (see the open circles in Figure 8.12 corresponding to equilibrium states after different magnitudes of unloading). A change in the initial conditions (occupying the same position against a different load, EP_1 and EP_2) led to a nearly parallel transfer of the $F(L)$ curve along the abscissa axis.

Threshold of the tonic stretch reflex as a control variable

Taken together, all these results suggest that the neural control of a muscle can be described with only one parameter corresponding to the location of the $F(L)$ curve along the abscissa axis. This parameter, the threshold of the tonic stretch reflex (λ), does not specify muscle length, muscle force, or muscle activation level. For a given value of λ, all these variables change depending on the external load magnitude (Figure 8.13). However, a value of λ specifies a relationship among these state variables corresponding to a $F(L)$ curve, which has also been addressed as the *tonic stretch reflex characteristic* and the muscle *invariant characteristic*. For a given value of λ and a given external load, the system "body + load" comes to an equilibrium characterized by certain values of muscle force and length, an *equilibrium point* (EP).

In the mid-1960s, Anatol Feldman formulated a hypothesis on the control of movements, which suggests that movements represent transitions between equilibrium points. These transitions may happen involuntarily, following a change in the external load without a change in the central command ($\lambda = $ const, as in Figure 8.14A), or voluntarily, following a change in the central command that can be adequately expressed as a change in the threshold of the tonic stretch reflex (λ_1 to λ_2, as in Figure 8.14B). A change in λ can lead to different actions depending on the external load. For example, in Figure 8.14B, the same shift in λ can lead to a movement (muscle length change), force production (muscle length is constant), or both, if the muscle works against an isotonic, isometric, or elastic load, as represented in that figure by a horizontal, vertical, and sloped dashed lines, respectively.

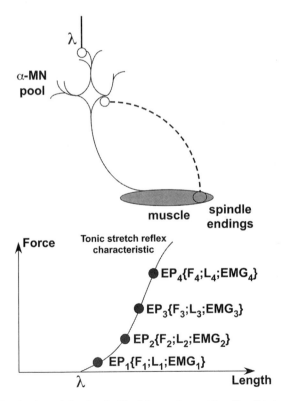

Figure 8.13 A fixed value of the threshold of the tonic stretch reflex (λ) does not specify muscle length, muscle force, or muscle activation level. For a given value of λ, all these variables change depending on the external load magnitude. Four equilibrium points are shown corresponding to four sets of these state variables.

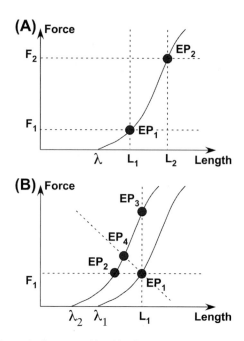

Figure 8.14 (A) A change in the external load leads to a movement, that is, a shift from an initial to a final equilibrium point (EP$_1$ and EP$_2$). (B) A change in the tonic stretch reflex threshold (from λ_1 to λ_2) may result in different peripheral consequences depending on the external load. In isometric conditions, muscle force changes (EP$_3$); in isotonic conditions, a movement takes place (EP$_2$); in mixed conditions (elastic load), both muscle force and length change (EP$_4$).

Three basic trajectories

Control of a single muscle may be associated with three trajectories (Figure 8.15). First, there is a time profile of the control variable $\lambda(t)$, which can be called the *control trajectory*. In some studies, $\lambda(t)$, or analogous joint-level variables, $r(t)$ and $c(t)$ (see later), have been referred to as the *virtual trajectory*, but this additional term is unnecessary and may be misleading. Second, at each moment of time, there exists an instantaneous equilibrium point (EP) defined by the current value of λ and the external load. A time series of these EPs is called the *equilibrium trajectory*, EP(*t*). The equilibrium trajectory involves changes of both muscle length and force with time. For example, in isotonic conditions, only muscle length changes, in isometric conditions only muscle force changes, while in most conditions both change (see Figure 8.14B). Third, there is *actual trajectory*, which can also involve changes in muscle length and force, $L(t)$ and $F(t)$, which is defined by both EP(*t*) and properties of the moving effector, for example its inertia. Note that only the control trajectory may be specified by the controller. The other two trajectories emerge given the control trajectory, the external forces and constraints, and the properties of the moving effector.

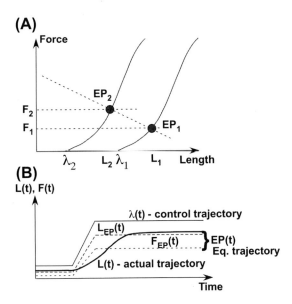

Figure 8.15 Voluntary movements are produced by a time shift of the control variable $\lambda(t)$, the control trajectory. At each moment of time, there exists an instantaneous equilibrium point (EP) defined by the current value of λ and the external load (for example EP_1 and EP_2 in panel A). A time series of EPs is the equilibrium trajectory, $EP(t)$ composed of length and force coordinates at EPs, $L_{EP}(t)$ and $F_{EP}(t)$. Actual trajectory involves changes in muscle length and force, $L(t)$ and $F(t)$, defined by both $EP(t)$ and properties of the moving effector, for example its inertia (B).

Control of a joint

Human joints are crossed by at least two muscles. So, control of a joint with only one axis of rotation that is crossed by only two muscles can be described with two parameters, for example with the two λs for the two opposing muscles, the agonist–antagonist pair. This general conclusion fits well with the everyday experience. What can a person do with a joint? Only two things: First, the person can move it to a new position if there is no resistance or produce torque if there is resistance. These are two different peripheral outcomes of basically the same command (as in Figure 8.14B). The other possibility is to co-contract the agonist–antagonist pair such that no net torque production (no net movement) takes place but the joint is "stiffened" (a term that is frequently used although the notion of joint stiffness is ill-defined, see Section 8.1). These two possibilities correspond to two combinations of shifts of the $F(L)$ curves for the two opposing muscles.

To consider joint control within the equilibrium-point hypothesis, one has to use mechanical variables that are adequate to describe rotations, such as joint angle (α) and joint torque (T). The two $F(L)$ curves for the two opposing muscles can be represented as $T(\alpha)$ curves (Figure 8.16). Since the muscles act against each other, one of them (the antagonist) produces negative T values. The two curves can shift in the same direction along the x-axis or in opposite directions. In the first case, a shift leads

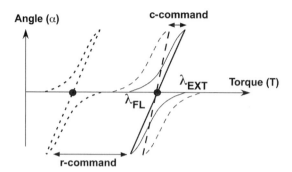

Figure 8.16 Control of a simple joint can be described using λ values for the muscles, for example λ_{FL} and λ_{EXT} for the flexor and extensor. Alternatively, two other variables may be used, r-command (reciprocal) and c-command (coactivation) corresponding to unidirectional and counter-directional changes in the two λ values. The joint characteristic, $T(\alpha)$ is effectively shifted by the r-command and rotated by the c-command.

to an increase in the activation level and force produced by one of the muscles and a decrease in the activation (force) produced by the other muscle. In the second case, the two muscles show parallel changes (increase or decrease) in their forces and levels of activation. Such changes in muscle activation are commonly addressed as *reciprocal* and *coactivation*. Correspondingly, a command leading to a parallel shift of the $F(L)$ curves may be called reciprocal (*r*-command), while the command that leads to curve shifts in opposite directions may be called coactivation (*c*-command).

In isotonic conditions, when the external load is zero, a change in the reciprocal command leads to a change in the joint angle (compare EP_1 and EP_2 in Figure 8.17A), while a change in the coactivation command leads to no joint motion, but the joint *apparent stiffness*, the slope of the $T(\alpha)$ line, changes (Figure 8.17A). If the external load is not zero, a change in the *c*-command can lead to joint displacement in addition to changes in the joint apparent stiffness (compare EP_1 and EP_3 in Figure 8.17B).

In isometric conditions, a change in the *r*-command produces net torque in one of the directions, while the effects of a change in the *c*-command both change the net torque and the apparent joint stiffness (compare EP_1, EP_2, and EP_3 in Figure 8.18).

The $\{r, c\}$ pair is equivalent to the $\{\lambda_1, \lambda_2\}$ pair. Simple relationships between the two pairs have been suggested: $r = (\lambda_1 + \lambda_2)/2$; $c = (\lambda_1 - \lambda_2)/2$; obviously, from these two equations one can express λ_1 and λ_2 as simple functions of r and c. It is natural to consider joint control as hierarchically higher than muscle control. The two variables, $\{r, c\}$, have clear spatial meanings; r defines the mid-point of a range of joint angular positions where both muscles are activated while c defines the size of that range. Since most joints are spanned by more than two muscles, the mapping of the $\{r, c\}$ pair on λ values is an example of the problem of redundancy. We will consider it in more detail in Chapter 9.

The alpha-model

A different version of the equilibrium-point hypothesis was suggested based on observations in experiments on deafferented monkeys by the group of Emilio Bizzi.

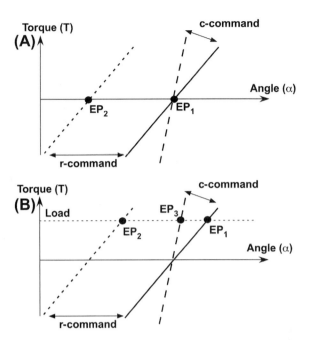

Figure 8.17 In isotonic conditions, when the external load is zero, a change in the r-command leads to a change in the joint angle (EP_1 and EP_2 in A), while a change in the c-command leads to no joint motion, but the slope of the $T(\alpha)$ line, changes. If the external load is not zero, a change in the c-command can lead to joint displacement in addition to changes in the joint apparent stiffness (compare EP_1 and EP_3 in B).

This version is commonly known as the *alpha-model*, in contrast to the original Feldman's *lambda-model*. In those experiments, the deafferented monkeys (that is, monkeys with no sensory information coming from the arms) were trained to produce accurate fast arm movements into a target under visual control. Further, they performed such movements without visual control, and sometimes a change in the

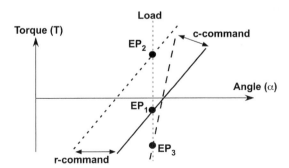

Figure 8.18 In isometric conditions, a change in the r-command produces net torque changes (compare EP_1 and EP_2). A change in the c-command changes both the net torque and the apparent joint stiffness (compare EP_1 and EP_3).

external torque was applied. The main finding was that if the torque change was transient, the monkey reached the target successfully, that is, it showed movement *equifinality*. Note that, since the monkey was deafferented, it could not feel the perturbation or its effects on arm trajectory; hence, it was safe to assume that the monkeys did not react to such perturbations. These results supported one of the main predictions of the equilibrium-point hypothesis.

Another important finding was that if the torque moved the monkey's arm into the target very quickly and released the arm there, the arm moved back from the target, then reversed, and moved to the target once again. This result shows that the equilibrium point does not jump from the initial to the final location but moves continuously over a certain time characteristic of the movement time.

Since the monkeys in those studies were deafferented, tonic stretch reflex (and all other reflexes) was absent. So, control with the tonic stretch reflex threshold (λ) was impossible. The authors interpreted the results as the consequence of an equilibrium point-type of control with a different control variable, the level of activation of the involved alpha-motoneuronal pools (hence, the alpha-model). Note that for a fixed level of muscle activation, the muscle shows spring-like properties (Figure 8.19). These properties differ significantly from those mediated by the tonic stretch reflex in intact animals. In particular, a change in λ leads to a shift of the force–length characteristic along the length axis (as in Figure 8.14). In contrast, a change in the level of muscle activation leads to rotation of the force–length characteristic with a major change in its slope and no major changes in its threshold (intercept), as illustrated in Figure 8.19. A shift in the α-command leads to a shift in the equilibrium point; for example, in isotonic conditions, a shift in the α-command leads to a motion (compare α_1, α_2, α_3 and L_1, L_2, L_3 in Figure 8.19). Such control is possible, as the mentioned experiments on deafferented monkeys demonstrate, but it is different from the control of intact muscles and joints. So, the alpha-model may be viewed as describing a special case of the equilibrium-point hypothesis, when no afferent feedback into the spinal cord is available.

Over the past 50 years or so, the equilibrium-point hypothesis has been developed to address such issues as movements at different speeds and in different loading conditions, movement variability, electromyographic patterns, single- and multi-joint

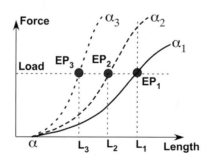

Figure 8.19 Within the α-model, a command to a muscle defines its activation level and a spring-like characteristic (compare the curves for α_1, α_2, and α_3). Different activation levels result in different combination of force and length—different equilibrium points (EP).

movements, and movements in persons with neurological disorders. It has survived waves of misunderstanding and attempts at disproving the hypothesis. As of now, it is the only hypothesis of motor control that incorporates basic neurophysiological principles (the threshold properties of neurons) and physical principles (movement as a shift of an equilibrium state).

8.4   Control with referent configurations

The development of the equilibrium-point hypothesis to the neural control of multi-joint movements has resulted in the notion of a referent configuration. By definition, *referent configuration* is a configuration of the body in which all the muscles are at the threshold of activation (their length values equal to the corresponding λ values). Note that, in real life, the referent configuration may not be achievable because of such factors as external forces and constraints, as well as constraints imposed by the body anatomy. As a result, it is virtually impossible to observe a person in whom all the muscles are completely quiescent. Non-zero levels of muscle activation reflect discrepancies between the actual muscle length and its threshold length ($L > \lambda$).

The idea of the referent configuration closely follows a basic physical principle that the magnitude of a variable is defined with respect to a referent value (measured within a frame of reference). Although commonly referent values are assumed to be zero, this does not have to be so. For example, although the threshold potential on the membrane may be constant, its activation threshold (the difference between the actual and threshold values of the potential) depends on the actual potential. So, the activation threshold is changed by changing the referent value from which the measurement is made.

The notion of the referent configuration does not imply that the central nervous system specifies all the λ values for all the participating muscles each time it tries to produce a movement. The controller is assumed to use control variables related to threshold parameters for salient variables, while the specific signals to individual joints, $\{r(t), c(t)\}$, and muscles, $\{\lambda(t)\}$, emerge given the control variables, the external forces, and the interactions within the body, which will be partly covered in Chapter 9.

Referent configuration defined by membrane depolarization

Imagine, for example, that the purpose of the controller is to specify three-dimensional coordinates for the endpoint of a limb with respect to the body (for example, as when pointing at the tip of one's nose). The idea of the referent configuration assumes that the control signal from an unknown hierarchically higher structure can be adequately expressed as subthreshold depolarization of a neuronal pool (N_1 in Figure 8.20), The output of this pool is further distributed among hierarchically lower neuronal pools, ultimately resulting in signals to alpha-motoneurons that innervate the muscles that can potentially move the endpoint towards the target. In a given external force field, an input to N_1 may be associated with a referent value of a potentially important mechanical variable, a value to which the system is attracted. The neuronal pool N_1

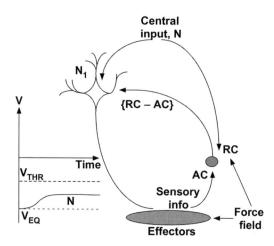

Figure 8.20 A scheme of control with referent configuration (RC) starts with setting subthreshold membrane depolarization in a neuronal pool (N_1). The central input, given external conditions, defines RC, at which all muscles would be silent. The difference between actual configuration (AC) and RC drives neurons N_1 and produces muscle activation.

receives another excitatory input from processed sensory signals from all the relevant peripheral receptors that carry information on the discrepancy between the actual configuration of the moving effector (AC) and its referent configuration (RC). If this signal is non-zero, it drives the neurons of N_1 to the threshold for activation, they generate action potentials, and the muscles are activated to move the effector towards the target. As soon as the effector reaches the target (AC − RC = 0), the sensory signal becomes zero, and the neuronal pool stops generating action potentials. The system comes to an equilibrium state.

Imagine that you grasp a small object between the thumb and index finger. The referent configuration may define the threshold aperture (the distance between the tips of the digits) but not referent coordinates for each of the digits. If this referent aperture is smaller than the actual one (constrained by the object rigid walls), active grasping force will be produced by both digits, ensuring sufficient friction at the contact sites. Now, the grasped object can be manipulated and, as long as the referent aperture remains unchanged, the grasping forces will be kept constant despite possible changes in the hand configuration. If the object is moved quickly, the referent aperture may change, leading to modulation of the grasping force that may be required by motion-dependent inertial and other forces (see Section 11.4).

Figure 8.20 illustrates an assumption that is present in virtually all studies of human movements but is rarely made explicit: For a selected level of analysis, it is assumed that physical and neurophysiological processes at hierarchically higher levels can be adequately represented as an input signal into elements at the level of analysis, and this signal may be assigned relevance to the task, intention of the person, etc. In other words, there is an assumption of a task- and intention-related "command" coming from hierarchically higher levels. It is important to always keep in mind that this signal is not computed by a smart, hierarchically higher neuronal structures but is a result of natural processes in those structures that obey the laws of physics, which are beyond the current level of analysis.

A moving system at an equilibrium may be characterized by its coordinates and forces (torques). However, this is an insufficient description. We know from everyday experience that the same limb configuration against the same external force field may be accompanied by different levels of muscle co-contraction. Such "stiffening" of a joint/limb may lead to no visible change in its position or net forces but it modifies reactions of the limb if the external force suddenly changes. Changing muscle co-contraction leads to changes not only in apparent stiffness of the effector, but also in its apparent damping. These terms imply that, in response to a small perturbation (a deviation from an equilibrium position), the effector generates forces that are proportional to the positional deviation (which can be measured in linear or angular units) and to velocity of this deviation:

$$F_{\text{RES}} = k\Delta x + b\Delta x/\Delta t, \tag{8.2}$$

where F_{RES} is force resisting the perturbation, Δx is positional deviation, and k and b are constants (apparent stiffness and damping).

Sometimes, the property of a mechanical system to resist positional deviations is described by the term *impedance*. In physics, this term is defined as the reaction of a system to a cyclic force input. The mechanical impedance is a function of the frequency of the applied force and can vary with the frequency of the force input. For example, at resonance frequencies, the mechanical impedance is low, meaning less force is needed to induce motion at a given velocity. Correspondingly, control based on establishing resistance of the system to deviations from equilibrium states is sometimes called *impedance control*.

Coactivation command

Within the referent configuration hypothesis, modulation of the resistance to deviations from equilibrium states is described with a set of variables that belong to the general notion of referent configuration. Earlier, when we discussed analysis of single-joint movements within the equilibrium-point hypothesis (Section 8.3), the notion of a coactivation command was introduced (*c*-command). Remember, this command reflects the range of joint positions within which both agonist and antagonist muscles can show non-zero activation. Changes in this command have strong effects of the joint apparent stiffness while having relatively small effects on its equilibrium position. For a single joint with only one kinematic degree-of-freedom, the *c*-command is one-dimensional.

Generalizing the notion of *c*-command to the motion of the endpoint of a multi-joint limb is non-trivial. Apparent stiffness of the endpoint of a kinematic chain can be characterized with six parameters corresponding to the directions and magnitudes of the main axes of the stiffness ellipsoid. Experiments have shown, however, that humans cannot voluntarily change each of the six parameters independently of each other. Note also that these parameters describe the overall mechanical effect of neurophysiological control signals that are subthreshold depolarizing inputs into hypothetical neuronal pools within the referent configuration hypothesis (as in Figure 8.20).

Self-test questions

1. What are the main challenges of applying classical physics to movements of biological objects?
2. Define stiffness according to classical mechanics.
3. What is Hooke's law?
4. What are the assumptions in using terms "muscle stiffness" and "joint stiffness"? Why is using a term "apparent stiffness" recommended?
5. Define natural frequency for an ideal oscillator (mass on a spring).
6. What is the main difference in movements of underdamped and overdamped systems?
7. Are human muscles underdamped, overdamped, or critically damped?
8. What are the main problems in using second-order linear models to describe human movements?
9. What is the main idea of threshold control? What are its challenges and advantages?
10. What are the effects of persistent inward currents on membrane properties?
11. How can persistent inward currents turn a membrane segment into a generator of action potentials?
12. What are the three main pillars of the equilibrium-point hypothesis?
13. Explain how human experiments under the "do-not-intervene" instruction support the equilibrium-point hypothesis.
14. Define equilibrium point. What can cause shifts of an equilibrium point?
15. What are the main differences in the isotonic movements and isometric contractions within the equilibrium-point hypothesis?
16. What are the three main trajectories within the equilibrium-point hypothesis?
17. Explain the difference between the control trajectory and the equilibrium trajectory.
18. How can joint apparent stiffness be controlled within the equilibrium-point hypothesis?
19. Define the reciprocal and coactivation commands.
20. Explain the main differences between the lambda-model and the alpha-model.
21. What experiments on deafferented monkeys proved that there is a gradual shift in the equilibrium point during fast movements?
22. Define referent configuration.
23. How can threshold properties of neurons be used to control movements with shifts in referent configurations?
24. What is impedance?
25. Define coactivation command within the scheme of control with referent configurations.

Essential references and recommended further readings

Bizzi, E., Accornero, N., Chapple, W., & Hogan, N. (1982). Arm trajectory formation in monkeys. *Experimental Brain Research, 46,* 139–143.

Bizzi, E., Hogan, N., Mussa-Ivaldi, F. A., & Giszter, S. (1992). Does the nervous system use equilibrium-point control to guide single and multiple joint movements? *Behavioral and Brain Science, 15*, 603–613.

Feldman, A. G. (1966). Functional tuning of the nervous system with control of movement or maintenance of a steady posture. II. Controllable parameters of the muscle. *Biophysics, 11*, 565–578.

Feldman, A. G. (1980). Superposition of motor programs. I. Rhythmic forearm movements in man. *Neuroscience, 5*, 81–90.

Feldman, A. G. (1986). Once more on the equilibrium-point hypothesis (λ-model) for motor control. *Journal of Motor Behavior, 18*, 17–54.

Feldman, A. G. (2009a). Origin and advances of the equilibrium-point hypothesis. *Advances in Experimental Medicine and Biology, 629*, 637–643.

Feldman, A. G. (2009b). New insights into action-perception coupling. *Experimental Brain Research, 194*, 39–58.

Feldman, A. G., & Latash, M. L. (2005). Testing hypotheses and the advancement of science: Recent attempts to falsify the equilibrium-point hypothesis. *Experimental Brain Research, 161*, 91–103.

Feldman, A. G., & Levin, M. F. (1995). Positional frames of reference in motor control: their origin and use. *Behavioral and Brain Sciences, 18*, 723–806.

Feldman, A. G., & Orlovsky, G. N. (1972). The influence of different descending systems on the tonic stretch reflex in the cat. *Experimental Neurology, 37*, 481–494.

Feldman, A. G., Goussev, V., Sangole, A., & Levin, M. F. (2007). Threshold position control and the principle of minimal interaction in motor actions. *Progress in Brain Research, 165*, 267–281.

Flash, T., & Hogan, N. (1985). The coordination of arm movements: An experimentally confirmed mathematical model. *Journal of Neuroscience, 5*, 1688–1703.

Fukson, O. I., Berkinblit, M. B., & Feldman, A. G. (1980). The spinal frog takes into account the scheme of its body during the wiping reflex. *Science, 209*, 1261–1263.

Giszter, S. F., Mussa-Ivaldi, F. A., & Bizzi, E. (1993). Convergent force fields organized in the frog's spinal cord. *Journal of Neuroscience, 13*, 467–491.

Gomi, H., & Kawato, M. (1996). Equilibrium-point hypothesis examined by measured arm stiffness during multijoint movement. *Science, 272*, 117–120.

Gribble, P. L., & Ostry, D. J. (2000). Compensation for loads during arm movements using equilibrium-point control. *Experimental Brain Research, 135*, 474–482.

Gribble, P. L., Ostry, D. J., Sanguineti, V., & Laboissiere, R. (1998). Are complex control signals required for human arm movements? *Journal of Neurophysiology, 79*, 1409–1424.

Gutman, A. M. (1991). Bistability of dendrites. *International Journal of Neural Systems, 1*, 291–304.

Hasan, Z. (1986). Optimized movement trajectories and joint stiffness in unperturbed, inertially loaded movements. *Biological Cybernetics, 53*, 373–382.

Heckman, C. J., Lee, R. H., & Brownstone, R. M. (2003). Hyperexcitable dendrites in motoneurons and their neuromodulatory control during motor behavior. *Trends in Neuroscience, 26*, 688–695.

Heckman, C. J., Gorassini, M. A., & Bennett, D. J. (2005). Persistent inward currents in motoneuron dendrites: Implications for motor output. *Muscle and Nerve, 31*, 135–156.

Kugler, P. N., & Turvey, M. T. (1987). *Information, natural law, and the self-assembly of rhythmic movement*. Hillsdale, NJ: Erlbaum.

Latash, M. L. (1993). *Control of human movement*. Urbana, IL: Human Kinetics.

Latash, M. L. (2008). *Synergy*. New York: Oxford University Press.

Latash, M. L. (2010). Motor synergies and the equilibrium-point hypothesis. *Motor Control, 14*, 294–322.

Latash, M. L., & Gottlieb, G. L. (1991). Reconstruction of elbow joint compliant characteristics during fast and slow voluntary movements. *Neuroscience, 43*, 697–712.

Latash, M. L., & Zatsiorsky, V. M. (1993). Joint stiffness: Myth or reality? *Human Movement Science, 12*, 653–692.

Latash, M. L., Aruin, A. S., & Zatsiorsky, V. M. (1999). The basis of a simple synergy: Reconstruction of joint equilibrium trajectories during unrestrained arm movements. *Human Movement Science, 18*, 3–30.

Malfait, N., Gribble, P. L., & Ostry, D. J. (2005). Generalization of motor learning based on multiple field exposures and local adaptation. *Journal of Neurophysiology, 93*, 3327–3338.

Matthews, P. B. C. (1959). The dependence of tension upon extension in the stretch reflex of the soleus of the decerebrate cat. *Journal of Physiology, 147*, 521–546.

Pilon, J.-F., De Serres, S. J., & Feldman, A. G. (2007). Threshold position control of arm movement with anticipatory increase in grip force. *Experimental Brain Research, 181*, 49–67.

Polit, A., & Bizzi, E. (1979). Characteristics of motor programs underlying arm movemnt in monkey. *Journal of Neurophysiology, 42*, 183–194.

Sainburg, R. L., Ghilardi, M. F., Poizner, H., & Ghez, C. (1995). Control of limb dynamics in normal subjects and patients without proprioception. *Journal of Neurophysiology, 73*, 820–835.

9 Coordination

9.1   Introduction

The *problem of motor redundancy* has already been mentioned in Section 3.5 as one of the central problems typical of the biological systems for movement production. This problem seems to emerge at any level of description of the neuromotor system. For example, there are more axes of joint rotation in the human limbs than absolutely necessary to perform typical movements; there are more muscles crossing each joint

Fundamentals of Motor Control. DOI: 10.1016/B978-0-12-415956-3.00009-9

than absolutely necessary to produce joint rotations and/or torques; each muscle consists of many motor units, which can be recruited in different patterns for the same overall level of muscle activation; and so on. In each of these examples, the controller seems to be confronted with a problem equivalent to solving a system of equations with fewer equations than unknowns. This is impossible unless more equations are available or some other constraints are introduced.

This traditional formulation of the problem of motor redundancy implies that the apparently redundant design of the human body is a source of computational problems for the central nervous system, and that the central nervous system solves these problems by performing computations and finding unique solutions each time it has to generate a motor action. This understanding of the problem follows the traditions set by Nikolai Bernstein, who emphasized that the main problem of motor control was the problem of elimination of redundant degrees of freedom.

Principle of abundance

An alternative view was developed based on a general idea that the apparently redundant design of the neuromotor system is in fact abundant (*principle of abundance*), not redundant. The change in the word implies that this design is not a source of computational problems but a rich and flexible apparatus that allows the central nervous system to facilitate several actions simultaneously based on the same set of elements (muscles, joints, etc.) without sacrificing the accuracy of any of the actions. The central nervous system is not looking for unique solutions but facilitates whole families of solutions that are equally able to solve the task. Selection of particular solutions from such families may be performed randomly or based on criteria that are not explicit in the task formulation. It would be more precise to speak about the emergence of solutions based on natural laws, not their selection.

In this chapter, first we will consider several approaches that follow the traditional formulation of the problem of motor redundancy. Then we will address the same problem starting from the principle of abundance. Ultimately, we will try to reconcile the two approaches.

9.2   Optimization

Cost function

One of the methods commonly used to address the problem of motor redundancy has been *optimization*. The general idea of this approach is to look for a solution for a problem of motor redundancy that both satisfies all the task constraints and optimizes (typically, minimizes or maximizes) a value of a particular function, known as a *cost function*. Cost functions have been applied to solve two groups of problems. First, to find a time profile of a variable among all possible time profiles that optimizes a cost function. A typical example would be defining the trajectory of the index finger during a pointing movement based on the initial position, target position, and sometimes also movement time. Second, to find a state of a redundant set of variables among all possible sets that optimizes a cost function. Typical examples would be producing a certain level of total force with several fingers or producing a certain moment of force in a joint by several muscles crossing the joint.

Minimal time

Within the first group of problems, let us consider three cost functions. The first is related to movement time. If the task is to move from one point to another as quickly as possible, the optimal solution is to apply the strongest possible acceleration and then, at an appropriate point, switch to the strongest possible deceleration. Peak acceleration and deceleration values are limited by maximal moment of force magnitudes achievable, given the muscle properties and the mechanical characteristics of the moving effector. If the accelerating and decelerating muscles (agonists and antagonists) are equally powerful and the moving system is purely inertial (both conditions are never met in real life), the switching time from acceleration to deceleration is exactly in the middle of the movement. This mode of control is known as *"bang-bang" control* (Figure 9.1). It leads to movement kinematics that is quite different from the smooth, bell-shaped velocity profiles observed in experiments with movements performed "as quickly as possible."

Minimal jerk

Arguably, the most commonly used cost function in studies of movement kinematics is an integral measure of squared jerk. Jerk in the third derivative of coordinate or the first derivative of acceleration. The so-called *minimum-jerk criterion* is commonly formulated as the requirement to minimize the following cost function:

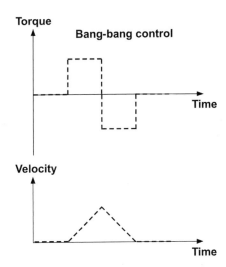

Figure 9.1 Torque and velocity profiles for "bang-bang control" applied to a purely inertial system.

$$J = \frac{1}{MT} \int_0^{MT} (da/dt)^2 dt,$$

where MT is movement time, and a is acceleration. This criterion leads to a polynomial solution for the trajectory, which corresponds to smooth kinematic functions similar to those observed in experiments (Figure 9.2). Minimum jerk is currently the method of choice if one wants to represent natural movement trajectories analytically. Note that the minimum-jerk criterion applied to the trajectory of the endpoint of a multi-joint limb does not necessarily generate minimum-jerk trajectories in individual joints. Moreover, individual joints may show large-amplitude non-monotonic trajectories, such that the initial and final joint positions may be very similar. Such trajectories definitely do not comply with the minimum-jerk criterion applied at the joint level.

There was an attempt to extend the minimum-jerk criterion to kinetic variables. This attempt resulted in the *minimum-torque-change model*. On the one hand, there is a degree of similarity between the two approaches because torque-change about a joint produces a change in its angular acceleration, that is, a jerk. So, for a purely inertial, one-joint system the minimum-torque-change and minimum-jerk criteria produce identical results. The two approaches differ when more realistic moving systems are considered, such as multi-joint systems that have not only inertial but also more complex mechanical properties, for example length- and velocity-dependent muscle force production.

Within the second group of problems, several approaches have been used based on mathematical, mechanical, and physiological considerations. For example, during multi-finger force production, a principle of *minimization of secondary moments* was suggested, based on observations that during such tasks, human subjects prefer to generate very small moments of force in pronation/supination. By itself, this principle is able to solve a problem of constant force production with only two fingers. Figure 9.3 illustrates the task of producing a constant level of total force with two fingers. This task has an infinite number of solutions that all belong to the line $F_1 + F_2 = C$ (open circles in Figure 9.3). Minimization of the total moment of force ($M_{TOT} = 0$) with respect to a pivot in-between the fingers (as in the insert) allows a single solution to be generated (shown by the black dot). If the number of fingers is larger than two, this principle introduces an additional constraint, which reduces the redundancy of the problem, but it does not lead to a single solution.

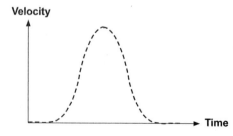

Figure 9.2 A smooth, bell-shaped velocity profile typical of natural movements can be produced by the minimum-jerk criterion.

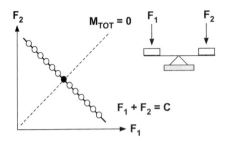

Figure 9.3 The task of producing a required force level with two effectors acting in parallel has an infinite number of solutions—points on the slanted line. If, in addition to this task, total moment of force is minimized with respect to a certain pivot (see the insert), a single solution emerges.

Minimal norm

Among mathematical approaches, let me mention minimization of the norm of the solution, that is minimization of the Eucledian distance between the initial and final states in the multi-dimensional space of elemental variables (for example, individual finger forces or individual joint rotations). Since forces of individual fingers are non-independent (all the fingers of the hand change their forces if a person tries to press harder with only one finger, see Section 11.4), norm minimization has also been applied to the space of hypothetical commands to individual fingers that can be changed one at a time, at least hypothetically. This approach produced data that matched better the experimental observations.

The principle of mechanical advantage is another method of reducing redundancy of a problem without necessarily finding a unique solution. The principle states that individual effectors are involved more in a common moment-of-force production task if their moment arms are larger. This allows required moment-of-force levels to be produced while reducing the total force produced by all the effectors.

A physiological criterion of minimum fatigue has been applied to the problem of torque sharing among muscles crossing a joint. This criterion has been used successfully to account for muscle force and activation patterns in complex tasks involving large muscle groups.

Pseudo-inverse

A common approach to finding an optimal trajectory for a redundant set of elements is to use a method developed in robotics known as *pseudo-inverse*. This method is based on finding a least squares solution to a system of linear equations that lacks a unique solution. This solution minimizes the sum of the squared deviations of elemental variables that are able to produce the required effect, for example deviations of joint angles that can move the limb endpoint into the target. The most common pseudo-inverse is the *Moore–Penrose pseudo-inverse*. If two fingers participate in the task of accurate total force production starting from zero force, the fingers have identical properties, and their forces can be changed by the neural controller independently of each other, Moore–Penrose solution predicts that the fingers will share the total force

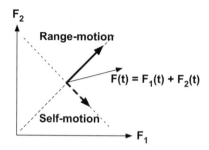

Figure 9.4 In a two-element system (F_1 and F_2) producing a common output, trajectory, $F(t)$ on the $\{F_1; F_2\}$ plane may be viewed as consisting of two components, one of which does not lead to changes in $F(t)$—self-motion, while the other one does—range-motion.

50 : 50. Within this approach, movement of a redundant system may be represented as the sum of two components, a movement along the "optimal" direction defined using the Moore–Penrose pseudo-inverse, and a movement orthogonal to that direction. These two components are commonly known as *range-space motion* and *self-motion*. By definition, self-motion of a system does not contribute to its motion towards the target but changes the values of the elemental variables. If you touch an object in space with an index fingertip and then move the arm joints without losing contact with the object, the joints will demonstrate self-motion with respect to the task of keeping the index fingertip coordinates unchanged.

Figure 9.4 illustrates the application of the pseudo-inverse optimization to a task of producing a linearly increasing total force with two fingers pressing on separate force sensors. At each force level, the trajectory of the system in the two-dimensional space of finger forces may be represented with a vector. One component of the vector will point along the shortest direction to the required force level (solid vector in Figure 9.4; range motion), while the other component will point along a line corresponding to no changes in the total force (dashed vector in Figure 9.4; self-motion).

All the mentioned optimization approaches share a common problem: They involve guessing a cost function, typically based on the available fragmented information, intuition, experience, and bias of the investigator. Relatively recently, attempts have been made to define cost functions objectively, based on experimental data distributions. Such approaches are termed *inverse optimization*. As of now, these approaches are applicable to only a limited set of systems. They are computationally very intense and/or involve complex mathematical operations.

9.3   Dynamical systems approach

Issues of terminology

There is a lot of confusion over the use of the term "dynamical system" (or "dynamic system") in biology in general and movement science in particular.

Mathematically, the dynamical system concept is formalization for any deterministic rule that describes the time dependence of a point's position in external space. So, any object that can change its location with time is, by definition, a dynamical system. Since this is true for any material object, from an elementary particle to the solar system and beyond, all of those are dynamical systems, including a brick in the wall of a house, a drop of oil on a hot skillet, a dripping faucet, and the human brain. So, the expression "the human brain is a dynamical system" is equivalent to stating that the human brain is a material object. From the subjective point of view of researchers, some of these objects are boring dynamical systems while others are exciting ones.

In movement science, commonly, only "exciting" systems are referred to as dynamical systems. In particular, systems that can potentially show loss of stability and qualitative changes in the patterns of variables that they produce are addressed as dynamical systems. Indeed, living on the edge of losing stability seems to be a common feature of many biological processes, including voluntary movements.

Stability of in-phase and out-of-phase patterns

A typical example of a dynamical system studied within the research on human movements would be two effectors such as, for example, two fingers, two limbs, or two joints. Consider a classical study by Scott Kelso and his colleagues, in which a person was asked to tap with two index fingers either synchronously (*in-phase*) or *out-of-phase* at a frequency defined by an external device, a metronome. This is a very easy task to perform. Imagine now that the frequency of the metronome is increased gradually. In the in-phase task, there were no dramatic changes in the movement pattern up to frequencies when the subject was unable to follow the metronome, and the pattern broke down completely. In the out-of-phase task, however, a more interesting pattern was observed. At a certain frequency, the two fingers showed an increase in variability of the relative phase of their taps and then they switched to the in-phase pattern (Figure 9.5). Prior to the switch, an increase in the standard deviation of the relative phase was seen. Note that this did not happen when the tapping was performed by two fingers of the same hand (for example, the index and middle fingers).

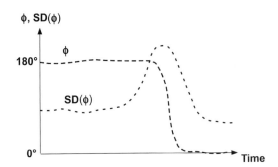

Figure 9.5 When two fingers tap out-of-phase (relative phase $\phi = 180°$), at some frequency, the pattern switches to in-phase. Prior to the switch, an increase in the standard deviation of the relative phase, $SD(\phi)$ is seen.

In natural sciences and engineering disciplines, the time evolution of dynamical systems is commonly given by a rule that allows the state of the system to be defined only a short time into the future. Such a rule is commonly expressed with a differential equation or a difference equation. To determine the state for all future times requires iterating the equation many times; this procedure is referred to as integrating the system or solving it. Once the system can be solved, given an initial state, it is possible to determine all its future states, that is, its trajectory.

Arguably, the best known equation proposed to describe effects of changes in movement frequency (and possibly other factors) on the stability of rhythmic movements is the so-called *Haken–Kelso–Bunz equation* (also known as the HKB model), which is a non-linear differential equation of motion:

$$d\phi/dt = -\sin\phi - 2k\sin2\phi, \tag{9.1}$$

where ϕ is the relative phase between movements of two effectors, and k is a parameter corresponding to the period of movement; when movement frequency increases, k decreases.

This equation is able to reproduce certain important, experimentally observed features of rhythmic movements. In particular, it suggests high stability (low variability of ϕ) of only two patterns, in-phase and out-of-phase. It shows that a drop in k (an increase in movement frequency) during an out-of-phase movement may be associated with a rather dramatic increase in variability of ϕ leading to a switch from the out-of-phase to an in-phase pattern.

Further studies have shown that stability of movement patterns depends crucially on the instruction to the subject, limb anatomical configuration, and the provided sensory feedback. For example, if a person is asked to perform a rhythmic two-joint shoulder–elbow task, flexing and extending both joints synchronously shows high stability with an increase in movement frequency (similarly to the in-phase tapping with two fingers). In contrast, a pattern when flexion of one joint is accompanied by extension of the other joint switches into the flexion–flexion, extension–extension pattern when movement frequency increases (it behaves similarly to the described out-of-phase finger tapping). However, if a subject is asked to imagine that he or she is a waiter with a horizontal tray on the palm and asked to move the imagined tray to and from the body, this movement never loses stability with an increase in its frequency, while it involves the flexion–extension, extension–flexion pattern.

Sensory information and stability of motor patterns

The importance of sensory information for phase relations between movements of two effectors was shown in experiments in which the subject could not see the moving effectors (hands) but saw motion of objects produced by hand motion. When in-phase hand motion corresponded to in-phase motion of the objects, it showed higher stability than out-of-phase motion. If frequency of motion increased, the in-phase motion remained in-phase while the out-of-phase motion could switch to the in-phase one. If now in-phase hand motion corresponded to out-of-phase object motion (and vice versa, out-of-phase hand motion produced in-phase object motion) the out-of-phase hand motion started to show higher stability as compared to the in-phase. Manipulating visual feedback even allowed movement patterns with the two effectors moving at different frequencies (with the frequencies related to each other as 2 : 3 or 3 : 5) to be turned into stable patterns. These patterns in conditions of natural visual feedback are typically very unstable.

The effects of anatomical factors can be observed, for example, when the effects of activation of muscle groups on the motion of the effector in the external space are changed by assuming a different posture in more proximal joints of the limb. This can be achieved, for example, in experiments with bilateral, rhythmic hand movements by pronating one of the hands and supinating the other hand. Such manipulations can also lead to changes in stability of motion patterns such that previously less stable patterns (such as flexion–extension/extension–flexion) become more stable than the previously more stable patterns (such as flexion–flexion/extension–extension).

Application to cyclic and discrete actions

Originally, the dynamical systems approach focused primarily on cyclic actions. A cyclic, sine-like motion of an object may be viewed as produced by a *limit cycle attractor*, a particular dynamical system that produces a cyclic trajectory, for example like the one illustrated in Figure 9.6 with solid, curved arrows. This plot shows the so-called *phase portrait* of the movement, that is, the dependence between an object's velocity (dX/dt) and coordinate (X). Setting the parameters of a limit cycle attractor allows generating a cyclic movement, which will continue until the parameters are changed. Discrete actions were viewed as fragments of a cyclic action stopped at an appropriate time. Alternatively a discrete movement may be viewed as a transition from

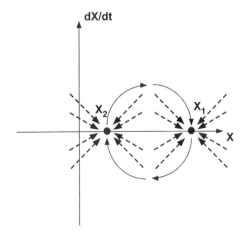

Figure 9.6 The solid curved arrows show a limit cycle trajectory on the phase plane $\{X; dX/dt\}$. The sets of dashed straight arrows show two point attractors.

one *point attractor* to another point attractor. The dashed lines in Figure 9.6 illustrate a phase portrait of two point attractors, which act to keep the system at coordinates X_1 and X_2. If a point attractor is moved to a new coordinate, the old coordinate becomes a deviation from the new one, and the system moves towards the new attractor (this description fits well with the earlier scheme of movement production by changing equilibrium points of the system and also is a trivial consequence of the definition of the "point attractor"). Further developments of this approach have led to the hypothesis that discrete and cyclic actions represent two basic types of action with distinctly different neurophysiological mechanisms and characteristics.

9.4   Synergy

The notion of "synergy" has been used in movement studies for over 100 years. In particular, Bernstein suggested that synergies represented means of alleviating the problem of motor redundancy by uniting *elemental variables* (those produced by elements of the system) into groups and then using one control variable per group. This general view implies under *synergy* something like "a group of variables that change synchronously." This definition of synergy has received experimental support in numerous recent studies that searched for groups of peripheral variables (such as joint displacements, muscle forces, or indices of muscle activation) that scaled linearly in the process of a movement or across movement repetitions with different parameters. Commonly, such groups of elemental variables were identified with methods of linear algebra (*matrix factorization methods*) such as *principle component analysis*, *factor analysis*, and *non-negative matrix factorization*. All these methods look for a smaller set of higher order variables that represent combinations of the original elemental variables and account for a substantial amount of variance in the original set. Quite commonly, a small set of such higher order variables (addressed as "synergies" or "modes" in different studies) was able to account for very large amounts of variance in the original data set.

However, reducing the number of variables with such methods is typically unable to eliminate motor redundancy completely. So, the controller is still facing the problem of selecting specific solutions from very large (infinite) sets of possibilities. Two approaches have been suggested to this problem. One of them assumes that a neural controller always selects a single solution, possibly based on an *optimization* criterion (see Section 9.2). The other one assumes that no single solution is ever selected, while families of solutions are allowed that are all equally able to solve the problem (perform the motor task). The latter approach is sometimes addressed as the *principle of abundance* since it views motor redundancy not as a source of compu-tational problems but as a rich (abundant) apparatus that allows the accuracy of performance to be combined with its stability (low variance across trials and/or relatively small effects of external perturbations) and flexibility (ability to switch to a different solution if task conditions change). For example, the opportunity to select different solutions from a family may be very helpful if one has to deal with changes in the environment (perturbations) or wants to perform another task at the same time.

Consider the earlier example of walking along holding a mug of hot coffee (Section 4.3). The mug has to be kept close to vertical to avoid spilling the contents. The kinematic redundancy of the arm offers an infinite number of joint configurations able to keep the mug vertical. Imagine now that you come to a closed door and have to press on the handle to open it. If the other hand is busy, a solution may be to press on the door handle with the elbow of the arm with the mug. If only one, optimal configuration were selected for the former task of keeping the mug vertical, the pressing action would lead to spilling the contents of the mug. So, the previous solution would have to be abandoned, and the problem of keeping the mug vertical would have to be solved many times (for the required sequence of elbow coordinates). If, in accordance with the principle of abundance, a family of solutions is selected, that is, a sub-space in the joint angle space within which the mug is always vertical, the task can be performed easily by moving across the sub-space in a direction corresponding to the required elbow motion.

Similarly, if the arm with the mug unexpectedly bumps into an external object, having a single solution would be disastrous. In contrast, having a family of solutions at one's disposal potentially allows channeling the mechanical effects of such a perturbation into a joint angle sub-space compatible with the task of keeping the mug vertical.

This last example links rather directly the principle of abundance with such important characteristics of human movements as their variability and stability. Human movements are always reasonably sloppy. This means that they combine variability in important performance variables (errors) with flexibility of motor patterns, that is, an ability to adjust to unexpected complicating factors such as changes in external forces, sensory signals, targets, etc.

Definition of synergy

The principle of abundance has allowed synergy to be defined as a neural organization that provides for low variability (high stability) of an important *performance variable* by co-varied adjustments of *elemental variables*. Such co-varied adjustments can be observed in response to a perturbation (external or internal) or across trials, as results of natural variability of the numerous elements involved in the production of any voluntary movement. This definition has several important features. First, to speak about synergies, one has to define a level of analysis (elemental variables). Second, synergies are always related to a potentially important feature of performance, they always do something. Third, synergies are linked to the mentioned universal features of movements, such as their variability and stability.

The earlier definition and the current one address two aspects of behavior of redundant systems—*sharing* and *co-variation*. The former reflects average across repetitive attempts contribution of elemental variables, while the latter deals with across-trials variability of elemental variables about this average pattern.

The uncontrolled manifold hypothesis

A computational method to identify and quantify synergies has been developed within the framework of the *uncontrolled manifold* (UCM) hypothesis. This hypothesis assumes that a neural controller acts in a space of elemental variables, forms in that space a sub-space (UCM) corresponding to a desired value of an important performance variable, and then acts to limit variability of the elemental variables to that sub-space.

Consider a simple example of producing a constant output (E_{TOT}) with two elements (E_1 and E_2), for example pressing with two hands on two force sensors with the task to produce a certain total force level (Figure 9.7). The task may be formulated as $E_1 + E_2 = E_{TOT}$. This is a typical problem of motor redundancy. This equation with two unknowns has an infinite number of solutions. All the solutions to this equation form a line, a one-dimensional sub-space in the two-dimensional space of elemental variables (the dashed line in Figure 9.7). As long as the values of the elemental variables belong to that line, the task is performed perfectly, and the controller does not have to interfere (assuming that there are no other tasks or constraints). This line is an example of the UCM for this particular task. That is why the term "uncontrolled manifold" has been introduced: It implies a sub-space, within which the controller does not have to interfere with the values of the elemental variables. In contrast, if the two elemental variables deviate from the UCM (along the slanted solid line in Figure 9.7), the task is violated, and the controller has to interfere to introduce a correction.

Good and bad variance

The UCM framework offers a method of quantifying synergies by comparing the amounts of variance within the UCM (that does not affect the performance variable) and orthogonal to it (that does). Such quantitative analyses use methods of linear algebra. They approximate the UCM with a linear space, which is the null-space of the Jacobian (remember, the Jacobian is a matrix that shows how very small changes in the elemental variables affect the performance variable). Within the null-space, changes in the performance variable are nil by definition. Variance within this space is sometimes called "good variance," since it allows the system to be flexible without

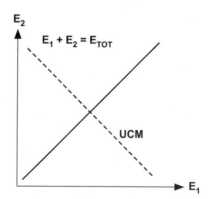

Figure 9.7 Consider a redundant task: $E_1 + E_2 = E_{TOT}$. All the solutions form a line (the dashed line), the uncontrolled manifold (UCM) for this task. Deviations from the UCM (for example along the solid line) lead to errors in performance.

violating the task, while variance orthogonal to this space is called "bad variance" because it introduces errors into performance. Both have to be quantified per dimension in each of the sub-spaces to be compared quantitatively. If "good" variance is significantly larger than the "bad" one, a conclusion can be drawn that the data reflect a synergy stabilizing that performance variable. Note that variance within the null-space is indeed "good," not irrelevant, because it allows the controller to use the same set of elements to perform other tasks and respond to perturbations as in the earlier example of walking with the mug of hot coffee.

One of the major advantages of the computational approach offered by the UCM hypothesis is the ability to analyze one and the same data set with respect to different performance variables. Different performance variables will correspond to different Jacobians and different UCMs within the space of elemental variables. Consequently, the relative amounts of "good" and "bad" variance are likely to differ. The method allows a string of questions to be asked to a data set: Is the set reflecting a synergy stabilizing performance variable PV_1? Is it reflecting a synergy stabilizing performance variable PV_2? And so on.

For example, consider the task of pressing with two fingers. Imagine that a subject performed the task many times, the forces of the two fingers were measured and plotted as points on the force–force plane (Figure 9.8). Two such clouds of data points are illustrated in Figure 9.8 with ellipses. The first cloud of data points (Figure 9.8A) is elongated approximately along the UCM for the total force (UCM_F). Analysis of these data will show significantly more "good" variance than "bad" variance, which can be interpreted as a two-finger synergy stabilizing total force. The second cloud (Figure 9.8B) is oriented orthogonally to the first one. Analysis of the second cloud with respect to the UCM_F will show that "good" variance is smaller than the "bad" one; so, there is no force stabilizing synergy. However, the same data can be analyzed with respect to another performance variable, the total moment of force with respect to a pivot in-between the two fingers. The data are elongated along that UCM (UCM_M), and a conclusion can be drawn that the data reflect a synergy stabilizing the total moment of force.

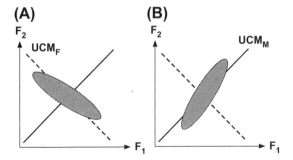

Figure 9.8 Examples of two clouds of data points in the task of pressing with two fingers. (A) The cloud is elongated mostly along the UCM for total force (UCM_F). (B) There is no force stabilizing synergy but the cloud of data points can be interpreted as a moment stabilizing synergy since it is elongated primarily along the UCM for total moment of force (UCM_M).

Synergies within a hierarchical system

Both the definition of a synergy and the UCM hypothesis assume a hierarchically organized control system with at least two levels. The upper level provides an input that specifies a desired value or a desired time profile of an important performance variable. The lower level distributes this input among a redundant set of elemental variables in such a way that the elemental variables are allowed to show high variability as long as their combined outcome produces the desired value of the performance variable. Figure 9.9 shows a hierarchy of such synergies that may be involved in tasks that require coordination of limbs, joints, and muscles.

As illustrated in Figure 9.9, elemental variables at one level of analysis may represent performance variables stabilized by synergies at another level. For example, individual joint rotations may be viewed as elemental variables for analysis of multi-joint kinematics during hand reaching or pointing movements. At a different level, individual joint rotations may be viewed as performance variables stabilized by a synergic organization of muscle forces (or activation patterns). At still another level, activation of a single muscle may be viewed as a performance variable stabilized by a synergy that uses firing patterns of individual motor units as elements. This example suggests that each voluntary movement may be viewed as built on a hierarchy of

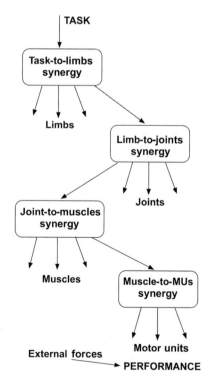

Figure 9.9 An illustration of a hierarchy of synergies. MU, motor unit.

synergies, within which outputs of higher hierarchical levels serve as inputs into lower hierarchical levels.

The two definitions of synergy, "variables that change together" and "co-variation that stabilizes performance," differ significantly. For example, if one places different weights on the top of a table and measures forces under the four legs, the four forces would change in parallel with the weight and, hence, qualify as a synergy according to the first definition, but not necessarily according to the second one. If a table is a synergy of its legs, any material object is a synergy of its parts. It is up to individual researchers to decide whether such a broad definition of synergy is useful.

9.5   Perception–action interactions

Interactions between motor and sensory processes are bi-directional. The importance of sensory information for motor control has been known for many years. Several infectious and metabolic disorders lead to problems with the transmission of sensory information to the central nervous system. In particular, before the invention of antibiotics, one of the common consequences of advanced syphilis was degeneration of the conduction pathways in the dorsal columns of the spinal cord (tabes dorsalis). These pathways carry information from proprioceptors in the lower body to the brain. In the absence of this information, patients showed significant balance problems even while standing with their eyes open, and could not stand at all with eyes closed. A common metabolic disorder leading to problems with sensory information transmission from distal parts of the body is diabetes. Although by itself diabetes is a metabolic, not a neurological disorder, its consequences can include a loss of sensory signals from the feet and lower legs. Such patients show impaired balance with eyes closed, although other sources of information, such as vision and even light finger touch, help improve stability of standing.

Movements in deafferented persons

There is a very rare disorder of the peripheral nervous system called large-fiber peripheral neuropathy (see Section 4.6). This disorder leads to disrupted conduction of action potentials along thick sensory fibers while conduction along motor fibers is unaffected. As a result, these patients do not show a significant loss in the ability to produce muscle force while they have a nearly complete lack of sensation in the affected areas. Such patients are sometimes imprecisely referred to as "deafferented." They show significant motor coordination problems over a variety of motor tasks including standing, walking, multi-joint arm movements, etc. For example, when a healthy person performs a multi-joint arm movement imitating cutting a loaf of bread, the knife follows a nearly straight trajectory. When a patient with large-fiber peripheral neuropathy tries to perform such a movement, the knife moves over a large arc and shows significantly different trajectories when moving towards the body and from the body (see Figure 4.10 in Section 4.6). These observations point at an important role of information from proprioceptors for multi-joint coordination.

Efferent copy and principle of reafference revisited

There are also effects of motor action on perception. Arguably, the first such effect was described by the famous German physicist and physician Hermann von Helmholtz (1821–1894). If a person closes one eye and moves the other eye, projection of the environment moves over the retina and produces an adequate perception of eye movement in the motionless environment. If the same person moves the eye by pressing on it with a finger, also producing motion of the projection of the environment over the retina, a strong illusion of a moving environment is typically perceived. The general idea that motor commands play a major role in perception was developed by von Holst who suggested that when the brain produces a motor command to an effector, a copy of this command, called the *efferent copy* (sometimes *efference copy*), plays a direct role in perception of motion of the effector.

The traditional view on the notion of the efferent copy is that it contains signals that are copies of the signals sent by alpha-motoneurons to the muscles. Von Holst used this idea to solve the famous posture–movement paradox described in an earlier section (see Section 4.2). He introduced a *principle of reafference* (Figure 9.10), according to which a copy of the command to muscles (efferent copy) is compared to changes in the afferent signals induced by movement (reafference), and the difference between the two is used to correct the command to muscles. This scheme, however, cannot explain how a person can relax at different joint positions. Indeed, all the muscles crossing a joint can be relaxed at a variety of joint positions (efferent copy of the commands to the muscles is the same), while afferent signals have to be different, in particular due to the position-dependent signals from muscle spindle sensory endings. The scheme in Figure 9.10 suggests that there will be a non-zero difference in the two signals, (EC−RA), and the process of muscle relaxation will have to be accompanied by joint motion to a new position.

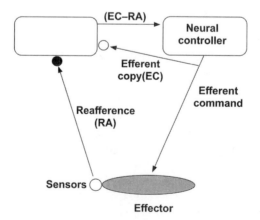

Figure 9.10 The principle of reafference of von Holst. A copy of the command to muscles (efferent copy) is compared to changes in the afferent signals induced by movement (reafference), and the difference between the two is used to correct the command to muscles.

Efferent copy within the EP hypothesis

An alternative view on efferent copy is compatible with the equilibrium-point hypothesis on motor control. Consider muscle states as points on a force–length plane (for simplicity, let us consider only steady-states). According to the equilibrium-point hypothesis, selecting a motor command to a muscle is associated with setting a value of the threshold of the tonic stretch reflex (λ). This results in a curve on the force–length plane, that is, a characteristic of the tonic stretch reflex for the muscle (Figure 9.11). Depending on external load, the muscle can be anywhere on that curve (at a steady-state!), but it cannot be anywhere else on the plane. This means that when a person sends a control signal to a muscle, this by itself already solves a big part of the problem of perception because only points on the tonic stretch reflex characteristic are allowed as steady-states (filled circles in Figure 9.11), while points off the curve are impossible (empty circles). In other words, selecting a value of λ links possible values of muscle length and force and reduces the problem of identifying a point in the two-dimensional space to a problem of finding a point along a one-dimensional line. Within this scheme, the efferent copy (a copy of λ used for perception purposes) has the physical meaning of a relation between muscle force and length.

Signals from peripheral receptors are necessary to define a point on that line. If one moves along a tonic stretch reflex characteristic from its threshold value to longer muscle length values (Figure 9.12), the activity of all major proprioceptive signals increases. This is because of an increase in both muscle length and muscle force. In addition, muscle activation level also increases along the curve and, given the well-known phenomenon of *alpha–gamma coactivation* (see Section 7.2), the level of activity of gamma-motoneurons also goes up. To summarize, all signals from major peripheral receptors show changes in the same direction along the tonic stretch reflex characteristic. Hence, such a set of signals becomes redundant (or rather abundant) and may be organized into a sensory synergy, stabilizing a point on the tonic stretch reflex characteristic that corresponds to the muscle's state. The abundance of signals from sensory receptors

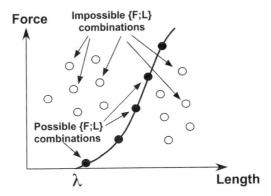

Figure 9.11 Defining a command to a muscle (a value of λ) helps solve the problem of perception because it limits solutions to points that are on the tonic stretch reflex characteristics (black points). The open circles are impossible force–length combinations.

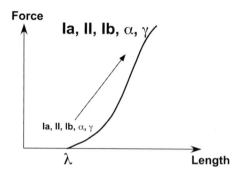

Figure 9.12 Activity of all major sensory receptors increases along the tonic stretch reflex characteristic in parallel with the activity levels of α- and γ-motoneurons.

allows stable, adequate perception to be expected even when one of the sources generates unreliable signals, for example as a result of an injury or inflammation.

This expectation is not always supported by facts. For example, application of low-amplitude (under 1 mm), high-frequency (over 50 Hz) vibration to a muscle may produce strong *kinesthetic illusions*. The direction of such an illusory motion is typically compatible with an increase in the length of the muscle subjected to vibration. Sometimes, even anatomically impossible joint positions may be perceived. If a muscle is involved in a complex task, vibration of the muscle may lead to major adjustments in the activation of other muscles. For example, if vibration is applied to the triceps surae muscle group while the person is standing with eyes closed, a major deviation of the body backwards is commonly observed—a *vibration-induced falling* (VIF). Such illusions and reactions have been interpreted as resulting from the vibration-induced extremely high level of activity of the primary muscle spindle endings that can be driven by vibration (this expression means that they generate action potentials in response to each vibration cycle).

These observations suggest that the central nervous system may fail to create an adequate perception of joint/body position if one of the sources of sensory information generates signals that are beyond the physiological range. Note that, in all the studies with vibration of a muscle, other sources of sensory information about the state of a joint crossed by the muscle produced veridical sensory information, which should have helped the central nervous system overcome the illusory perception. Interpretation of the effects of vibration on perception is complicated by motor effects of the vibration (it produces tonic muscle contraction, the *tonic vibration reflex*) and also its possible effects on the efferent copy.

9.6   Perception–action coupling

Ecological psychology

James Gibson (1904–1979) is commonly considered the father of an area called *ecological psychology*. In particular, Gibson introduced the notion of *direct perception*, suggesting that sensory signals could be coupled to motor commands directly without first using these signals to update the picture of the world and one's own body. This statement is trivial for spinal reflexes, but more complex, voluntary actions have been traditionally viewed as mediated by some kind of complex sensory information processing in the brain, resulting in computed *motor commands.*

The idea of action–perception coupling (without a stage of neural computation) has been developed by the group of the British–American psychologist Michael Turvey, who combined the idea of direct perception with the *dynamical systems* approach to motor control. Studies of this group focused mostly on patterns of natural coordination during simultaneous motion of two effectors when, typically, no other instruction was given to the subjects beyond "move naturally." As in many other studies within the dynamical systems field, stabilization of the relative phase has been shown under such an instruction. However, the exact phase value being stabilized was found to depend on the physical properties of the moving effectors. Those were manipulated, in particular, by changing the mechanical properties of the two effectors, for example by modifying the natural frequencies of the two pendulums swung by the two hands of a person. The importance of sensory information for creating a stable phase relation between two trajectories has been demonstrated by studies of pairs of persons who looked at each other while swinging pendulums. Phase stabilization was observed in this case as well, even though the brains of the two participants could not share any information and were linked by vision only.

Other studies of perception–action coupling focused on the effects of manipulating a particular sensory input on a movement pattern. It has been shown, in particular, that natural postural sway (which typically looks like a noisy process without a clear pattern; see Section 11.1) can be entrained by a visual stimulus, for example a picture of dots projected on the screen in front of the standing subject that oscillates back-and-forth. Postural sway can also be entrained by cyclic sensory stimuli of another modality, for example when a person stands, lightly touches a touch-pad, and the pad starts to move rhythmically in a horizontal direction. Hence, both voluntary and involuntary movements show natural coupling to sensory signals. Taken together, these studies have demonstrated that movement adjustments can occur even when the participant is unaware of changes in the conditions and tries to perform "the same action" naturally.

Phenomena of perception–action coupling are not limited to movements of two effectors performed by a person or by two persons who look at each other. They can also be seen when a person performs a rhythmic movement while looking at a computer-generated image of a movement with parameters coupled to the corresponding parameters of his or her own movement.

Self-test questions

1. Suggest examples for the problem of motor redundancy at different levels of movement analysis.
2. Formulate the principle of abundance.

3. What is a cost function? Present examples of typical cost functions in movement studies.
4. Explain what bang–bang control is.
5. Define jerk.
6. What is minimized within the minimum-jerk criterion?
7. For what systems do minimum-jerk and minimum-torque-change criteria produce identical results?
8. Define the principle of minimization of secondary moments.
9. What is minimum norm?
10. Define range–space motion and self-motion.
11. What is a dynamical system?
12. What happens when a person performs out-of-phase tapping with the two index fingers and then increases the tapping frequency?
13. Suggest an explanation of why people switch to in-phase tapping (from out-of-phase) but not to hopping (from walking) with frequency increase.
14. What results of the tapping experiments can be accounted for by the Haken–Kelso–Bunz model?
15. Present examples of the importance of sensory information for stability of coordination patterns.
16. How are discrete and cyclic actions viewed within the dynamical systems approach?
17. Present two definitions for "synergy" commonly used in movement studies.
18. Define the uncontrolled manifold?
19. What is "good variance"?
20. What does a statement "the four fingers form a synergy" mean?
21. What observations on patients prove the importance of sensory information for motor coordination?
22. What motor deficits are observed in persons with large-fiber peripheral neuropathy?
23. Formulate the reafference principle as suggested by von Holst.
24. Interpret the notion of efferent copy within the equilibrium-point hypothesis.
25. How does selecting a motor command help perception within the equilibrium-point hypothesis?
26. What are the typical effects of muscle vibration on perception?
27. Explain the notion of direct perception.
28. Suggest examples of perception–action coupling.

Essential references and recommended further readings

Berkinblit, M. B., Feldman, A. G., & Fukson, O. I. (1986). Adaptability of innate motor patterns and motor control mechanisms. *Behavioral and Brain Science, 9,* 585–638.

Bernstein, N. A. (1967). *The co-ordination and regulation of movements.* Oxford: Pergamon Press.

Bizzi, E., Giszter, S. F., Loeb, E., Mussa-Ivaldi, F. A., & Saltiel, P. (1995). Modular organization of motor behavior in the frog's spinal cord. *Trends in Neuroscience, 18,* 442–446.

Crowninshield, R. D., & Brand, R. A. (1981). A physiologically based criterion of muscle force prediction in locomotion. *Journal of Biomechanics, 14,* 793–801.

Danion, F., Schöner, G., Latash, M. L., Li, S., Scholz, J. P., & Zatsiorsky, V. M. (2003). A force mode hypothesis for finger interaction during multi-finger force production tasks. *Biological Cybernetics, 88,* 91–98.

d'Avella, A., Saltiel, P., & Bizzi, E. (2003). Combinations of muscle synergies in the construction of a natural motor behavior. *Nature Neuroscience, 6*, 300–308.

Feldman, A. G., & Latash, M. L. (1982). Afferent and efferent components of joint position sense: Interpretation of kinaesthetic illusions. *Biological Cybernetics, 42*, 205–214.

Flash, T., & Hogan, N. (1985). The coordination of arm movements: An experimentally confirmed mathematical model. *Journal of Neuroscience, 5*, 1688–1703.

Fukson, O. I., Berkinblit, M. B., & Feldman, A. G. (1980). The spinal frog takes into account the scheme of its body during the wiping reflex. *Science, 209*, 1261–1263.

Gelfand, I. M., & Latash, M. L. (1998). On the problem of adequate language in movement science. *Motor Control, 2*, 306–313.

Gelfand, I. M., & Tsetlin, M. L. (1971). On mathematical modeling of the mechanisms of the central nervous system. In I. M. Gelfand, V. S. Gurfinkel, S. V. Fomin, & M. L. Tsetlin (Eds.), *Models of the structural–functional organization of certain biological systems* (pp. 9–26). Cambridge, MA: MIT Press.

Gibson, J. J. (1979). *The ecological approach to visual perception.* Boston, MA: Houghton Mifflin.

Gorniak, S., Zatsiorsky, V. M., & Latash, M. L. (2007). Hierarchies of synergies: An example of the two-hand, multi-finger tasks. *Experimental Brain Research, 179*, 167–180.

Haken, H., Kelso, J. A. S., & Bunz, H. (1985). A theoretical model of phase transitions in human hand movements. *Biological Cybernetics, 51*, 347–356.

Hogan, N. (1984). An organizational principle for a class of voluntary movements. *Journal of Neuroscience, 4*, 2745–2754.

Ivanenko, Y. P., Poppele, R. E., & Lacquaniti, F. (2004). Five basic muscle activation patterns account for muscle activity during human locomotion. *Journal of Physiology, 556*, 267–282.

Kang, N., Shinohara, M., Zatsiorsky, V. M., & Latash, M. L. (2004). Learning multi-finger synergies: An uncontrolled manifold analysis. *Experimental Brain Research, 157*, 336–350.

Kelso, J. A. S. (1995). *Dynamic patterns: The self-organization of brain and behavior.* Cambridge, MA: MIT Press.

Koshland, G. F., Gerilovsky, L., & Hasan, Z. (1991). Activity of wrist muscles elicited during imposed or voluntary movements about the elbow joint. *Journal of Motor Behavior, 23*, 91–100.

Krishnamoorthy, V., Latash, M. L., Scholz, J. P., & Zatsiorsky, V. M. (2003). Muscle synergies during shifts of the center of pressure by standing persons. *Experimental Brain Research, 152*, 281–292.

Kugler, P. N., & Turvey, M. T. (1987). *Information, natural law, and the self-assembly of rhythmic movement.* Hillsdale, NJ: Erlbaum.

Latash, M. L., Aruin, A. S., & Shapiro, M. B. (1995). The relation between posture and movement: A study of a simple synergy in a two-joint task. *Human Movement Science, 14*, 79–107.

Latash, M. L., Scholz, J. P., & Schöner, G. (2002). Motor control strategies revealed in the structure of motor variability. *Exercise and Sport Science Reviews, 30*, 26–31.

Latash, M. L., Shim, J. K., Smilga, A. V., & Zatsiorsky, V. (2005). A central back-coupling hypothesis on the organization of motor synergies: a physical metaphor and a neural model. *Biological Cybernetics, 92*, 186–191.

Latash, M. L., Scholz, J. P., & Schöner, G. (2007). Toward a new theory of motor synergies. *Motor Control, 11*, 276–308.

Müller, H., & Sternad, D. (2004). Decomposition of variability in the execution of goal-oriented tasks: Three components of skill improvement. *Journal of Experimental Psychology: Human Perception and Performance, 30*, 212–233.

Nelson, W. (1983). Physical principles for economies of skilled movements. *Biological Cybernetics, 46*, 135–147.

Prilutsky, B. I. (2000). Coordination of two- and one-joint muscles: Functional consequences and implications for motor control. *Motor Control, 4*, 1–44.

Rosenbaum, D. A., Engelbrecht, S. E., Busje, M. M., & Loukopoulos, L. D. (1993). Knowledge model for selecting and producing reaching movements. *Journal of Motor Behavior, 25*, 217–227.

Saltzman, E. L., & Kelso, J. A. S. (1987). Skilled actions: A task-dynamic approach. *Psychological Reviews, 94*, 84–106.

Santello, M., & Soechting, J. F. (2000). Force synergies for multifingered grasping. *Experimental Brain Research, 133*, 457–467.

Scholz, J. P., & Schöner, G. (1999). The uncontrolled manifold concept: Identifying control variables for a functional task. *Experimental Brain Research, 126*, 289–306.

Scholz, J. P., Schöner, G., & Latash, M. L. (2000). Identifying the control structure of multijoint coordination during pistol shooting. *Experimental Brain Research, 135*, 382–404.

Schöner, G. (1990). A dynamic theory of coordination of discrete movement. *Biological Cybernetics, 63*, 257–270.

Schöner, G. (1995). Recent developments and problems in human movement science and their conceptual implications. *Ecological Psychology, 8*, 291–314.

Schöner, G. (2002). Timing, clocks, and dynamical systems. *Brain and Cognition, 48*, 31–51.

Ting, L. H., & Macpherson, J. M. (2005). A limited set of muscle synergies for force control during a postural task. *Journal of Neurophysiology, 93*, 609–613.

Turvey, M. T. (1990). Coordination. *American Psychologist, 45*, 938–953.

Uno, Y., Kawato, M., & Suzuki, R. (1989). Formation and control of optimal trajectory in human multijoint arm movement. *Biological Cybernetics, 61*, 89–101.

Van Deursen, R. W., & Simoneau, G. G. (1999). Foot and ankle sensory neuropathy, proprioception, and postural stability. *Journal of Orthopedics, Sports, and Physical Therapy, 29*, 718–726.

Von Holst, E. (1954). Relation between the central nervous system and the peripheral organs. *British Journal of Animal Behaviour, 2*, 89–94.

10 Neurophysiological structures

Chapter Outline

Fundamentals of Motor Control. DOI: 10.1016/B978-0-12-415956-3.00010-5

10.1   The spinal cord

As far as movements are concerned, the spinal cord is an essential part of the central nervous system. It ensures transmission of signals from peripheral receptors to the brain and also from the brain to output elements, motoneurons that send action potentials to muscles. The spinal cord also houses the neuronal machinery that ensures the functioning of a variety of muscle reflexes. Besides, the spinal cord can control certain rather complex actions that play an important role in the everyday motor repertoire. The importance of the spinal cord for motor function is reflected in the severe motor pathologies that follow spinal cord injury.

Anatomy of the spinal cord

The spinal cord is an elongated structure that joins the *medulla* at its rostral end and spreads until the lumbar vertebrae. At all levels, the anatomical structure of the spinal cord is relatively standard (Figure 10.1A): There is a butterfly-like gray area in the center that contains the bodies of the neurons and some of the shorter fibers. The *gray matter* is surrounded by the *white matter* consisting of long neural fibers (axons) that carry information both up to more rostral (closer to the head) parts of the central nervous system and down to more caudal (closer to the "tail") areas of the spinal cord.

The spinal cord can be viewed as consisting of *segments*—8 cervical segments, 12 thoracic segments, 5 lumbar segments, and 5 sacral segments (Figure 10.1B). Each segment receives sensory information from a particular area of the body; this information is delivered through the *dorsal* (closer to the back) *roots* via the axons of the sensory neurons (Figure 10.1C). The bodies of the sensory neurons are located outside the spinal cord, in the *spinal ganglia*. Each segment innervates muscles in an area of the body, which is more or less the same as the one from which this segment receives sensory information. The axons of the motoneurons exit the spinal cord via the *ventral* (closer to the stomach) *roots*. The segmental structure of the spinal cord is commonly illustrated using pictures of the body with zebra-looking stripes.

The pairs of dorsal and ventral roots enter the spinal cord through the gaps between adjacent vertebrae. The spinal cord segments, however, do not match the vertebrae one-to-one. This is particularly pronounced at the lower thoracic–upper lumbar level, where the *lumbar enlargement* houses many lumbar and sacral segments within a relatively small anatomical space (Figure 10.1B). As a result, the lower portion of the spine contains no spinal cord, only the dorsal and ventral roots from the accumulated segments. This part is called *cauda equina* (horse tail) because of the resemblance of the strings of roots to the tail of a horse.

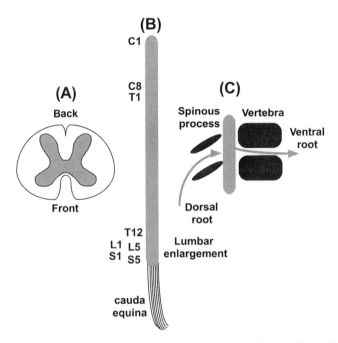

Figure 10.1 (A) At all anatomical levels, the cross-section of the spinal cord looks like a butterfly with the gray matter in the middle surrounded by white matter. (B) There are eight cervical segments (C1–C8), twelve thoracic segments (T1–T12), five lumbar segments (L1–L5), and five sacral segments (S1–S5). Segments T12–S5 are packed within a relatively small space called the lumbar enlargement. Below the lumbar enlargement there is no spinal cord, only dorsal and ventral roots that form the cauda equina. Dorsal roots enter the spinal canal in-between adjacent spinous processes, while ventral roots exit the spinal canal in-between adjacent vertebrae.

The output elements of the spinal cord, the *motoneurons*, are located mostly in the ventral area of the gray matter (Figure 10.2). Larger motoneurons (*alpha-motoneurons*) send their axons to muscles and induce muscle fiber contractions leading to tendon force production and movements. Smaller motoneurons (*gamma-motoneurons*) send their axons to muscle fibers within special sensory organs called muscle spindles. The activity of gamma-motoneurons, by itself, does not induce movements or tendon force production; it modulates the sensitivity of sensory endings in muscle spindles to muscle length and velocity. Alpha-motoneurons have been viewed as the point of convergence of all movement-related neural signals; the renowned British neurophysiologist Sir Charles Sherrington called them "the final common path" of the motor control processes.

Most neurons within the spinal cord are *interneurons*. They receive signals from and send their axons to other neurons. Only a handful of interneurons have been described in sufficient detail meaning that the main sources of their input signals and their primary target neurons are known. Much of the spinal cord neuronal machinery is described as a "black-box," using input–output characteristics.

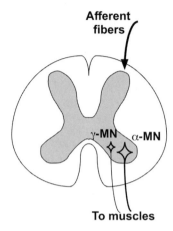

Figure 10.2 Afferent (sensory) fibers enter the spinal cord from the back. Motoneurons (MN) (both α- and γ-) are located close to the ventral horns.

Functional role of reflexes

The argument about the role of spinal reflexes in the control of natural movements is very old. Sir Charles Sherrington viewed movements as results of modulation of muscle reflexes. Another great physiologist of the late nineteenth and early twentieth century, Ivan Pavlov used a broader definition of reflexes and considered all animal (and human) actions as combinations of *inborn* and acquired (*conditioned*) *reflexes*. Their opponents, including such famous scientists as Graham Brown and Nikolai Bernstein, claimed that the central nervous system was not a reactive but an active system, and movements were initiated by neuronal structures within the central nervous system, not caused by sensory stimuli. Some of these hypothetical structures have been termed *central pattern generators*. Recently, the argument about the relative role of central and reflex processes in movement production has been raised to a new level of sophistication: Researchers developing the *dynamical systems* approach have emphasized the coupling between sensory and motor variables (see perception–action coupling approaches, Sections 9.3 and 9.6), that is, reactive nature of movements. In contrast, champions of the *motor programming* and *internal model* approaches (Sections 5.1 and 5.3) emphasize computational processes within the central nervous system resulting in movements.

Some of the better known reflexes have been described in Section 2.4. There is an ongoing argument whether spinal reflexes play a functional role in natural movements. Let us look at a couple of observations relevant to this argument and supporting the point of view that spinal reflexes do contribute to the movement control (some of the observations have been mentioned earlier).

1. Imagine that you ask a person to press as hard as possible with the hand against a stop such that the activity of biceps brachii is close to maximal (see Figure 6.2 in Section 6.1). Now imagine that the stop has been unexpectedly removed. The arm will show a quick flexion motion while

the activation level of biceps will drop to zero for some time. This disappearance of muscle activity is called the *unloading reflex*. Its time delay is very short, suggesting its reflex, likely spinal, origin. This observation suggests that reflex effects are anything but small: They can lead to transient disappearance of the maximal voluntary muscle activation level.

2. Consider a person after a spinal cord injury that led to a complete transection of the spinal cord at an upper thoracic level. Such patients commonly display a pathological state called *spasticity* (described in more detail later). It is characterized by increased resistance of joints to externally imposed motion, increased reflex responses to muscle stretch (particularly to a quick stretch), and muscle spasms that can be induced by a variety of stimuli, even by a simple touch. These reflex responses are seen in the absence of voluntary movements since all the descending pathways have been interrupted. The phenomenon of spasticity suggests that reflexes are indeed very powerful and require signals from the brain structures to be kept under control.

Reciprocal inhibition

One of the best-known reflex loops is *reciprocal inhibition* (described in Section 3.4). This mechanism plays a clear functional role. Imagine that you perform a voluntary movement of a joint, for example flexion. The extensor muscle (the antagonist) is going to be stretched and, because of the length and velocity sensitivity of the muscle spindles, the extensor will show an increase in its activation, thus resisting the movement. Sherrington suggested that the mechanism of reciprocal inhibition allowed scaling down the antagonist resistance, thus allowing movements to be performed more efficiently (Figure 10.3). There are descending pathways from the brain to the interneurons (*Ia-interneurons*) that mediate the reciprocal inhibition loop. These pathways may be used to scale the gain of reciprocal inhibition, thus varying the natural resistance of the antagonist muscle.

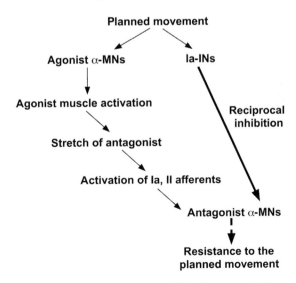

Figure 10.3 Central control of Ia-interneurons (Ia-INs) allows use of the mechanism of reciprocal inhibition to reduce resistance of antagonist muscles. MN, motoneuron.

Recurrent inhibition

There is a feedback loop within the spinal cord that plays an important role in defining characteristics of recruitment of alpha-motoneurons. This loop involves small neurons located in the ventral horns of the spinal cord called *Renshaw cells* (Figure 10.4). Renshaw cells are inhibitory interneurons. They project back to the alpha-motoneurons of the same pool. They also make inhibitory projections to alpha-motoneurons of synergistic muscles and to gamma-motoneurons, innervating the muscle. Renshaw cells may be viewed as components of a system that unites alpha-motoneurons of a pool into a *synergy* stabilizing output of the pool (see Section 9.4).

Imagine that alpha-motoneurons of a pool produce a certain level of muscle activation. Now imagine that one of the activated motoneurons for an unknown reason stops generating action potentials (Figure 10.5). The Renshaw cell that was activated by that motoneuron will lose its major excitatory input and stop firing. As a result, its target motoneurons will receive less inhibition and may be expected to increase their firing frequency. If a motoneuron was not active, removing part of the inhibitory input may bring its membrane to the threshold for action potential generation. Overall, turning a Renshaw cell off will increase the overall level of activation of the pool, which will (partly) compensate for the lack of contribution from the motoneuron that stopped producing action potentials.

H-reflex, flexor reflex, and crossed extensor reflex

Muscle spindles house two kinds of sensory endings—*primary* and *secondary*. The primary endings are sensitive to muscle length and velocity. They are innervated by very large, fast-conducting (up to 100–120 m/s) myelinated axons, called *Ia-afferents*, which produce a variety of reflex effects. These involve the monosynaptic reflex excitation of alpha-motoneurons innervating the muscle that houses the spindle (H-reflex and T-reflex, described in Section 3.4), the abovementioned reciprocal inhibitory reflex effects, and the polysynaptic tonic stretch reflex (Sections 4.1 and 8.3). The *secondary endings* are sensitive to muscle length only; they are innervated by

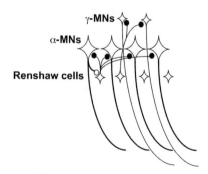

Figure 10.4 Recurrent inhibition. Renshaw cells are small interneurons that receive excitatory projections from alpha-motoneurons (α-MNs) and inhibit the motoneurons of the same pool as well as gamma-motoneurons (γ-MNs).

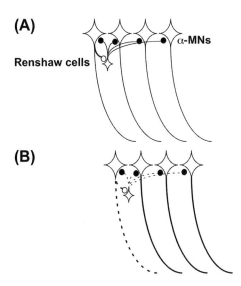

Figure 10.5 The Renshaw cell system may be viewed as stabilizing the output of a moto-neuronal pool. If an alpha-motoneuron (α-MN) stops firing, the Renshaw cell it used to excite (A) stops firing as well. Its inhibition of other neurons of the pool is removed, and the pool, as a whole, increases its activity, (partly) compensating for the lack of activity from the α-MN that stopped producing action potentials (B).

thinner myelinated fibers with a slower conduction velocity (about 30 m/s). They are part of the *flexor reflex afferents* (FRA) group that produces excitatory effects on flexor muscles (*flexor reflex*) and inhibitory effects on extensor muscles within the same extremity. These afferents also show opposite effects on muscles of the contralateral extremity: Their projections excite extensor alpha-motoneurons (*crossed extensor reflex*) and inhibit flexor alpha-motoneurons within that extremity (Figure 10.6).

Observations on the flexor and crossed extensor reflexes led Sherrington to a hypothesis that locomotion represented a sequence of those reflexes. Indeed, if you imagine the paw of a limb touching the ground and accepting much of the weight of the animal, receptors in the skin of the paw (that are also part of the FRA group) will start generating action potentials. This sensory activity will lead, after a certain delay, to activation of flexor muscles of that limb (its lifting off the ground) with simultaneous activation of extensor muscles of the contralateral limb. As a result, the contralateral paw will touch the ground and the weight will be transferred to that limb. Then, the cycle will repeat itself. This was indeed a very clever hypothesis that happened to be wrong (see Section 11.2 on locomotion).

Reflexes from Golgi tendon organs

The reflex effects of force-related sensory signals have attracted much attention lately. Receptors sensitive to tendon force are called *Golgi tendon organs*. They are mostly located close to the junction between the muscle fibers and the tendon. Golgi tendon organs are innervated by thick, myelinated axons (*Ib-afferents*) with a conduction

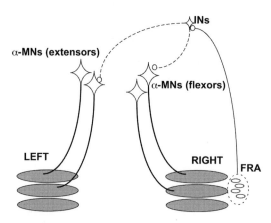

Figure 10.6 Flexor reflex afferents (FRA) produce activation of flexors within the same extremity (flexor reflex) and activation of extensors in the contralateral extremity (crossed extensor reflex). MN, motoneuron; IN, interneuron.

velocity of about 80 m/s. Their reflex effects on the muscle that houses the receptor (agonist) and the antagonist muscle are opposite to the effects of the primary spindle afferents. In particular, Ib-afferents exert inhibitory effects on alpha-motoneurons innervating the agonist muscle, mediated by *Ib-interneurons* (Figure 10.7). There are also facilitatory effects on alpha-motoneurons innervating the antagonist muscle mediated by Ib-interneurons and another pool of interneurons.

During natural movement, reflex effects of both Ia- and Ib-afferents can typically be described as negative feedback loops. Indeed, imagine that you produce voluntary elbow flexion. The flexor muscle will shorten while the extensor muscle will stretch. Shortening of the flexor muscle will reduce signals from the primary endings of flexor

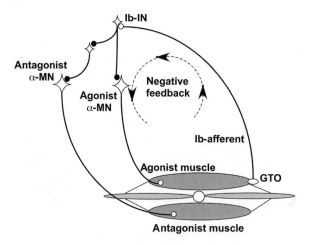

Figure 10.7 Activity of Golgi tendon organs (GTO) induces reflex suppression of the alpha-motoneurons (α-MNs) innervating the muscle of origin (via one inhibitory interneuron, Ib-IN) and disinhibition (excitation) of the antagonist muscle α-MNs (via two inhibitory interneurons).

spindles, resulting in less excitation received by flexor alpha-motoneurons and less inhibition received by extensor alpha-motoneurons. Stretching of the extensor will lead to higher activity of its primary spindle endings, resulting in a similar effect—higher activation of extensor alpha-motoneurons and stronger reciprocal inhibition of flexor alpha-motoneurons. As a result, activation of the flexor muscle will produce reflex effects that reduce this activation and facilitate activation of the antagonist. The overall effect will try to stop the movement (negative feedback). Higher voluntary flexor force during this movement will also contribute to the same effect, that is, inhibition of flexor alpha-motoneurons and facilitation of extensor alpha-motoneurons.

Interaction of reflexes

In some conditions, in particular during reflex effects produced by a passive limb motion (produced by an external force, for example by another person), the reflex effects of Ia- and Ib-afferents can be opposite to each other. An example is the so-called *clasp-knife phenomenon* observed in some patients after spinal cord injury. If a clinician tries to move a spastic limb of a patient in a certain direction, the stretched muscle resists strongly because of the hyperexcitable tonic stretch reflex. This resistance can become very strong. It results in a very large force produced by the muscle, leading to a correspondingly high activity level of the force-sensitive Ib-afferents. These afferents have an inhibitory reflex effect on the agonist alpha-motoneurons. When these inhibitory effects overpower the excitation received from primary spindle endings, the muscle may suddenly become silent and stop resisting the external effort. As a result, the joint collapses like a pocket knife.

In natural conditions, an increase in muscle force leads to activation of many receptors of different types. For example, muscle contraction leads to a change in the geometry of muscle fibers affecting the length-sensitive receptors in muscle spindles. There are also effects of muscle contraction on a variety of cutaneous and subcutaneous receptors and on joint receptors (mediated by changes in the joint capsule tension). Studies of the overall effects of force-related sensory signals, in particular by the group of T. Richard Nichols, have documented complex patterns that include inter-muscle and inter-joint effects. In particular, such reflex effects differ between one-joint and two-joint muscles that are commonly viewed as agonists (for example, the soleus, gastrocnemius medialis, and gastrocnemius lateralis). The organization of these reflexes suggests a relation to functional limb actions via a complex synergic mechanism.

Reflexes and the equilibrium-point hypothesis

Spinal reflexes play a very important role within the equilibrium-point hypothesis. Indeed, within this hypothesis, the main control variable for a single muscle is the threshold of its *tonic stretch reflex* (λ, see Section 8.3). If the reflex effects are eliminated, for example as a result of cutting the dorsal roots (*deafferentation*), this mechanism of control becomes impossible.

After deafferentation, the animal has to learn how to use its limbs in the absence of the tonic stretch reflex. It is indeed possible as demonstrated in experiments on deafferented monkeys, although movements become clumsy and poorly coordinated. In the absence of reflexes, descending signals from the brain become the only input into the alpha-motoneuronal pools. To produce movements, this input has to be modified, leading to different level of activation of the pool. The muscles will still produce force that shows length and velocity dependence, but these dependences will be defined not by the tonic stretch reflex (which has been eliminated by the procedure) but by peripheral muscle properties. Note that the length and velocity dependences of muscle force are modulated strongly by muscle activation level. A particular version of the equilibrium-point hypothesis, the *alpha-model*, used these features of muscle force production to describe the control of movements of deafferented animals (see Section 8.3).

The alpha-model assumes that different activation levels (different commands) result in different slopes of the force–length relationship. An equilibrium point is achieved when the forces produced by an agonist–antagonist muscle pair and the external load balance each other. Movements are generated by changes in the alpha-command, resulting in a shift of the equilibrium point. Experiments on deafferented monkeys confirmed such features of this mode of control as equifinality in cases of transient unexpected perturbations and gradual shifts of the equilibrium point during voluntary movements.

The tonic stretch reflex is not the only reflex input into an alpha-motoneuronal pool. A few other inputs have already been mentioned, including those from sensory receptors located in other muscles of the limb and even from sensory receptors in another limb. So, descending commands are not the only input that defines depolarization of the target alpha-motoneurons and sets the threshold of the tonic stretch reflex, λ. These will also depend on a few other factors such as signals from the abovementioned remote sensory organs, the history of activation of the alpha-motoneuronal pool, and the rate of the muscle length change mediated by the velocity sensitivity of primary spindle endings. The combined action of these factors can be summarized as:

$$\lambda = \lambda^* + \mu V + f(t) + \rho, \tag{10.1}$$

where λ is the threshold of the tonic stretch reflex defined by the depolarization of the motoneuronal pool, λ^* is the descending contribution to λ, μV is a factor reflecting the velocity sensitivity of primary spindle endings, $f(t)$ is a history-dependent factor, and ρ reflects effects from sensory receptors in other muscles. Figure 10.8 illustrates the dependence between muscle length and the number of recruited alpha-motoneurons (α-MN) as defined by a parameter λ. It emphasizes that λ is not defined exclusively by descending signals but also by the abovementioned factors (λ^*, μV, $f(t)$, and ρ).

The fact that λ is not under exclusive descending control does not create a problem for the equilibrium-point hypothesis. Descending commands, such as λ^*, are tools that are used by the central nervous system to produce movements. The action of a tool is commonly modified by environmental factors. For example, a moment of force applied to the steering wheel of a car by the hands of the driver may have different effects on wheel turning motion depending on the friction between the

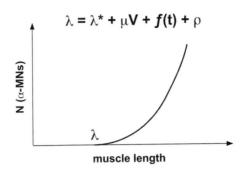

$$\lambda = \lambda^* + \mu V + f(t) + \rho$$

Figure 10.8 A dependence of the number of recruited alpha-motoneurons (α-MNs) on muscle length. Threshold (λ) of the tonic stretch reflex is a function of a descending input (λ^*), velocity-dependent feedback (μV), a history-dependent term [$f(t)$], and reflex input from other muscles (ρ). Reproduced by permission from Feldman, A. G., & Latash, M. L. (2005). Testing hypotheses and the advancement of science: Recent attempts to falsify the equilibrium-point hypothesis. *Experimental Brain Research, 161*, 91–103.

pavement and the wheels and presence or absence of a power-assisted steering mechanism. Nevertheless, one can control direction of car motion with sufficient precision. The control is organized about important performance variables such as car motion direction. Effects of other factors are compensated for.

10.2 Central pattern generators

It has been known for centuries that the beheaded chicken runs for some time and flaps its wings rhythmically. This observation by itself suggests that locomotor patterns, both running and flying, can be produced by the spinal cord deprived of its natural input from the brain. On the other hand, experiments by Graham Brown early in the twentieth century showed that animals could generate locomotor behaviors even when the dorsal roots into the corresponding segments of the spinal cord had been cut. This means that locomotion does not require an input from peripheral receptors, that is, it is not reflex-based. Taken together, these two groups of observations suggested that the spinal cord isolated from neural inputs, both from the brain and from the periphery, can produce rhythmic patterns of activity of alpha-motoneurons.

The term *central pattern generator* (CPG) has been used to denote a neural system that is able to produce a pattern of activity in an autonomous regime, that is, without a patterned input from either hierarchically higher neural structures or peripheral apparatus. This notion has been used to describe neural control of a variety of actions, typically rhythmic ones, such as locomotion, breathing, chewing, and scratching. Additional experimental support for the existence of CPGs came from studies of locomotor-like rhythms (and rhythms resembling other activities) generated by the central nervous system of animals whose movements were suppressed by agents such as *kurare* (a poison suppressing neuro-muscular transmission of action potentials that was originally used by hunters in Central and South America).

Half-center model

Early CPG schemes were very simple, consisting of small sets of neuron-like elements that could, by themselves, generate rhythmic activity. A very simple example of the so-called *two half-center model* is shown in Figure 10.9. Two groups of neurons are assumed to interact and suppress the activity of the cells in the other group (for example, via inhibitory interneurons); they also generate output directed at the executive apparatus, for example, to motoneurons of muscles involved in a rhythmic activity. The scheme in Figure 10.9 presents a typical positive feedback loop. Imagine that one group of neurons becomes slightly more active. The other group of neurons will receive a stronger inhibitory input and will generate lower activity. This will decrease the inhibition of the neurons of the first group. Their activity will go up and increase the inhibition of the second group. After a short time, the second group of neurons will become silent, while the first one will show a very high level of activity.

To avoid getting the system stuck in a state where only one of the two neuronal half-centers is active, it is assumed that the neurons in the main two pools fatigue quickly and turn off after a brief period of high activity. So, after a period of time, neurons of the first group will fatigue and turn-off, and the other group of neurons will be released from the inhibition and become active. Then, those neurons will get fatigued and so on. This will result in a rhythmic activity, which will continue until an external influence turns both neuronal groups off or they run out of important substances, for example neuromediators or sources of energy (such as ATP). The two half-centers are assumed to receive an input from a hierarchically higher group of neurons that can initiate, terminate, or modulate the rhythmic process inherent to the scheme shown in Figure 10.9.

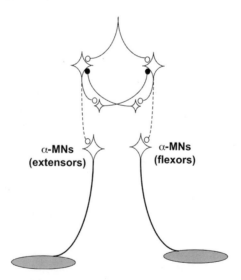

Figure 10.9 A scheme of a simple central pattern generator (a two-half-center model). Excitatory projections are shown by open circles, while inhibitory projections are shown with filled circles. MN, motoneuron.

The CPG also receives inputs from peripheral sensors such as *visual receptors*, *vestibular receptors*, and *proprioceptors* and possibly other structures within the central nervous system. The afferent input into a CPG is able to bring about changes in the pattern of its activity, leading, for example, to changes in *gait* (from walking to trotting to galloping, see Section 11.2). Such changes can also be induced voluntarily (i.e. by changing the input from the assumed hierarchically higher center).

Actual neuronal schemes of CPGs have been deciphered only for animals with a relatively simple central nervous system; the most complex among those animals is the lamprey. Actual CPG schemes are much more complex than the cartoon scheme consisting of two half-centers illustrated in Figure 10.9. They involve many neuronal pools with sophisticated connections linking CPGs for different subsets of effectors (legs, fins, wings, etc.).

Wiping reflex in frogs

Much of the important information about the spinal cord has come from studies of frogs. These animals were the favorite object of experimental physiological studies in the nineteenth century, and this interest was revived in the second half of the twentieth century. In particular, in the middle of the nineteenth century, the great German physiologist Eduard Pflüger described the wiping reflex that could be observed in a decapitated (headless) frog. After decapitation, the frog's body was suspended by its shoulders, and a small piece of paper soaked in a weak acid solution was placed on the back of the body. After a short latent period, the ipsilateral hindlimb (the hindlimb on the side of the stimulus placement) performed a coordinated movement and wiped the stimulus off the back. This observation demonstrates that the spinal cord can generate coordinated multi-joint movements of the extremities to a spatial target.

In the second half of the twentieth century, a group of physiologists in Moscow repeated Pflüger's experiment using not decapitated but *spinalized frogs*. In those animals, the head was left intact but the spinal cord was cut at a high cervical level. As a result, no signals could come from the brain to the extremities. Spinalized frogs also showed the wiping reflex. Important new features of the reflex were described. In particular, the hindlimb of the frog produced a series of wiping movements targeting the same area of the back (where the stimulus was placed); individual movements within the series produced wiping of the back in different directions. This means that the movements were organized to wipe the same spatial location but at different angles. In other words, the spinal cord was able to organize a multi-joint coordinated action that preserved the location of the spot to be wiped (a multi-joint synergy stabilizing the important endpoint coordinate, see Section 9.4) while allowing the direction of the wiping movement to vary.

Another important observation was made with the stimulus placed not on the back of the body but on a forelimb. Accurate wiping was observed for various positions of the forelimb with the stimulus with respect to the body. This implies that the spinal cord is "aware" of changes in body configuration and is able to use this information for movement production.

The synergic organization of the hindlimb joints was confirmed in experiments with hindlimb loading and joint fixation. In the loading studies, a heavy (lead) bracelet was placed on one of the distal joints of the hindlimb, thus changing dramatically the inertial properties of the limb. Movement kinematics was changed. Nevertheless, the hindlimb was able to wipe the target successfully at the first attempt. Successful wiping was also observed, also at the first attempt, when one of the hindlimb joints was blocked mechanically. These observations suggest powerful *error compensation* among the joints within the duration of the wiping movement, resulting in accurate endpoint location. The wiping action was very quick at the room temperature and it slowed down if the frog was cooled down: A frog taken from the refrigerator showed very similar wiping actions but performed the wiping as if it were filmed in slow motion.

An elegant, simple kinematic model was suggested by Israel Gelfand, Michael Berkinblit, and Anatol Feldman to account for the effects of error compensation among joint rotations. Within this model, joint rotational velocity was defined as the cross-product of two vectors, one pointing from the joint to the spatial target ($\mathbf{R}$), and the other pointing from the joint to the endpoint ($\mathbf{R_1}$) (Figure 10.10):

$$\omega = a|\mathbf{R}| \times |\mathbf{R_1}| \cdot \sin(\alpha), \tag{10.2}$$

where ω is the vector of angular velocity $|\mathbf{R}|$ and $|\mathbf{R_1}|$ are the magnitudes of the two mentioned vectors, α is the angle between those two vectors, and a is a constant. Naturally this model continues generating joint rotations until the endpoint comes into the target. Then, within all the $\{\mathbf{R}; \mathbf{R_1}\}$ vector pairs, the vectors become parallel to each other, all the $\sin(\alpha)$ values become zero, and the movement stops.

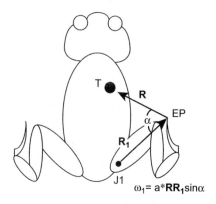

$$\omega_1 = a*\mathbf{RR_1}\sin\alpha$$

Figure 10.10 An illustration of a model by Gelfand, Berkinblit, and Feldman of multi-joint coordination during the wiping reflex movement by the frog. Angular joint velocity (ω) is defined by a product of two vectors, one pointing from the endpoint to the target ($\mathbf{R}$) and the other pointing from the joint to the endpoint ($\mathbf{R_1}$). Reproduced by permission from Gelfand, I. M., & Latash, M. L. (1998). On the problem of adequate language in motor control. *Motor Control, 2,* 306–313.

Effects of spinal cord stimulation

There have been several attempts to explore the neurophysiological basis of coor-dinated limb actions controlled by the spinal cord. A series of studies by the group led by Emilio Bizzi explored the effects of electrical stimulation applied directly to structures within the spinal cord on hindlimb endpoint action. Stimulation at a mid-thoracic level led in many cases to a hindlimb motion that brought the endpoint into a new spatial position. Less frequently, an anatomically extreme posture, for example, complete extension of the limb, was observed. These results are readily compatible with the equilibrium-point hypothesis and the idea of *multi-joint synergies*. Indeed, if one assumes that stimulating a certain structure in the spinal cord defines an equi-librium state of the endpoint, this point is going to be achieved, possibly with different joint trajectories, if the stimulation is applied in slightly different initial joint configurations. These observations are also compatible with the abovementioned kinematic model of wiping (see Equation 10.2).

The results of the experiments with spinal cord stimulation are not that easy to interpret in terms of neurophysiological mechanisms because of a number of factors. The most important one is that the exact structures that were subjected to stimulation were unknown. If one assumes, for example, that the stimulation produced changes in reflex loop gains (by changing the excitability of the corresponding interneurons), a movement to an equilibrium is expected where all the reflex actions balance each other. Sometimes such an equilibrium point may not exist; then, movement to an anatomically extreme position may be expected where the unbalanced reflex action produces non-zero forces/torques.

The same group studied the effects of electrical spinal cord stimulation on the force produced at the endpoint of the hindlimb when the limb was prevented from moving. These experiments resulted in force maps, that is families of force vectors produced by a standard stimulation applied when the limb was held at different spatial locations. All the force fields could be classified as belonging to three groups: (1) converging to a point in space; (2) forming a circular pattern about a point in space; and (3) leading in a certain direction.

These and some other studies led to an idea of the spinal cord containing motor primitives, that is, neural structures producing relatively simple blocks for complex actions. Any action was supposed to be built of a number of motor primitives recruited with appropriately selected scaling coefficients.

Spinal cord injury

Injury to the spinal cord is unfortunately a rather common consequence of a variety of accidents and acts of violence. It can also be produced by other factors such as malformations and pathological changes in intervertebral disks. Spinal cord injury can lead to a variety of sensory, motor, and autonomic consequences. Injury to pathways that carry information to the brain (ascending pathways) leads to disruption of the sensory function, while injury to descending pathways (from the brain to the spinal structures) leads to a loss in the ability to produce voluntary movements.

Besides, spinal cord injury frequently leads to pathological changes in the neuronal machinery of the spinal cord, resulting in changed spinal reflexes.

Depending on the level and severity of the injury, its consequences can include impairment of the motor function in different parts of the body (Table 10.1). This impairment may or may not involve a phenomenon termed *spasticity*. The brilliant British neurologist Hughlings Jackson (1835–1911) defined spasticity as a state characterized by positive and negative signs. Positive signs included phenomena that are seen in spastic patients but not in healthy persons. Examples of positive signs are *flexor and extensor spasms*, *clonus*, the *clasp-knife phenomenon*, the *withdrawal reflex* (sometimes imprecisely referred to as "Babinski reflex"), and elements of *dystonia*. Negative signs include phenomena that are missing in patients with spasticity, for example, *weakness* and *discoordination*. More recently, a strong velocity-dependent component in reflexes to muscle stretch has been emphasized as an important feature of spasticity.

Another frequently mentioned sign of spasticity is increased *muscle tone*. Muscle tone is a poorly defined term commonly used to describe the motor function, particularly impaired motor function. There is no objective measure for muscle tone (actually, there are tools that claim to be measuring muscle tone, but they all produce the highest readings for a dead person whose muscles are in rigor mortis). Typically, tone is assessed by a clinician who asks the patient to be relaxed and then moves one of the joints (typically, one of the major joints in the arms and legs). The clinician feels resistance to this imposed motion, and assigns to it an index corresponding to this feeling in comparison to what is expected in a typical healthy person. Obviously, resistance to such an imposed motion would depend on a variety of factors, such as inertia of the body segment, length- and velocity-dependence of forces produced by peripheral tissues, presence or absence of changes in muscle activation, etc. The latter factor may be particularly important.

Figure 10.11 illustrates a typical dependence of active muscle force on muscle length (tonic stretch reflex). A relaxed person has the threshold for muscle activation set at a value of muscle length longer than the current muscle length. The muscle can be relaxed for different values of λ (compare λ_1 and λ_2 in Figure 10.11). When the muscle is stretched by an externally imposed motion (L_2 in Figure 10.11), its resistance will depend on the degree of initial muscle relaxation, that is, on the distance between the initial muscle length (L_1) and its initial threshold of the tonic stretch reflex. For example, persons with Down syndrome are commonly described as *hypotonic*. This is likely to reflect the fact that they obey the instruction "to relax"

Table 10.1 Likely consequences of spinal cord injury

Level of injury	Symmetry of symptoms	Affected extremities	Spasticity
Supraspinal	Unilateral	Arms and legs	Present
Cervical	Bilateral	Arms and legs	Present
Thoracic	Bilateral	Legs	Present
Lumbar (upper)	Bilateral	Legs	Present
Lumbar (low), Sacral	Bilateral	Legs	Absent

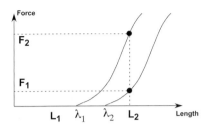

Figure 10.11 When a person is relaxed, the threshold for active muscle force generation, λ, may have different values (λ_1 and λ_2) larger than the length of the muscle (L_1). When the muscle is stretched by an externally imposed motion (L_2), its resistance ("tone," compare F_1 and F_2) depends on the degree of initial muscle relaxation, that is, on the distance between the initial muscle length (L_1) and its initial threshold of the tonic stretch reflex.

better than persons without Down syndrome: They shift the threshold for muscle activation further away from the current muscle length.

The equilibrium-point hypothesis offers a unified description of both positive and negative signs of spasticity. Figure 10.12 illustrates the muscle force–length characteristics within the whole anatomical range of natural muscle length changes. A healthy person can relax a muscle at any anatomically accessible muscle length. This means that the threshold of the tonic stretch reflex, λ, can be shifted outside the anatomical range (the rightmost curve in Figure 10.12A). On the other hand, a person can produce high muscle forces, even if the muscle is close to its shortest possible length. This implies that the range of λ shifts is larger than the anatomical muscle length range. In spasticity, the controller loses the ability to shift λ over the whole range of its values, and large λ shifts can be produced by sensory feedback signals. This leads to two consequences. First, voluntary control of the muscle force becomes impaired. Second, sensory signals can lead to involuntary burst of muscle activation (spasms, for example, produced by a shift of λ from λ_1 to λ_2 in Figure 10.12B). The scheme in Figure 10.12 suggests that normalizing the range of λ shifts may be expected to lead to an improvement in both positive and negative signs of spasticity, a prediction confirmed by several recent studies.

10.3   The brain: A general overview

Representation of functions in the brain

The issue of representation of major functions of the body in the brain has been debated over centuries. It looked as though a pendulum were swinging between two polar views with a period of about 50 years. By the middle of the nineteenth century, the predominant view was that different functions were localized in different brain structures that represented their control centers. This view was based on numerous clinical observations of people with brain injury that showed reproducible patterns of functional loss associated with injury to specific brain structures. The logic behind

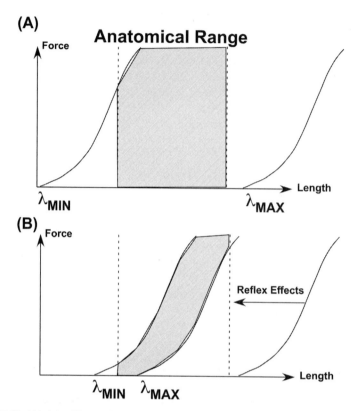

Figure 10.12 (A) A healthy person can shift the threshold of the tonic stretch reflex, λ, outside the anatomical range for muscle length. (B) In a person with spasticity, the range of voluntarily produced λ shifts is reduced, leading to both impairment of voluntary force production and a possibility of muscle spasms. The accessible ranges of active force–length combinations are shown as shaded areas.

this view was straightforward: If an injury to a brain area leads to a severe deterioration of a brain function, this means that that particular area contains a control center for that particular function. Of course, this logic is flawed. Nobody would claim that the control center of important functions of a TV set is in its wires, even though cutting a wire can lead to elimination of sound, image, or both. The idea of strict function localization in the brain led, in particular, to *phrenology*, the science of bumps on the human skull that were supposed to reflect features of one's mind.

By the end of the nineteenth century, an alternative view started to dominate. Once again, the main source of evidence was observations in patients after brain injury. However, the emphasis shifted from reproducible patterns of functional loss to observations of *functional recovery*, even after severe injuries to brain areas that had been assumed to contain control centers for those functions. Along similar lines, observations of children with inborn brain abnormalities showed that even severe pathologies to certain brain areas failed to eliminate some of the basic functions apparently controlled by those areas. Several experiments on animals, in particular by Karl Lashley (1890–1958), a prominent American psychologist, showed that aspects of a learned function remained after removal of large portions of the relevant brain tissue as long as a certain amount of tissue remained intact (and it did not matter what portion of the tissue was spared). The alternative view—that the anatomical structures of the brain were not assigned to specific functions but could contribute to any function depending on the functioning of other areas, external signals, etc.—started to dominate. The typical apparent distribution of functions among the brain structures in the adult was viewed as an emergent pattern based on the similar anatomy (defined by the genetic material) and similar experiences during typical development.

In his very first book written in the early 1930s, Bernstein argued with the then dominant view of the Pavlov school that all behaviors were based on combinations of *inborn* and *conditioned reflexes*. In that book, Bernstein reviewed all the pros and cons regarding the two mentioned views on the representation of function in the brain and concluded that both views contained only parts of the truth. He used the terms "atomism" for the function localization approach (in our times, this approach would likely be called *reductionism*) and "wholism" for the idea of the lack of specialization of neural structures. He used the term "dynamics" to address the ability of the brain structures to adjust their function with injury and experience; the more commonly used contemporary term is *plasticity* (see Section 10.4). Here are a couple of quotations from that book:

> *It would be incomparably harder to imagine how the neural process in all the nerves could be the same (as claimed by academician I.P. Pavlov), disregarding all the morphological differences among the nerves, their peripheral apparata and intrinsic systemic interactions, than to accept that more diverse morphology is expected to produce more diverse dynamic phenomena. This sounds as if someone would try to persuade me that the bassoon, the violin, the double-bass, and the tam-tam produce absolutely identical sounds, and the only difference is in that some of these instruments are to the left of the conductor, while others are to the right, and they play different notes (p. 315).*

> *Neither atomism, nor wholism (accepted as postulates) can provide a comprehensive interpretation of the nervous system, primarily because they can exist separately only as abstractions. The nervous system will be explained only when we are able to express the factual inseparability of the two principles and find terms to express processes reflective of the dynamics of their interaction (p. 325).*

These quotations summarize the currently dominant view on the relations between brain structures and functions. Most researchers would agree that there are no "places" in the brain where particular functions are located; rather, functions are distributed among many anatomical structures in the brain. In cases of injury or specialized training, there is marked neural plasticity, which will be discussed in more detail later. Of course, this does not mean that any part of the brain can do anything; plastic changes are limited in their ability to contribute to recovery of a lost function.

Operators in the brain. Distributed processing modules

Later in his career, Bernstein in collaboration with two of his younger colleagues, Phillip Bassin and Lev Latash, suggested an idea that there might be localized *operators* in brain structures. The term "operator" meant a specific input–output transformation of neural signals that could be used as a brick for building various functions, including very dissimilar ones. Recently, this idea has been developed by the American neurophysiologist James Houk and his colleagues, who introduced and developed the notion of *distributed processing modules* (DPMs). Two types of DPM have been introduced, those based on loops involving the *basal ganglia* and the *cortex* and those involving the *cerebellum* and the cortex (in addition to other brain structures such as the *thalamus*). The notions of Bernstein's operators and Houk's DPMs seem to be very similar. One can suggest a notion of a multi-neuronal system, which uses neurophysiological processes to link physical variables at the input and at the output of the system, and this definition would probably fit both operators and DPMs.

Given this broad definition, the mechanism of the tonic stretch reflex qualifies as a DPM or operator that links such physical variables as muscle length (and velocity) and force as described in Section 4.4. The operation performed by this module is stabilization of the equilibrium point (a combination of muscle length and force where the system "muscle + its reflex feedback loops + load" is in an equilibrium) with a synergy among the motor units. Indeed, if one motor unit stops generating action potentials (for an unknown reason), the load will become higher than muscle force, the muscle will stretch, and the tonic stretch reflex will lead to additional motor unit recruitment and/or increased frequency of action potentials. This will result in partial *error compensation*, which is a distinctive feature of synergies.

Ascending and descending pathways

The motor control function of the brain is inseparable from its sensory function. The two functions, sometimes referred to as a single sensorimotor function, rely on information transmission from the brain to the spinal cord (and to the nuclei of the cranial nerves) and from the peripheral receptors to the brain. This information is transmitted along the *descending* and *ascending pathways*. There are certain common features of all the pathways within the CNS. These features include, in particular, the presence of *relay nuclei* where information from different sources may be combined (Figure 10.13). Arguably, the best-known relay structure is the thalamus, which receives both sensory and motor information, processes it, and sends it to the cortex of the large hemispheres.

Sensory pathways display a feature called *topographic organization*. This feature means that neighboring receptor cells project to neighboring cells in relay nuclei, which in turn project to neighboring cells in their target nuclei and so on (as illustrated in Figure 10.13). Similarly, axons that originate from neighboring cells of a brain area that is the source of a descending pathway are more likely to project onto neurons in the spinal cord that ultimately result in contractions of muscles controlling movements of neighboring body segments. As a result, there are many *motor maps* and *sensory maps* within the central nervous system. These maps, however, may be rather mosaic with no one-to-one correspondence to anatomical body structures.

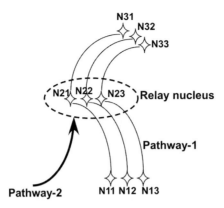

Figure 10.13 Pathways within the central nervous system are characterized by the presence of relay nuclei, integration of information from several pathways, and preservation of somatotopy.

Only a few of the major descending pathways will be mentioned in the following sections. More information may be found in textbooks on anatomy and neurophysiology of the central nervous system.

10.4 Cortex of the large hemispheres

The upper layer of the large hemispheres, called the *cortex*, plays a major role in the voluntary motor function in addition to its role in many other sensory and cognitive functions. An injury to the cortex, for example following a stroke, typically leads to severe consequences for voluntary motor control, including a combination of weakness or even complete paralysis in certain body areas and uncontrolled muscle contractions that interfere with voluntary movements.

The cortex of a single hemisphere is traditionally described as consisting of five *lobes*—frontal, parietal, temporal, occipital, and insular. Another classification uses anatomical landmarks to divide the cortex into 52 zones, which are called *Brodmann areas* after the German physiologist Korbinian Brodmann (1868–1918). The two hemispheres are directly connected via two major pathways, the *corpus callosum* and the *anterior commissure*.

Neural organization of the cortex

The neural organization of the cortex shows a typical laminar structure with six layers and two major groups of neurons—the *stellate cells* and the *pyramidal cells* (Figure 10.14). The stellate cells play the role of interneurons within the cerebral cortex; their axons do not leave the cortex. The axons of pyramidal cells leave the cortex and project to a variety of other structures within the central nervous system. Some of the dendrites of pyramidal cells are oriented towards the surface of the cortex (*apical dendrites*). Other dendrites are oriented horizontally in layers 2, 3, and 4, and

Cortical Surface

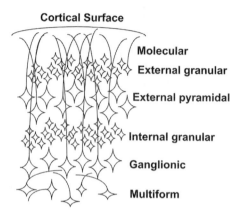

Figure 10.14 Typical structure of the cortex with the six main layers.

may be a few millimeters long. The uppermost layer of the cortex is called the *molecular layer*. It is composed mostly of axons and apical dendrites and contains only a few cell bodies. The next is the *external granular layer*, containing a large number of small pyramidal and stellate cells. It is followed by the *external pyramidal layer*, which contains mostly pyramidal cells. The next layer, the *internal granular layer* is composed of stellate and pyramidal cells. The fifth, *gangionic layer* contains large pyramidal cells. And the last, sixth layer, the *multiform layer*, consists of different neurons many of whose axons leave the cortex.

The pyramidal tract. The corticospinal tract

One of the best-known output tracts of the cortex is the *pyramidal tract* with the long axons of the cortical cells projecting onto different structures participating in the control of movements (Figure 10.15). The human pyramidal tract consists of about one

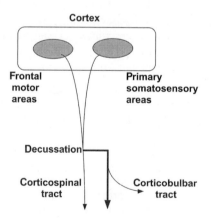

Figure 10.15 The corticospinal tract. Note that most of the fibers cross (decussate) at the level of pyramids. Some of the fibers form the corticobulbar tract and innervate cranial nerve nuclei.

million fibers that originate primarily from cortical neurons in the frontal motor areas (Brodmann areas 4 and 6) with a contribution from neurons in the parietal somato-sensory areas. Most of these fibers are myelinated (more than 90%); however, only a fraction of those fibers conduct action potentials at very high velocities (over 50 m/s). The pyramidal tract consists of two major groups of axons. The first group includes the axons of cortical neurons that form the *corticospinal tract* that goes down to the spinal cord. The second group includes fibers innervating the motor nuclei of the cranial nerves (the *corticobulbar tract*) that control the muscles of the face and the neck.

Most of the fibers (over 80%) of the corticospinal tract cross the midline of the body at the brainstem level (*decussation of pyramids*) and travel in the contralateral dorsolateral column of the spinal cord to the spinal segments. A smaller number of fibers do not cross the midline and descend within the ventromedial part of the spinal cord. The uncrossed fibers innervate mostly proximal muscles, including muscles that control trunk movements. As a result, an injury to a cortical area related to motor function leads to most pronounced motor impairments in the contralateral extremities.

Somatotopic cortical representations. The homunculus

In the 1950s, a famous Canadian neurosurgeon, Wilder Graves Penfield (1891–1976), used electrical stimulation of different cortical neurons during surgeries on the open brain and observed motor responses in different body parts. Based on these responses, he compiled maps showing a distorted human figure (a *homunculus*) drawn on those brain areas, in particular, on the motor area of the cortex. The homunculus drawings typically show a human-like figure with exaggerated representations for the hand (and particularly for the thumb), the face, and the tongue, while the representation of the trunk is relatively small. Later, similar distorted body representations were drawn for other animals.

More recently, however, studies using more sophisticated methods of brain stim-ulation, in particular studies by the American neurophysiologist Marc Schieber, have shown that the cortical representations of different body parts do not form a human-like figure. Rather, these representations are mosaic, with neurons representing different body parts intermixed within a single area of the cortex. These studies have documented widespread phenomena of *divergence* and *convergence* in the cortico-spinal projections (Figure 10.16). The phenomenon of divergence implies that a single neuron (for example, N1 in Figure 10.16) can induce muscle contractions in different body parts (muscles M1 and M3), while convergence implies that two (or more) neurons (N1 and N3), which may be located rather far away from each other in the cortex, may produce contractions of the same muscle (M1) or motion of the same body part. So, the currently dominant view is that the somatotopic organization of the motor cortex does not imply a one-to-one map of body parts, muscles, or movements.

Cortical plasticity

Numerous studies have documented changes in the strength and patterns of projec-tions of the cortical neurons onto peripheral effectors, muscles, and body parts. Such

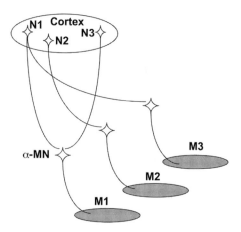

Figure 10.16 The phenomena of convergence (N1 and N3 on the α-MNs of M1) and divergence (N1 to α-MNs innervating M1 and M3). MN, motoneuron.

changes have been observed following major brain injury (for example, after stroke), amputation of a body part, recovery after a brain injury, and as a result of specialized practice (for example, learning how to play a musical instrument or how to read Braille). Such effects of neural plasticity have been documented using *transcranial magnetic stimulation* of the brain and various methods of brain imaging, including *magnetic resonance imaging* and *positron emission tomography* (more on these methods in Sections 13.5 and 13.6).

Neural plasticity has been documented following relatively short practice episodes, lasting for about an hour. Most commonly, practice led to an enlarged representation of the effector and a decrease in the threshold of its response to brain stimulation. However, less straightforward and more task-specific effects of practice were observed in studies that required coordination of several effectors. Practicing such tasks could lead to a decrease of the response to brain stimulation (see Section 12.4).

Cortical activity during movement preparation

When a person produces a voluntary movement, changes in the neuronal activity can be observed in several cortical areas. If a unilateral arm or hand movement is produced in a self-paced manner (at a self-selected time), early changes in the cortical activity include bilateral changes in the electrical potential recorded over the *supplementary motor area* (SMA) and *primary motor area* (M1). The amplitude of this potential (called the *readiness potential* or the *Bereitschaft potential*) grows over more than 1 s. The readiness potential is followed by a unilateral change in the potential over the appropriate region of the M1 contralateral to the moving body part. If a movement is performed in response to a visual signal, neurons in the premotor area show a substantial increase in their activity level in addition to the activity in the SMA and M1.

Variables reflected in neuronal activity

A number of studies have tried to link neuronal activity in cortical areas related to movement production to kinematic, kinetic, and electromyographic characteristics of the movement. Classical studies performed in the USA by Edward Vaughn Evarts (1926–1985) and his colleagues suggested that activation of individual cortical neurons immediately prior to action initiation was related to forces produced by the corresponding effectors (or muscle activation levels). A number of later studies, however, documented relations between indices of activity of cortical neurons, particularly in the M1 area, and a variety of mechanical characteristics of voluntary movements. Those characteristics involved both kinetic and kinematic indices such as force applied by an effector, rate of force change, movement direction, and movement velocity.

An important paradigm switch from focusing on activation patterns of individual cortical neurons to analysis of characteristics of activation of *neuronal populations* was made in the remarkable experiments pioneered by the group of the American–Greek neurophysiologist Apostolos Georgopoulos. These studies were performed on monkeys trained to produce hand movements in different directions of the workspace. Arrays of electrodes were implanted into the projection of the arm in the M1 cortical area to record the activity of many cortical neurons simultaneously. Depending on the direction of the arm movement, individual neurons showed modulation of their baseline activity level. This modulation was smooth (cosine-like) with a peak corresponding to a particular direction termed the *preferred direction* of that particular neuron (Figure 10.17A). Preferred directions were found for a large number of neurons. Then, each neuron was assigned a spatial vector of a unitary length pointing in its preferred direction in the external coordinate frame with the origin in the initial hand location. The *neuronal population vector* was computed as the sum of all the individual neuronal vectors multiplied by coefficients equal to the total number of action potentials those neurons generated during a brief time interval about the movement initiation. This vector pointed in the movement direction (Figure 10.17B).

Many later studies of neuronal populations and their relations to performance of motor tasks followed a similar scheme. First, a variable was identified, typically directly related to performance of an explicit motor task. Such performance variables could involve direction of movement of a limb, force vector applied by the limb onto a stationary object (a handle), velocity vector, and so on. Then, activity of a population of neurons was recorded using arrays of implanted electrodes. The relations between the level of activity of each individual neuron and the identified performance variable were computed. Commonly, such relations looked like smooth, cosine-like functions with a preferred direction of the performance variable vector corresponding to a peak increase in the activity of the neuron (as in Figure 10.17A). Moving in the direction opposite to the preferred direction could lead to a drop in the baseline neuron activity. Further, each neuron was assigned a vector pointing in its preferred direction and the neuronal population vector was computed as described in the previous paragraph. Such studies have shown relations of cortical neuronal population vectors to a variety of performance variables such as the spatial trajectory of

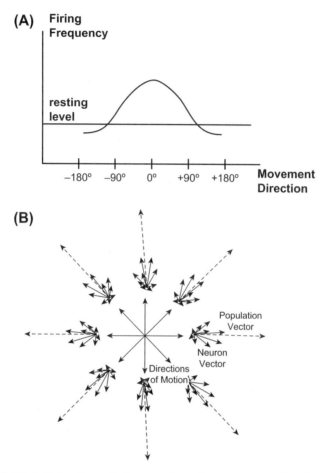

Figure 10.17 (A) Activity of a cortical neuron depends on movement direction as a cosine function with one of the directions showing the maximal increase in the activity (preferred direction). (B) When neuronal activity vectors are summed up over a pool of cortical neurons, the resultant vector (dashed lines) points close to the movement direction. A cartoon illustrating results by Georgopoulos and colleagues. Reproduced by permission from Latash, M. L. (2008). *Neurophysiological basis of movement*, 2nd edn. Urbana, IL: Human Kinetics.

the effector's endpoint, or the force vector applied by an end-effector, or derivatives of these variables.

The demonstrated relations between activation patterns of populations of cortical neurons and mechanical variables in the external world present a unique opportunity to use such signals to substitute for or improve a disordered motor function in persons with a variety of movement disorders. Indeed, if a population of M1 neurons can reliably encode important variables for motor behavior, recording such neuronal activity, deciphering it with appropriate analyses, and using the output to drive a robotic device may be able to help paralyzed people to perform certain actions. Such approaches have been actively developed recently using studies of both animals (typically monkeys) and paralyzed patients. The current rate of technological advances suggests that soon there will be devices able to substitute for impaired or impossible movements in patients using neuronal population activity of the patient's brain.

It seems appropriate to present another couple of quotations from Bernstein. First: "No area of the cortex can currently be viewed as the origin or the final destination of a neural process . . . Every area and every layer of the cortex represent only transit points of the neural process" (p. 326). In other words, Bernstein suggests that the motor cortex plays the role of a hidden layer (in the artificial *neural network* parlance) where information is expected to be garbled. Any correlations of neuronal activation with mechanical movement characteristics may reflect specific conditions within each specific study. Another quotation: "In the higher motor centers of the brain (very probably in the cortex of the large hemispheres) one can find a localized reflection of a projection of the external space in a form in which the subject perceives the external space with motor means" (quoted after Bongaardt 2001, p. 80) explains why different studies ended up with different variables reflected in neuronal cortical populations: Depending on the task, the animal "perceived the external space with motor means" via different salient sets of mechanical variables, and those variables were reflected in the activation patterns of the cortical neuronal pools.

Cortical control and the equilibrium-point hypothesis

All the studies that try to link cortical activity to performance mechanical variables bypass an important step—the identification of variables that may be specified by descending signals to the spinal cord. Chapters 5–8 present a variety of such potential variables. I hope that the reader would agree that descending signals cannot in principle specify any of the following mechanical variables: trajectories, velocities, forces, torques, etc., only neurophysiological variables that translate into mechanics with an important contribution of the external force field and related sensory signals. So far, there has been only one hypothesis, namely the equilibrium-point hypothesis, that specifies such hypothetical neurophysiological variables as subthreshold depolarization of the neuronal (including motoneuronal) pools that translates into changes of the tonic stretch reflex threshold of the corresponding muscles (Sections 8.2 and 8.3). So, a question can be asked: Do changes in the activity along the corticospinal pathway encode changes in λ values for the involved muscles?

Several recent studies have provided evidence in favor of this hypothesis. According to the equilibrium-point hypothesis, the corticospinal signals produce only one component that affects activation of the alpha-motoneurons (Figure 10.18). The other component is excitation along the tonic stretch reflex loop. If a muscle is stretched (as in Figure 10.18B), the contribution of the tonic stretch reflex is expected to increase (shown by the thicker line). So, if the same level of muscle background activation is produced at two values of muscle length, the contribution

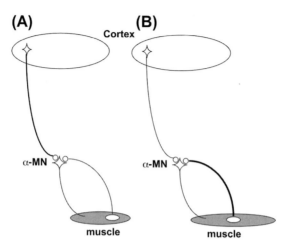

Figure 10.18 When muscle length is increased (as in B compared to A), the contribution of spindle ending activity to excitation of alpha-motoneurons (α-MNs) is increased (shown with the thicker line). To reach the same muscle activation level, less excitation is needed from the descending (in particular, corticospinal) pathways.

of the corticospinal tract has to be higher for the shorter muscle (Figure 10.18A). Since the response of cortical neurons to transcranic magnetic stimulation (TMS) increases with background activity level, this simple analysis suggests that muscle stretch should lead to smaller responses of the muscle to the TMS observed at similar levels of muscle activation. This prediction of the equilibrium-point hypothesis has been confirmed experimentally.

Mirror neurons

Much attention has been drawn recently to *mirror neurons* in the brain. These neurons were discovered by a group led by an Italian scientist, Giacomo Rizzolatti, in experiments performed on the ventral premotor cortex of the macaque monkey. The experiments showed that some cortical neurons increased their activation level when the monkey performed a particular hand-arm action and when the monkey observed an experimenter performing this action. Later, it was proposed that the human *Broca's region* (involved in speech production) was the homologue region of the monkey ventral premotor cortex. Functional magnetic resonance imaging (see Section 13.6) allowed large brain areas to be examined during action observation and action performance. Those studies have suggested that a wide network of brain areas in humans have mirror neurons. Those areas include, in particular, the somatosensory cortex. There has been much speculation about the possible involvement of mirror neurons in action–perception coupling, motor learning, speech production, imagery of actions, and many other phenomena. As of now, the role of these neurons in motor control remains unknown.

10.5   Loops through the basal ganglia

The basal ganglia represent a constellation of paired nuclei that have been the focus of attention for researchers, partly because of a number of motor disorders associated with dysfunction of particular neural projections within the basal ganglia. Perhaps, the best known one is *Parkinson's disease*. Based on typical clinical consequences of the major disorders of the basal ganglia, their function has been commonly associated with the motor function, particularly with movement initiation and sequencing movement fragments. More recently, however, evidence has been accumulating pointing at an important role of the basal ganglia in motor learning as well as in cognitive processes not directly associated with movement.

Neuroanatomy of the basal ganglia

The basal ganglia consist of ten large subcortical nuclei shown in Figure 10.19, five on each side, right and left. These nuclei do not receive direct inputs from, and do not send direct outputs to, the spinal cord. Three of the nuclei of the basal ganglia lie deep in the cerebrum, laterally to the thalamus. The phylogenetically oldest nucleus is the *globus pallidus*, also known as the *paleostriatum*. The globus pallidus consists of two parts—*internal* (GP_i) and *external* (GP_e). Two nuclei—the *caudate nucleus* and the *putamen*—form the neostriatum, or just *striatum*. The other two nuclei of the basal ganglia—the *subthalamic nucleus* and the *substantia nigra*—are located in the midbrain. The substantia nigra is divided anatomically into two parts; its dorsal region is called *pars compacta* while its ventral region is called *pars reticulata*. Pars reticulata and GP_i are the main output structures of the basal ganglia; they project to the thalamus and to the brainstem.

The striatum receives most of the inputs to the basal ganglia, in particular excitatory inputs from many of the cortical areas. These projections are modulated by *dopaminergic* inputs from substantia nigra (pars compacta). There are two major

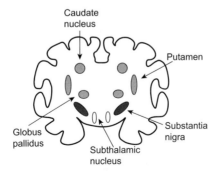

Figure 10.19 The five paired main nuclei forming the basal ganglia. Reproduced by permission from Latash, M. L. (2008). *Neurophysiological basis of movement*, 2nd edn. Urbana, IL: Human Kinetics.

outputs of the striatum. One of them targets output structures of the basal ganglia, GP$_i$ and substantia nigra, pars reticulata, which project on the ventral nuclei of the thalamus. The other output projects on GP$_e$, involves the subthalamic nucleus, and also ends up projecting on GP$_i$ and substantia nigra, pars reticulata. The two *pathways* are sometimes referred to as *direct* and *indirect*. Since thalamic nuclei project on the cortex, there are two *cortico-basal-thalamo-cortical loops* through the basal ganglia. The two loops are shown schematically in Figure 10.20. In this scheme, excitatory connections are shown with solid arrows and open circles, while inhibitory connections are shown with dashed arrows and filled circles. Counting the number of inhibitory synapses in the two loops suggest that the direct loop is a *positive feedback* (two inhibitory synapses) while the indirect loop is a *negative feedback* (three inhibitory synapses). Positive feedback systems are prone to getting out of control (see Section 7.1); hence, proper functioning of the basal ganglia requires accurate balance of the gains in the two loops.

Another output of the basal ganglia is directed at *superior colliculus* and then at brainstem nuclei that are known for their role in initiation of locomotion (*parapontine nuclei*). Changes in this output in Parkinson's disease may be associated with the well-known problems with gait initiation, called episodes of *gait freezing*.

Motor disorders associated with dysfunctions of the basal ganglia

A number of motor disorders are associated with problems within the basal ganglia. These may result in both excessive movements (*hyperkinetic* disorders) and movement poverty (*hypokinetic* disorders). The best known hypokinetic disorder,

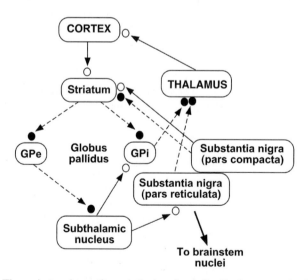

Figure 10.20 The main two loops through the basal ganglia. Excitatory projections are shown with open circles and solid arrows. Inhibitory projections are shown with filled circles and dashed arrows. GP$_e$, globus pallidus external; GP$_i$, globus pallidus internal.

Parkinson's disease, is a consequence of progressive death of dopamine-producing neurons within the substantia nigra (pars compacta). Projections of those neurons to the striatum modulate both direct and indirect loops. The lack of dopamine is associated with a dysfunction of both loops, resulting in excessive inhibition of the thalamus. This leads to difficulty with movement initiation and modification, and slowness of movements typical of Parkinson's disease. Other motor problems typical of Parkinson's disease are *tremor* (involuntary cyclic movements at 5–6 Hz, typically postural), *rigidity* (excessive resistance to externally imposed motion), and *postural instability*. Unlike spasticity, rigidity does not have a strong velocity-dependent component; commonly, it is accompanied by a phenomenon of intermittent episodes of increased resistance called *cogwheel rigidity*. Postural instability is characterized by two components—delayed and reduced *anticipatory postural adjustments* and poorly modulated, high-amplitude long-latency responses to perturbations (see Section 11.1).

Hyperkinetic disorders include *Huntington's chorea*, *hemiballismus*, and *dystonia*. Huntington's chorea is a genetically defined disorder associated with degeneration of projections from the striatum to GP_e (i.e. a dysfunction of the indirect loop). It leads to poorly coordinated excessive movements, in particular a dance-like gait (which is the origin of the term *chorea*). Somewhat similar, poorly coordinated movements are observed in cases of injury to one of the subthalamic nuclei, which is also involved in the indirect loop. Since the two subthalamic nuclei are relatively far from each other, it is very rare to have an injury to both in one person. As a result, large amplitude movements of *ballism* are limited to one side of the body, contralateral to the site of the injury (hence, *hemiballism*).

Dystonia is arguably the least understood hyperkinetic disorder. It is characterized by clumsy posturing of the affected effectors with a characteristic twisting component of involuntary movements. Pathological examination of patients with dystonia shows changes in the basal ganglia in a substantial percentage of cases; however, in many other cases, there are no clear problems with the basal ganglia.

Hyperkinetic disorders may also develop in patients who have been taking certain medications for a long time. Such disorders are known as *tardive dyskinesias*. They may be seen in patients with Parkinson's disease who have been taking large doses of dopaminergic drugs for years.

The role of the basal ganglia in movements

Despite the obvious motor problems in patients with dysfunction of the basal ganglia, their role in motor control remains unclear. There seems to be agreement only on the importance of the basal ganglia for movement initiation and sequencing. However, the neural activity in different parts of the basal ganglia correlates only weakly with potentially important characteristics of voluntary movements such as its speed and amplitude. So, the basal ganglia seem to be the middle-men of the brain structures involved in motor control: They do not define movement parameters but facilitate tasks performed by other structures that may be more directly involved in defining movement characteristics.

Several recent studies have linked the activity of the basal ganglia to the formation of *synergies* (or modes, see Section 9.4). In particular, the basal ganglia have been implicated in uniting the postural and the locomotor synergies (Sections 11.1 and 11.2) into a single functional synergy and in the control of multi-joint reaching. It has also been suggested that the basal ganglia play an important role in the formation of a synergy between gripping force and lifting force during manipulation of hand-held objects (see Section 11.4).

Cortico-basal-thalamo-cortical loops play a central role in the scheme suggested by James Houk. Within that scheme, control of movements is performed with distributed processing modules (DPMs, see Section 10.3). DPMs involving the basal ganglia are assumed to participate in making choices among tasks based on experience and prediction of future success (reward).

10.6   Loops involving the cerebellum

The cerebellum is one of the most conspicuous structures of the brain. It contains more neurons than the rest of the central nervous system combined. There are only five types of neurons in the cerebellum, and their connections create an impression of a very regular network. As a result, the cerebellum has been arguably the favorite structure for neural models.

Neuroanatomy of the cerebellum

Cerebellar neurons receive inputs from other parts of the central nervous system via two pathways—the *mossy fibers* and the *climbing fibers*. The organization of the two pathways is strikingly different (Figure 10.21). The mossy fibers originate from a variety of neural structures including those in the spinal cord and other brain

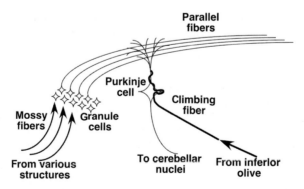

Figure 10.21 The two main inputs into the cerebellum. The mossy fibers project on small granule cells whose axons form the parallel fibers system. The climbing fibers project on Purkinje cells, wrap around the cell body and proximal dendrites and make numerous synapses on a single target cell.

structures, in particular the cortex of the large hemispheres. Their target cells are the granule cells that send their axons towards the outer layer of the cerebellum where these fibers form the parallel fiber system. The parallel fibers make excitatory synapses on the huge dendritic trees of *Purkinje cells*, which are the output cells of the cerebellum. When a Purkinje cell is excited via those synapses, it generates a typical action potential called a *simple spike* (Figure 10.22A).

The source of the other input into the cerebellum, the *climbing fibers*, is a single nucleus, the *inferior olive* in the brainstem. The climbing fibers project directly onto the Purkinje cells, typically one climbing fiber per one Purkinje cell, where a single climbing fiber can make numerous excitatory synapses with the target Purkinje cell on its body (soma) and proximal dendrites. As a result, a single action potential along a climbing fiber forces the target Purkinje cell to generate an unusual action potential called the *complex spike* (Figure 10.22B).

The Purkinje cells make inhibitory projections on *cerebellar nuclei*, which in turn project on several target structures within the central nervous system. There are three pairs of the cerebellar nuclei—the *fastigious*, the *dentate*, and the *interpositus nuclei* (the last one is composed of two nuclei—*globose* and *emboliform*). The cerebellar nuclei project on basically all the structures related to the motor function, including the spinal cord, the vestibular and reticular nuclei, the red nucleus, the superior colliculus, and the cortical areas (via the thalamus).

The philogenetically oldest, central part of the cerebellum, the *vermis*, receives most of its input from the spinal cord and the brainstem. Its output projects on the fastigial nucleus, which in turn makes projections to the spinal cord and brainstem structures, including the vestibular nuclei. The area of the cerebellum adjacent to the vermis (the paravermal area) receives inputs from the spinal cord, the brainstem, and the cortex of the large hemispheres. The Purkinje cells in the paravermal area project on the interpositus nucleus, which projects on brainstem structures and the cortex (via the thalamus). The lateral zone of the cerebellum receives most of its input signals from the cortex. Its Purkinje cells project on the dentate nucleus. The output of the dentate nucleus is directed at both cortical areas and nuclei in the brainstem. Unlike the motor areas of the cortex of the large hemispheres, the cerebellar nuclei participate in the control of movements of the ipsilateral part of the body.

(A)   **(B)**

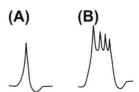

Figure 10.22 The Purkinje cells can generate simple spikes (A) and complex spikes (B). Reproduced by permission from Latash, M. L. (2008). *Neurophysiological basis of movement*, 2nd edn. Urbana, IL: Human Kinetics.

Two major loops involving the cerebellum

Two major brain loops involve the cerebellum. The first loop involves projections from the cortex to the cerebellum, which are mediated by nuclei in the pons and the mossy fiber system, projections of the Purkinje cells to the dentate nucleus, projections of the dentate nucleus to the thalamus, and thalamic projections to the cortex. The other loop involves projections from the inferior olives to the cerebellum via the climbing fibers, projections of the Purkinje cells to the interpositus nucleus, projections of the interpositus on the red nucleus, and red nucleus projections on the olives. Note that the two loops involve structures that are the sources of two major descending pathways, the *pyramidal tract* and the *rubrospinal tract*, taking part in the control of voluntary movements.

Consequences of cerebellar disorders

Much of the information on the functional role of the cerebellum comes from observations of patients with cerebellar disorders and animals with experimental injuries to the cerebellum. In animals, complete removal of the cerebellum leads to surprisingly mild consequences, given that over 50% of the neural cells within the central nervous system have been removed: The animal may show recovery of the motor and non-motor functions to a substantial degree.

Cerebellar injuries have been known to lead to major postural and movement abnormalities including problems with balance, movement timing, and coordination. As a result, until relatively recently, the cerebellum was considered a "motor organ" of the brain. At the end of the twentieth century, however, researchers became aware of the contribution of the cerebellum to sensory and cognitive processes, and the notion of a *cerebellar cognitive affective syndrome* was introduced. The cerebellum has also been implicated in a number of disorders associated with atypical development, such as *Down syndrome* and *autism*.

One of the most common motor consequences of cerebellar disorders is *ataxia*, that is, loss of coordination among joint involvement during both whole-body tasks (standing and stepping) and tasks involving one extremity (such as reaching). *Cerebellar tremor* is relatively slow; it has both *postural* and *kinetic* components. The last term means that it may show an increase during a purposeful movement (unlike Parkinsonian tremor), particularly when the moving effector approaches the target (*intentional* tremor). Problems with movement timing in cerebellar patients include poor ability to keep rhythm in both externally paced and self-paced movements.

Typical disorders associated with cerebellar lesions are illustrated in Figure 10.23. Based on typical clinical consequences of such disorders, earlier hypotheses on the role of the cerebellum in movements were mostly focused on movement timing, coordination of multi-joint actions, and motor learning.

The cerebellum, interaction torques, and motor adaptation

Mechanical analysis of the different components of joint torques (see Sections 5.1 and 5.2) during two-joint elbow–shoulder pointing actions has shown that patients with

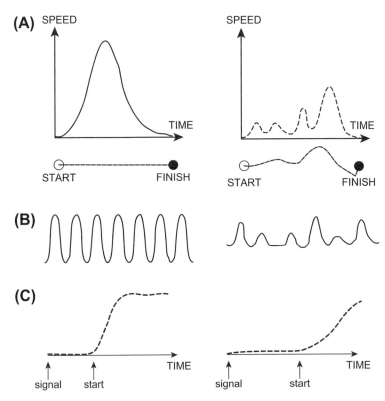

Figure 10.23 Typical features of movements in cases of cerebellar disorders. The left panels show typical patterns in a healthy person. (A) Movements are less smooth with many velocity peaks and directional errors. (B) There is a pronounced inability to produce rhythm. (C) Movements take more time to initiate (longer reaction time), and they are slower. Reproduced by permission from Latash, M. L. (2008). *Neurophysiological basis of movement*, 2nd edn. Urbana, IL: Human Kinetics.

severe cerebellar disorders might have lost the ability to compensate for the action of *interaction torques* on joint motion. As a result, total torque at the elbow joint could closely follow the interaction torque due to the motion of the shoulder joint, while the muscle elbow torque modulation was minimal. In contrast, healthy subjects showed rather dissimilar patterns of the interaction and total torques, which were produced with substantial contribution of the muscle elbow torques. These observations may be considered within the *leading-joint hypothesis* (see Section 5.2), which assumes that the controller is involved in two processes: The production of an action in a leading joint (the shoulder joint in the mentioned example) and adjustment of the interaction torques in other joints of the limb to fit the task requirements. The abovementioned results suggest that patients with cerebellar disorders can produce an appropriate action in the leading joint but their ability to modify the interaction torques is impaired, leading to inaccurate movements.

The importance of the cerebellum for *motor adaptation* has been demonstrated in experiments with prismatic glasses. When a person puts such glasses on, they distort the image of the environment on the retina. In particular, the environment can be perceived as shifted by a fixed angle as compared to reality. If a person is asked to produce a quick pointing movement with the glasses on, the movement is typically inaccurate, pointing at the perceived (wrong) target location. If the person repeats the movement again and again, after a handful of repetitions, the motor control system recalibrates itself, and the movements become accurate. After this adaptation processes, taking the glasses off leads to a pointing error in the opposite direction (after-effect). A person with a cerebellar disorder is likely not to show adaptation to prismatic glasses, even after many repetitions of the pointing movement, and no after-effect after the glasses have been taken off.

Long-term potentiation and long-term depression

The importance of the cerebellum in motor learning and adaptation has received support from a series of studies that showed the phenomena of *long-term potentiation* (LTP) and *long-term depression* (LTD). These terms reflect a long-lasting change in efficacy of a synaptic connection following a vigorous activation through that synapse or a particular combination of inputs into the target neuron. In particular, the combination of activation of a Purkinje cell via both the parallel fibers and the climbing fiber was shown to lead to a depression of the efficacy of parallel fiber synapses on the Purkinje cell. This process was hypothesized to play a major role in the adaptation of the *vestibulo-ocular reflex* (reflex eye rotation to preserve gaze direction when the head turns).

The cerebellum and synergies

At the end of the nineteenth century, a hypothesis was proposed by the French neurologist Joseph Francois Felix Babinski (1857–1932) that the cerebellum played an important role in controlling movement synergies. Babinski implied under synergies coordinated actions of large muscle groups. If one implies under a synergy a neural organization of a large set of elements with the purpose of producing a reliable (stable) action (see Section 9.4), the hypothesis of Babinski sounds very attractive. Indeed, many of the typical disorders associated with cerebellar lesions may be described as *poor coordination* of various elements. Poor coordination of muscles, joints, and limbs may lead to ataxia. Poor coordination of words may result in problems with language skills, while poor coordination of objects in the environment may result in an impaired ability to draw or copy complex pictures, both typical components of the cognitive cerebellar affective syndrome. Finally, poor coordination at an inter-personal level may be viewed as a substantial contributor to autism.

Internal models in the cerebellum

Researchers who prefer to use the idea of internal models for motor control commonly consider the cerebellum as the likely site in the brain where such models are created, updated, and refined. In particular, several hypotheses have been offered that the cerebellum contained *predictors* of future body states (direct internal models). A number of experimental studies of learning to move in novel environments have shown changes in neural activation in certain areas of the cerebellum. As mentioned earlier, the importance of the cerebellum for motor learning and adaptation has been known for many years. So, such results by themselves neither contradict nor prove that the cerebellum contains internal models.

The cerebellum and distributed processing modules

Loops through the cerebellum play a central role in the scheme of motor control suggested by James Houk and based on the notion of distributed processing modules (DPMs, see Section 10.3). According to Houk's theory, DPMs through the basal ganglia and the cerebellum are involved in two types of processes. First, the selection and initiation of an action. Second, specification of parameters of the action such as its direction, magnitude, and speed. The first group has been assigned to loops through the basal ganglia (compare to the well-documented problems with movement initiation in Parkinson's disease). The second group has been mostly assigned to loops through the cerebellum (compare to *dysmetria*, an inability to produce actions of appropriate magnitude, typical of cerebellar disorders). Houk and his colleagues hypothesized that, in the course of learning, the cerebellar neural structures learn to modulate activity of Purkinje cells in a predictive fashion, and further, this signal from Purkinje cells is combined with a cerebral cortical signal in the production of natural movements.

Self-test questions

1. What are the main functions of the spinal cord?
2. How many segments are there in the spinal cord? How many of those are in the lumbar enlargement?
3. Where in the spinal cord are the motoneurons located?
4. Are spinal reflexes weak or strong? Give a couple of examples in support of your answer.
5. What is reciprocal inhibition?
6. What is the function of Renshaw cells?
7. Describe the flexor reflex and the crossed extensor reflex.
8. Describe spinal reflex effects of afferents from Golgi tendon organs.
9. What is the clasp-knife phenomenon? Why does it happen?
10. What is the role of reflexes within the equilibrium-point hypothesis?
11. What factors, beyond descending signals from the brain, can modulate the threshold of the tonic stretch reflex?
12. What observations support the idea that the spinal cord contains central pattern generators?
13. Describe the half-center model.
14. Can the spinal cord organize multi-joint synergies stabilizing trajectory of the endpoint of a limb? Give examples.
15. What results with spinal cord stimulation support the idea that the spinal cord contains motor primitives?

16. Define spasticity. Give examples of positive and negative signs of spasticity.
17. Define muscle tone. What factors can contribute to tone as estimated in a typical clinical testing?
18. What observations support the idea that the brain contains representations of different functions?
19. What observations support the idea that the brain does not contain representations of different functions?
20. Define neural plasticity.
21. What is a distributed processing module?
22. Describe the main features of ascending and descending pathways.
23. Describe the main cortical layers.
24. How are the corticospinal and corticobulbar tracts organized?
25. Explain the notions of convergence and divergence in descending projections from the cortex.
26. What are the main characteristics of the readiness potential?
27. What is preferred direction of a cortical neuron?
28. What is the neuronal population vector?
29. What are the mirror neurons? What could be their functional role?
30. Describe the direct and indirect loops through the basal ganglia.
31. What are the main output structures of the basal ganglia?
32. Present examples of hypokinetic and hyperkinetic disorders associated with dysfunction of the basal ganglia.
33. What is the likely role of the basal ganglia in voluntary movements?
34. Describe the main differences between the two main inputs into the cerebellum.
35. What is the source of the parallel fibers?
36. What neurons do the climbing fibers make synapses on?
37. Can a single action potential along a mossy fiber produce a response from the cerebellum?
38. What is a complex spike? What neurons are capable of producing complex spikes?
39. What are the two main loops involving the cerebellum?
40. What are the main features of movement disorders associated with cerebellar dysfunction?
41. What are LTP and LTD?
42. What findings do support the idea that the cerebellum contains internal models?
43. What is the role of the cerebellum in distributed processing modules?

Essential references and recommended further readings

Amirikian, B., & Georgopoulos, A. P. (2003). Motor cortex: Coding and decoding of directional operations. In M. A. Arbib (Ed.), *The handbook of brain theory and neural networks* (2nd ed.). (pp. 690–701) Cambridge, MA: MIT Press.

Asanuma, H. (1973). Cerebral cortical control of movements. *Physiologist, 16*, 143–166.

Barto, A. G., Fagg, A. H., Sitkoff, N., & Houk, J. C. (1999). A cerebellar model of timing and prediction in the control of reaching. *Neural Computing, 11*, 565–594.

Bastian, A. J., Martin, T. A., Keating, J. G., & Thach, W. T. (1996). Cerebellar ataxia: abnormal control of interaction torques across multiple joints. *Journal of Neurophysiology, 76*, 492–509.

Berkinblit, M. B., Feldman, A. G., & Fukson, O. I. (1986a). Adaptability of innate motor patterns and motor control mechanisms. *Behavioral and Brain Science, 9*, 585–638.

Berkinblit, M. B., Gelfand, I. M., & Feldman, A. G. (1986b). A model for the control of multijoint movements. *Biofizika, 31*, 128–138.

Bernstein, N. A. (1996). On dexterity and its development. In M. L. Latash, & M. T. Turvey (Eds.), *Dexterity and its development* (pp. 1–244). Mahwah, NJ: Erlbaum Publishers.

Bizzi, E., Giszter, S. F., Loeb, E., Mussa-Ivaldi, F. A., & Saltiel, P. (1995). Modular organization of motor behavior in the frog's spinal cord. *Trends in Neuroscience, 18*, 442–446.

Bongaardt, R. (2001). How Bernstein conquered movement. In M. L. Latash, & V. M. Zatsiorsky (Eds.), *Classics in movement science* (pp. 59–84). Urbana, IL: Human Kinetics.

Celnik, P. A., & Cohen, L. G. (2004). Modulation of motor function and cortical plasticity in health and disease. *Restorative Neurology and Neuroscience, 22*, 261–268.

Evarts, E. V. (1968). Relation of pyramidal tract activity to force exerted during voluntary movement. *Journal of Neurophysiology, 31*, 14–27.

Feldman, A. G. (1986). Once more on the equilibrium-point hypothesis (λ-model). for motor control. *Journal of Motor Behavior, 18*, 17–54.

Fukson, O. I., Berkinblit, M. B., & Feldman, A. G. (1980). The spinal frog takes into account the scheme of its body during the wiping reflex. *Science, 209*, 1261–1263.

Georgopoulos, A. P. (1986). On reaching. *Annual Review of Neuroscience, 9*, 147–170.

Georgopoulos, A. P., Schwartz, A. B., & Kettner, R. E. (1986). Neural population coding of movement direction. *Science, 233*, 1416–1419.

Giszter, S. F., Mussa-Ivaldi, F. A., & Bizzi, E. (1993). Convergent force fields organized in the frog's spinal cord. *Journal of Neuroscience, 13*, 467–491.

Graybiel, A. M. (2005). The basal ganglia: learning new tricks and loving it. *Current Opinions in Neurobiology, 15*, 638–644.

Graziano, M. S., Aflalo, T. N., & Cooke, D. F. (2005). Arm movements evoked by electrical stimulation in the motor cortex of monkeys. *Journal of Neurophysiology, 94*, 4209–4223.

Hallett, M. (2001). Plasticity of the human motor cortex and recovery from stroke. *Brain Research Reviews, 36*, 169–174.

Holdefer, R. N., & Miller, L. E. (2002). Primary motor cortical neurons encode functional muscle synergies. *Experimental Brain Research, 146*, 233–243.

Houk, J. C. (2005). Agents of the mind. *Biological Cybernetics, 92*, 427–437.

Houk, J. C., Buckingham, J. T., & Barto, A. G. (1996). Models of the cerebellum and motor learning. *Behavioral and Brain Sciences, 19*, 368–383.

Ito, M. (1989). Long-term depression. *Annual Reviews of Neuroscience, 12*, 85–102.

Ivry, R. B., & Spencer, R. M. (2004). The neural representation of time. *Current Opinions in Neurobiology, 14*, 225–232.

Jankowska, E. (1979). New observations on neuronal organization of reflexes from tendon organ afferents and their relation to reflexes evoked from muscle spindle afferents. In R. Granit, & O. Pompeiano (Eds.), *Reflex control of posture and movement* (pp. 29–36). Amsterdam: Elsevier.

Latash, M. L. (2008). *Neurophysiological basis of movement* (2nd ed.). Urbana, IL: Human Kinetics.

Levin, M. F., & Feldman, A. G. (1994). The role of stretch reflex threshold regulation in normal and impaired motor control. *Brain Research, 657*, 23–30.

Matthews, P. B. C. (1959). The dependence of tension upon extension in the stretch reflex of the soleus of the decerebrate cat. *Journal of Physiology, 47*, 521–546.

Miller, L. E., Holdefer, R. N., & Houk, J. C. (2002). The role of the cerebellum in modulating voluntary limb movement commands. *Archives Italiennes de Biologie, 140*, 175–183.

Mussa-Ivaldi, F. A., Giszter, S. F., & Bizzi, E. (1994). Linear combinations of primitives in vertebrate motor control. *Proceedings of the National Academy of Sciences USA, 91*, 7534–7538.

Nichols, T. R. (1994). A biomechanical perspective on spinal mechanisms of coordinated muscular action: an architecture principle. *Acta Anatomica, 151*, 1–13.

Nichols, T. R. (2002). Musculoskeletal mechanics: a foundation of motor physiology. *Advances in Experimental and Medical Biology, 508*, 473–479.

Orlovsky, G. N., Deliagina, T. G., & Grillner, S. (1999). *Neuronal control of locomotion. From mollusc to man.* New York: Oxford University Press.

Penfield, W., & Rasmussen, T. (1950). *The cerebral cortex of man. A clinical study of localization of function.* New York: Macmillan.

Prochazka, A., Clarac, F., Loeb, G. E., Rothwell, J. C., & Wolpaw, J. R. (2000). What do reflex and voluntary mean? Modern views on an ancient debate. *Experimental Brain Research, 130*, 417–432.

Rizzolatti, G., & Craighero, L. (2004). The mirror-neuron system. *Annual Reviews in Neuroscience, 27*, 169–192.

Rizzolatti, G., Fogassi, L., & Gallese, V. (2001). Neurophysiological mechanisms underlying the understanding and imitation of action. *Nature Reviews in Neuroscience, 2*, 661–670.

Rothwell, J. C. (1994). *Control of human voluntary movement* (2nd ed.). London: Chapman & Hall.

Schieber, M. H., & Santello, M. (2004). Hand function: peripheral and central constraints on performance. *Journal of Applied Physiology, 96*, 2293–2300.

Sherrington, C. S. (1910). Flexion reflex of the limb, crossed extension reflex, and reflex stepping and standing. *Journal of Physiology, 40*, 28–121.

Smith, A. M. (1993). Babinski and movement synergism. *Revue Neurologique (Paris), 149*, 764–770.

Thach, W. T. (1998). A role for the cerebellum in learning movement coordination. *Neurobiology of Learning and Memory, 70*, 177–188.

Watts, R. L., & Koller, W. C. (Eds.). (2004). *Movement disorders. Neurological principles and practice* (2nd ed.). New York: McGraw-Hill.

11 Exemplary behaviors

Fundamentals of Motor Control. DOI: 10.1016/B978-0-12-415956-3.00011-7

11.1   Posture

Posture can be defined as a combination of the relative positions of body segments or of the whole body with respect to a *reference frame*. Postural control may refer to keeping the position of a body segment with respect to an external reference frame, for example to the environment or to an external object moving in the environment (consider holding the handles while riding a bicycle). Postural control may also refer to keeping the position of a segment with respect to the body itself. Here are a few examples of these aspects of postural control: (1) A ballet dancer or a figure skater maintaining a beautiful arm configuration while moving over the floor or the ice rink. (2) A waiter carrying a loaded tray on one of the hands through the crowded restaurant. (3) A carpenter holding a nail with a hand while hitting it with the hammer held by the other hand.

This chapter, however, will focus on another aspect of posture, that is, maintaining position of the whole body with respect to a particular direction in the environment, most commonly the direction of gravity. Examples of this aspect involve whole-body movements during standing, such as swaying, turning, stepping, etc.

Problems associated with standing

The mechanical stability of a stationary object in the field of gravity requires the projection of the *center of mass* to be kept within the support area. Human vertical posture is inherently unstable because of the relatively high center of mass location (about 1 m over the ground) and the relatively small effective area of support (on the order of 0.1 m^2). Sometimes, a standing person is compared to an inverted pendulum, an inherently unstable mechanical object. There are several joints between the center of mass of the body and the support area. This may be considered as an additional complicating factor since joint motions have to be coordinated, while each joint has to avoid occupying an uncomfortable position. Apparently, keeping the projection of the center of mass within the support area is possible only for certain combinations of positions in the individual joints. This is a *kinematically redundant problem*: Consider the task of keeping the center of mass coordinate in the anterior–posterior direction at a certain location by a three-joint system (ankle, knee, and hip) (Figure 11.1). Each of the joints is spanned by several muscles, which present another apparent problem of motor redundancy.

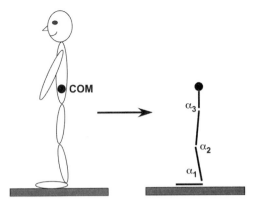

Figure 11.1 Vertical posture is inherently unstable because of the relatively high center of mass (COM) location, relatively small support area, and the joints between the COM and the support surface. The main joints are the ankle, knee, and hip (B).

Traditionally, three aspects of postural control are considered related to three typical tasks: quiet standing, performing quick actions while standing, and keeping vertical posture when an unexpected mechanical perturbation acts on the body. In other words, answers to the following three major questions are being searched for: How does a standing person manage not to fall down? How does a standing person prepare posture to a predictable perturbation associated with an action by the person? How is the fragile vertical posture protected from being destroyed by unexpected external forces?

Center of pressure

Postural studies typically consider a number of mechanical variables that can be measured using a force platform, a common tool that allows measurement of the forces and moments of force acting on the body (see Section 13.2). One of the most commonly used variables in postural studies is coordinate of the *center of pressure* (COP). The COP is the point of application of the resultant vertical force acting on the body from the supporting surface. Shifting the COP leads to changes in the moment of force acting on the body. COP shifts, therefore, may be viewed as the means of moving the COM, which has to follow the COP since the body can be in an equilibrium only when the projection of the COM on the support surface and the COP position coincide. Controlling COP by changing the activity of postural muscles is commonly viewed as a major mechanism that allows us to keep the COM projection within a safe area. COP coordinates can be computed if the moment of force acting on the body and the two forces that contribute to this moment of force are known. These force and moment components are measured by a typical force platform, as shown in Figure 11.2:

$$M_Y = COP_X \cdot F_Z + F_X \cdot d_X, \tag{11.1}$$

where X, Y, and Z are orthogonal directions of the coordinate system (Z is the vertical coordinate), M stands for moment of force, F stands for force, d_X stands for the lever

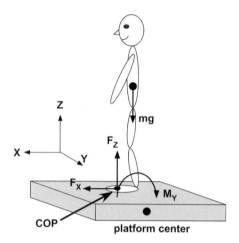

Figure 11.2 An illustration of computation of the center of pressure (COP) coordinate based on forces and moments of force measured by a typical force platform.

arm of the horizontal (shear) force F_X (note that d_X is measured along the z axis), and COP_X is the COP coordinate along the x axis. A similar equation can be written for the moment of force about the anterior–posterior axis (M_X): $M_X = COP_Y \cdot F_Z + FY \cdot d_Y$. Rearranging the two equations produces:

$$COP_X = (M_Y - F_X \cdot d_X)/F_Z, \tag{11.2}$$

$$COP_Y = (M_X - F_Y \cdot d_Y)/F_Z.$$

Postural sway

When a person tries to stand quietly and not to move, the center of mass projection demonstrates small, seemingly chaotic deviations from some average coordinate. These unintentional deviations are called *postural sway*. The term is also applied to unintentional deviations of the COP. When a young, healthy person stands quietly with open eyes, COP deviations in both anterior–posterior and medio-lateral directions are on the order of 5–10 mm. Center of mass displacements are smaller, on the order of a couple of millimeters. Closing the eyes leads to a substantial increase in the sway amplitude as well as in other variables commonly used to describe sway such as its average speed, area covered by the COP trajectory, etc.

Many studies have viewed postural sway as oscillation of an inverted pendulum about the ankle joint produced by the spring-like properties of the joint. According to this view, time changes of the ankle joint stiffness produce time changes in the body oscillation. The natural frequency (ω) of such a system in a sagittal plane, assuming no damping and small-amplitude oscillations, is:

$$\omega = \sqrt{[(K - W \cdot COM_Z)/I_A]}, \tag{11.3}$$

where K is the angular stiffness of the assumed joint spring, W is the weight of the body, COM_Z is the coordinate of the center of mass in the vertical direction, and I_A is the moment of inertia with respect to the ankles. The product $W \cdot COM_Z$ multiplied by $\sin\alpha$ (or simply by α for small deviations) yields a moment of gravity force.

This very simple model has several problems. First, the notion of joint stiffness is poorly defined (see Section 8.1). Stiffness can be used to describe deformable objects that produce force against deformation and store potential energy. Joints do not deform. Muscles and tendons do deform and can be assigned stiffness values. However, reducing a system with several muscles and tendons to a single spring is a gross simplification. Besides, *apparent stiffness* of a muscle changes with its activation level. Second, experimental estimations of the apparent ankle joint stiffness have produced conflicting results, typically much lower than necessary to stabilize the inverted pendulum representing the body. Third, it has been shown that the length of muscle fibers may change in the opposite direction to what could be concluded by observation of joint motion. In particular, body sway forward (stretching the plantarflexors) is, at certain phases, associated with shortening of the muscle fibers in the triceps surae group. This means that muscle fiber length changes may be in the opposite direction to the changes in the "muscle + tendon" complex. As a result, these changes are unable to produce restoring spring forces necessary to keep the body from falling. One obvious source of the mentioned problems is that they do not consider possible changes in the zero length of the muscle "springs." Such changes may be expected from changes in the threshold of the tonic stretch reflex according to the *equilibrium-point hypothesis* (Section 8.3).

The idea of a single-joint inverted pendulum has been developed assuming a neurally controlled torque generator at the ankle joint, acting in parallel to the "ankle joint spring," with torque magnitudes computed and implemented using feedback loops typical of control theory approaches. Such control schemes are sometimes rather complex, involving several loops acting in parallel driven by sensory signals of different modalities, with different time delays and adjustable gains. An example of such a scheme suggested by Robert Peterka is presented in Figure 11.3.

Rambling and trembling during standing

One of the important sources of problems of the abovementioned approach is the assumption that posture is stabilized with respect to a fixed coordinate corresponding to the unstable equilibrium of the inverted pendulum. A number of studies have provided strong evidence that the body sways not about a fixed point but about a migrating point. This approach views sway as a more complex phenomenon than previously thought; sway is assumed to represent the superposition of at least two processes. The two processes have been identified and quantified during quiet standing using the so-called *rambling–trembling decomposition* of postural sway.

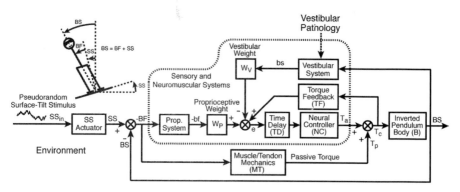

Figure 11.3 A typical scheme for postural control based on a single-joint inverted pendulum approximation. In this particular case, the analysis is focused on the roles of the vestibular and somatosensory signals in response to pseudorandom surface tilt; visual feedback is absent because the subject is assumed to stand with eyes closed. Reproduced by permission of the authors from Peterka, R. J., Statler, K. D., Wrisley, D. M., & Horak, F. B. (2011). Postural compensation for unilateral vestibular loss. *Frontiers in Neurology, 2*, 57.

The rambling–trembling decomposition is based on the idea that the body oscillates about a moving coordinate (*rambling*). The decomposition is considered separately for the two main sway directions, anterior–posterior and medio-lateral. When the COP coordinate happens to coincide with the current rambling coordinate, the body is at an instantaneous state of equilibrium. Because of its inertial (and other) properties, it moves through this state (oscillates about it, *trembling*). Rambling coordinates can be identified at time instants when the horizontal force acting on the body in the selected direction is zero. These points can be interpolated, that is connected with a smooth line, to produce the rambling trajectory, Rm(t) (Figure 11.4A). Trembling is defined as the difference between the COP(t) trajectory and Rm(t): Tr(t) = COP(t) − Rm(t) (see Figure 11.4B).

The idea of rambling–trembling decomposition fits well with the equilibrium-point hypothesis (see Section 8.3). Indeed, if one assumes that a neural controller defines a trajectory of the referent body position, the actual body trajectory is expected to follow the referent trajectory with a time delay characteristic of the body's mechanical properties, such as inertia, and the external force field. The actual body trajectory can also show oscillations, which may be absent in the referent trajectory, because of the inherently unstable vertical posture and both peripheral and reflex-defined length and velocity dependence of muscle force.

The latter interpretation of body sway views it not as noise in the system of postural control but as a combined mechanical outcome of a purposeful shift of the COP and peripheral properties of the neuromotor system. This view differs qualitatively from the control theory schemes, within which any deviation of the body from a position typical of quiet standing is viewed as the source of error signals. To illustrate the idea that the referent body position can change, note that humans can stand in a non-vertical posture (for example, leaning forward or backwards), and no corrective adjustments in the muscle activation levels are seen.

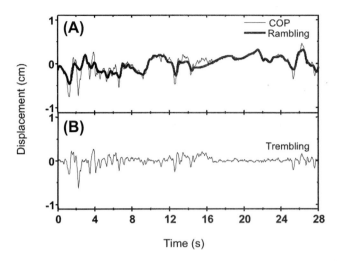

Figure 11.4 (A) Time profiles of the center of pressure (COP, thin line) and rambling (thick line) during quiet stance. (B) The corresponding trembling trajectory. Reproduced by permission from Latash, M. L. (2008). *Neurophysiological basis of movement*, 2nd edn. Urbana, IL: Human Kinetics.

Sway and postural stability

The relation between postural sway and postural stability is not trivial. *Mechanical stability* is typically defined as an ability to keep a state following a perturbation that takes the system away from that state. For example, a metal rod placed on one of its flat ends on the ground may show zero sway but it is very unstable, because even a slight push will make it fall to the ground. In some cases, *postural stability* (defined as an ability to keep balance when posture is perturbed) shows changes that are parallel to changes in the sway. For example, elderly persons show increased sway and worse postural stability. However, there are opposite examples. The most striking one is the reduced postural sway in some patients with Parkinson's disease, while postural instability is one of the cardinal features of this neurological disorder (see Section 10.5).

In addition to the involuntary postural sway seen under the instruction to stand quietly, humans can also produce voluntary sway. Whether the two are different reflections of basically the same control process is unknown, although the *Occam razor* (a simpler explanation of a phenomenon should be preferred over a more complex one) suggests that this is likely to be true. When body sway happens over substantial amplitude, joint deviations can be quantified with reasonable accuracy. Several typical patterns of joint motion can be observed during voluntary sway. If a person is asked to sway very slowly, much of the motion happens at the ankle joints. When the sway frequency increases, more and more involvement of the hip joints can be seen. The predominance of a limited number of joint motion patterns during voluntary sway has suggested that these patterns are preferred because of mechanical or neural reasons.

Joint equations of motion can be written using different variables. The most natural way is to write them using individual joint rotations and moments of force acting at the joints as the basic variables. The motion equation of a three-joint system in the field of gravity can be written in a matrix form as:

$$\mathbf{C}(\phi) \cdot d^2\phi/dt^2 - \mathbf{D}(\phi) \cdot \phi + \mathbf{A}(\phi, \, d\phi/dt) = \mathbf{T}, \qquad (11.4)$$

where $\mathbf{C}$ and $\mathbf{D}$ are inertial and gravitational matrices, $\mathbf{A}$ is a matrix reflecting centripetal and Coriolis forces, $\mathbf{T}$ is the vector of joint torques, and ϕ is the vector of joint angles. In a linear approximation, the equation can be simplified into:

$$\mathbf{C} \cdot d^2\phi/dt^2 - \mathbf{D} \cdot \phi = \mathbf{T}. \qquad (11.5)$$

This set of equations has all individual joint torques and motions dependent on each other. The equations can be re-written using a different set of variables that correspond to linear combinations of joint angles in such a way that motion along each of the new variables depends only on the torque vector component along that variable and does not depend on torque vector components along other variables. Such linear combinations of joint angles have been termed *eigenmovements*. A team of three neurophysiologists, two Russians, Alexander Frolov and Alexey Alexandrov, and one French, Jean Massion, performed analysis of whole-body movements by standing persons. They showed that frequently such movements were limited to a single eigenmovement performed with a certain amplitude.

Posture–movement paradox and the equilibrium-point hypothesis

In an earlier section, the posture–movement paradox has been mentioned (see Section 4.2). With respect to vertical posture, two body configurations were considered—vertical and leaning forward (see Figure 4.2). The question was: What kind of muscle activation pattern will be observed in the second (leaning) posture? There is no unambiguous answer. If a person occupies the vertical body configuration and then an unexpected push moves the body into the second, leaning forward, configuration (as in Figure 4.2A), large bursts of muscle activation will be observed trying to bring the body back to the original position. In contrast, if a person stands quietly while leaning forward (Figure 4.2B), a combination of relatively low, steady-state muscle activation levels will be observed with higher activation of the dorsal muscles that counteract the natural tendency of the body to fall forward. How does the central nervous system "know" when to produce bursts of muscle activation and when not to do this for the same posture of the body?

There is only one hypothesis in the area of motor control that handles the posture–movement paradox naturally. This is the equilibrium-point (referent configuration) hypothesis. According to this hypothesis, neural control results in setting a *referent configuration* of the body. If an actual body configuration coincides with the referent one, no muscle activation is observed. So, if a person occupies a posture (vertical or not) voluntarily, a new referent body configuration is established. Muscle activation in this configuration is minimal given the external force field. If a body is moved away from the referent configuration, muscles show relatively large changes in the activation levels directed at moving the body back to its original posture. For example, if a person who stands voluntarily while leaning forward (Figure 11.5) is pushed backwards, towards the more vertical posture, there will be bursts of activation of the ventral muscles trying to bring the body back to the original posture.

Within the referent configuration hypothesis, performing a voluntary movement, for example sway or sit-to-stand, is associated with a time shift of the referent configuration that results in muscle activation changes leading to a new body posture. This type of control is associated with a few non-trivial predictions. For example, if a person performs a rhythmic body movement, referent configuration is also expected to move rhythmically but not in phase with the body (the difference between the referent and actual configuration is driving the action). However, at certain phases the two configurations are expected to coincide. At those phases, all the muscles participating in the action are expected to show a global minimum in their activation levels (EMG). This prediction has been confirmed experimentally.

Vertical posture is protected against potentially destabilizing factors (perturbations) by several lines of defense. Posture-stabilizing mechanisms differ in their relative timing with respect to a perturbation and efficacy. They are summarized in Table 11.1.

Anticipatory postural adjustments

If a person performs an action that is expected to compromise posture, changes in the steady-state activation levels of postural muscles occur in anticipation of the action.

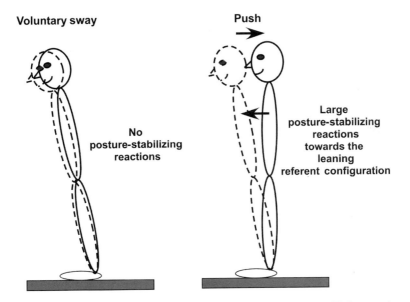

Figure 11.5 When a person sways voluntarily (left panel), no posture-stabilizing reactions are seen. If a similar deviation of the body from the vertical is produced by an external force (right panel), large posture-stabilizing reactions are seen in postural muscles.

Table 11.1 Main posture-stabilizing mechanisms

	Time delay	Positive features	Negative features
Anticipatory postural adjustments (APAs)	<0	Feed-forward; allow preparation to a perturbation	Based on prediction; always suboptimal
Muscle/tendon elasticity	0	Act instantaneously; always against the local perturbation	Not strong enough; not task-specific
Reflexes	30 ms	Act after a short delay; negative feedback loops	Poor central control; jerky
Pre-programmed reactions (long latency reflexes, M_{2-3})	70 ms	Act after a short delay; task-specific	Produce approximate correction
Voluntary corrections	150 ms	Task-specific	Long time delay

Such *anticipatory postural adjustments* (APAs) are commonly seen about 100 ms prior to activation of muscles that initiate the intended, focal action. Examples of such actions include fast arm movements performed by a standing person, pushing against an object, lifting, catching, and dropping objects, etc.

The traditional view on APAs is that they represent consequences of neural commands generated in anticipation of a predictable perturbation (in a *feed-forward* manner) based on the estimated effects of the perturbation on posture. The purpose of APAs has been assumed to generate forces and moments of force that would counteract the perturbing forces and moments of force and, in the best-case scenario, cancel them out. This rarely happens because APAs are based on predicted mechanical effects of perturbations, which may differ substantially from their actual effects. As a result, APAs are always mechanically suboptimal. APAs are associated with reproducible shifts of the COP that are most commonly compatible with the hypothesis that their role is to counteract the expected effects of the action on posture. Note that "not falling down" may be only one of the purposes of APAs; these postural adjustments may also be associated with keeping posture in individual joints and avoiding large movements of the head, for example to preserve constancy of visual perception and to avoid large changes in the vestibular signals.

Three main factors define the pattern and magnitude of APAs (Figure 11.6). First, APAs scale with the expected direction and magnitude of the *perturbation*. This is not surprising given their assumed functional purpose. Second, APAs scale with the magnitude of *voluntary action* performed by the subject. This is less obvious. In most everyday situations, stronger actions are associated with stronger expected postural perturbations. Examples include performing faster and slower movements and lifting heavy and light objects. However, in some cases, action magnitude does not scale with the perturbation magnitude. For example, if a standing person shoots a rifle, the recoil may be very strong although the action (pressing the trigger) is minimal. In

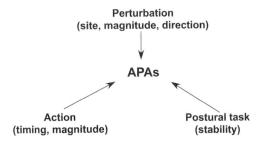

Figure 11.6 Anticipatory postural adjustments (APAs) depend on the magnitude (and other characteristics) of the expected perturbation, the magnitude of the action associated with the perturbation, and postural stability.

such cases, APAs are scaled down with the magnitude of the action, and a major postural perturbation is observed. Compare the effects of the recoil on the trunk in an inexperienced person (who may nearly lose their balance) and in an experienced marksman or biathlon expert (who may show next to no visible effects on posture). In addition, APAs depend on the time available to make a decision. For example, compared to self-paced actions performed at a self-selected time, in simple reaction time conditions (the person is asked to move as quickly as possible following an auditory or visual signal), APAs start closer to the time of action initiation or even simultaneously with the action. Third, APAs scale with *postural stability*. This scaling is non-trivial: APAs are reduced when a person stands in very stable conditions (for example, while leaning against the wall) and also in very unstable conditions (for example, while standing on a board with reduced support area). The former effect is easier to interpret: Indeed, if the posture is well protected against perturbations, APAs may become unnecessary. The latter effect is less trivial. It is associated with the fact that, in certain conditions, the APAs may themselves turn into sources of postural perturbations. APAs are associated with shifts of the COP and changes in the shear forces. If the area of support is narrow, a large COP shift may move outside this area and trigger loss of balance. Similarly, if one stands on a low-friction surface (for example, on ice), a large shear force may lead to slippage and fall.

In certain conditions, APAs can actually act not against the expected perturbation but with it. This happens when a person performs an action that triggers APAs in conditions where it is much safer to move the body in the direction of the perturbation than against it. For example, if one stands on the edge of a precipice and performs an action that by itself perturbs the body away from the precipice, typical APAs acting against the perturbation may be too dangerous (imagine that the perturbation is expected but it does not come!). In such a situation, APAs may be seen moving the body from the edge.

Length and velocity dependence of muscle force, co-contraction, and preflexes

If a perturbation comes unexpectedly, no APAs can be produced. Then, the body has to rely on reactive mechanisms to counteract the effects of the perturbation on balance. An important, and frequently overlooked, line of defense is the length- and velocity-dependence of muscle force. As a result, force changes are directed against the changes in muscle length at a close to zero time delay. As such, they always act against the perturbation. Stronger perturbations produce larger muscle length changes and lead to stronger peripheral length- and velocity-dependent responses. These properties of muscle force can be modified by the central nervous system by changing the background level of muscle activation: More active muscles show higher apparent stiffness. So, if one knows that a perturbation may come but does not know when or in what direction, it is possible to prepare for the perturbation by *co-contracting* agonist–antagonist postural muscle groups. This may not be the most efficient method of stabilizing posture; nevertheless, it is seen in certain situations. The instantaneous muscle reactions to perturbations modulated via their pre-activation have been termed *preflexes* in contrast to reflexes that are always mediated by the central nervous system and come after a substantial time delay.

Posture-stabilizing role of reflexes

APAs and preflexes are only able to produce approximate and typically insufficient changes in muscle forces. The next line of defense is reflex and reflex-like responses mediated by the central nervous system. As mentioned in Section 3.4, reflexes are typically *negative feedback loops*, which means that they always act to reduce the effects of a factor that caused them. Monosynaptic reflexes are rarely produced by postural perturbations because they require a very quick muscle stretch. This does not mean that monosynaptic projections of Ia-afferents on alpha-motoneurons are not functioning or unimportant. Simply, by themselves, these projections do not lead to motor unit recruitment.

Polysynaptic reflexes, in particular the tonic stretch reflex, represent major posture-stabilizing mechanisms. They are assumed to be the main mechanism of ensuring an equilibrium state given a referent configuration of the body and the external force field. However, if a perturbation is strong, these mechanisms turn out to be insufficiently strong because their gain is relatively low.

Pre-programmed reactions to postural perturbations

The next group of neurally mediated muscle responses has a variety of names. Among the most commonly used ones are long-latency responses, pre-programmed reactions, and triggered reactions. General features of these responses have been described briefly in Section 3.4. They occur at intermediate latencies, about 50–70 ms, which are longer than the typical latencies of spinal reflexes (20–40 ms) and shorter than the quickest simple reaction time (>90 ms). These responses are context-dependent. In particular, they can be modulated by instruction to the subject whether to react to a perturbation or to let the perturbation move the effector (or the body).

Two commonly seen patterns of long-latency responses to the perturbation of body equilibrium have been described by Lewis Nashner and Fay Horak as the *ankle strategy* and the *hip strategy* (Figure 11.7). The former pattern is observed in young,

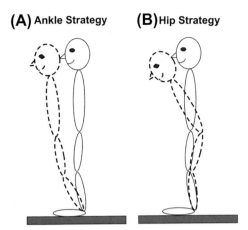

(A) Ankle Strategy   **(B)** Hip Strategy

Figure 11.7 An illustration of changes in joint configuration during postural adjustments using the ankle strategy (A) and hip strategy (B).

healthy persons who stand quietly, and a relatively small perturbation is applied unexpectedly (Figure 11.7A). This pattern starts with major changes in the activation of muscles crossing the ankle joint and involves body motion mostly about the ankle joints. For example, if a person stands on a platform, and the platform moves forward unexpectedly, there will be an initial deviation of the body backwards from the vertical posture. The quickest reaction, at a delay of about 70 ms (depending on the length of the subject's legs), will be observed in the tibialis anterior leading to a body sway forward about the ankle joint, thus correcting the perturbation-induced deviation. If the platform moves backwards, the initial reaction is seen in the triceps surae muscle group.

The hip strategy can be seen in young subjects standing on a surface with reduced support area and/or in response to a stronger perturbation (Figure 11.7B). This strategy involves the earliest and strongest changes in the activation of hip muscles leading to a large-amplitude hip motion. The hip strategy can also be seen in elderly persons standing naturally without any complicating factors. The kinematic patterns of the two strategies resemble two of the three eigenmovements as introduced earlier. The predominance of these strategies provides additional support for the idea of eigenmovements as building blocks for typical postural actions and reactions.

Patterns of long-latency responses are strongly context-specific: The same perturbation can lead to such responses in different muscle groups depending on the initial posture and other factors. For example, if a person stands in a bus and holds onto a rail, an unexpected movement of the bus will produce posture-stabilizing responses in the arm muscles in addition to more typical responses in the leg and trunk muscles. If the person is holding a mug of hot coffee in the right hand, the same unexpected bus motion will produce a very different pattern of arm muscle responses, stabilizing the position and orientation of the mug. These examples suggest that posture-stabilizing mechanisms mediated by long-latency responses are directed not at individual muscles or joints but at a task-specific set of variables that describe body configuration in the most salient way. *Referent body configuration* at the highest level of the hierarchical system involved in postural control may be viewed as a combination of referent values for those most salient variables. In the example of a person with a mug of coffee in the hand, the referent configuration may include the orientation of the hand with the mug with respect to the vertical.

Role of sensory information in postural control

Effective postural control is impossible without sensory information. For example, patients who suffer from a very rare disorder called *large-fiber peripheral neuropathy* lose sensation in their limbs, while the axons of the motoneurons are not affected. Such patients can produce sufficient muscle forces, but they are unable to stand with eyes closed. Opening the eyes makes standing and other activities associated with vertical posture, such as walking, possible. Similar postural problems, but less dramatic, may be seen in persons who suffer from advanced stages of diabetes. These persons frequently lose sensory information from the distal portions of the legs. Although information from more proximal body parts is preserved, standing with eyes closed in nearly impossible. These observations point out the crucial importance of two sources of information for postural control—somatosensory signals from the legs, particularly from the feet, and visual information. In contrast, vestibular information that is unaffected in both abovementioned groups of patients is unable by itself to allow balance to be maintained.

The last statement may sound unexpected because *vestibular information* has been shown to have a strong effect on postural control. This information is produced by sensory receptors located in the inner ear that are sensitive to linear and rotational acceleration. In particular, these receptors are expected to signal head orientation with respect to gravity. Signals from the vestibular apparatus act on *vestibular nuclei*, which also receive inputs from the cerebellum. Four paired nuclei form the vestibular nuclei group; these are called the *superior, lateral, medial,* and *inferior nuclei*. The lateral vestibular nucleus is also known as the *Deiters' nucleus*. The vestibular nuclei are the origins of the *vestibulospinal tracts* that play a major role in the neural control of both body and head posture. In particular, the lateral vestibular tract that originates from the Deiters' nucleus produces ipsilateral facilitatory effects on both alpha- and gamma-motoneurons innervating limb muscles. This tonic input helps to maintain the background activity of antigravity muscles. Observations of patients with vestibular disorders support the important role of the vestibular system in the control of vertical posture.

Recently, a German scientist, Thomas Mergner, and his colleagues have suggested a hypothesis that vestibular information produces a reference frame within which information from other sensory receptors is evaluated. Obviously, in the absence of information from non-vestibular receptors, the intact reference frame by itself is next to useless for balance control. On the other hand, having signals from non-vestibular receptors without a reference frame makes it impossible to quantify those signals and extract relevant information.

The importance of visual information for postural control has already been illustrated with examples of patients who are able to stand with eyes open, but not with eyes closed. Manipulations of visual information have been shown to lead to major effects on posture. For example, if a standing person looks at a screen or wears goggles that display a projection of an artificially created environment (a so-called *virtual environment*), movement of an image on the screen or of the virtual environment produces major postural deviations from the vertical.

Effects of light touch on posture

Somatosensory information can be used for postural control in two ways. First, it signals the distribution of pressure under the feet, joint positions, and muscle forces. This information is important for both quiet stance and postural reactions to perturbations. Second, it can help identify body position and orientation in space in the absence of vision. This second role of somatosensory information has been demonstrated in studies of the effects of light touch on posture performed by James Lackner and his colleagues. When a person stands with eyes closed, body sway increases substantially. However, if a standing person is allowed to touch a stationary object with a finger, the sway magnitude is reduced dramatically. In such studies, the force produced by the finger on the external object was always kept under 1 N, which is insufficient to produce mechanical stabilizing effects. Hence, it has been concluded that the main effect of finger touch is mediated by sensory information provided by the finger pressure-sensitive receptors and maybe other receptors in the hand.

The importance of touch information for postural control has been confirmed in studies when a person stood with eyes closed and touched lightly a touch-pad that could move slowly in one of the two main directions—anterior–posterior and mediolateral. Motion of the touch-pad entrained the body sway: The body started to move in-phase with the motion of the touch-pad.

Light touch has also been shown to attenuate APAs. This observation is far from obvious. Since the purpose of the APAs is to counteract expected external perturbations, light touch is not expected to help because it is mechanically inefficient. The touch, however, allows the central nervous system to be more confident in the current location of the body and the safety margin, that is, the distance from the center of mass projection to the edge of the support area. Hence, as compared to standing without touching an object, standing while touching an external object may be compared to standing in more stable conditions, and APAs are known to be reduced under more stable conditions.

This brief review suggests that sensory signals of various modalities play important roles in postural control. The importance of signals from different sources may be task-specific and may also change with practice. These effects have been referred to as *sensory reweighting*. Most commonly, sensory reweighting has been discussed within the control theory approach: Vertical standing has been modeled as the task of balancing an inverted pendulum by a control system with several feedback loops acting in parallel that are characterized by different gains, time delays, and other characteristics, such as the frequency response, which reflects the dependence of the gain in the feedback loop on the frequency of the incoming signal.

Muscle synergies in postural tasks

During standing, postural control requires coordinated changes in the activation levels of numerous muscles. Since the classical studies of the great British neurologist Hughlings Jackson, researchers have agreed that the brain is unlikely to specify activation levels of individual muscles. Rather, muscles are united into task-specific groups and one control variable is used to adjust the muscle activation levels within each group. This idea is illustrated in Figure 11.8.

Several methods have been used to identify such muscle groups. All these methods belong to the group of matrix factorization methods (see Section 6.4). They analyze correlations or co-variations between activation indices of all possible pairs of muscles and then look for linear combinations of such indices (referred to as *synergies* or *muscle modes*) that allow a relatively large amount of variance in the original data set to be described with a relatively small number of muscle groups. Typical methods include principal component analysis, factor analysis, non-negative matrix factorization, and independent component analysis. These methods have been used to analyze multi-muscle systems in various tasks not limited to posture, such as locomotion, grasping, and hand force production.

According to the definition offered earlier (see Section 9.4), synergies represent neural organizations that stabilize important features of performance by co-varied adjustments of elemental variables. Based on this definition, groups of muscles with linear scaling of activation levels do not immediately qualify as synergies. However, they do qualify as elemental variables manipulated by the controller. Under this assumption, a multi-muscle (more exactly, multi-muscle mode) synergy is co-variation of muscle-mode magnitudes across trials that stabilizes a value or a time profile of an important mechanical variable. Several studies have shown that muscle-mode magnitudes do co-vary across trials to stabilize shifts of the COP (and also shear force magnitude) during a variety of tasks performed by standing subjects. Such tasks involve

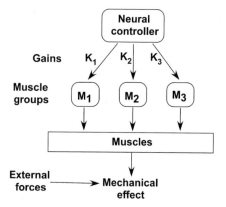

Figure 11.8 Hierarchical control of multi-muscle systems. The controller unites the muscles into groups (muscle modes, M_1–M_3) and uses one variable per mode (k) to produce parallel changes in the muscle activation.

postural preparation to quick arm movement and to load release from extended arms, voluntary sway, and preparation to making a step.

Preparation to making a step

The issue of postural preparation to stepping is intermediate between the control of posture and locomotion. When a person stands quietly with the weight distributed evenly between the two feet, it is impossible to lift a leg without losing balance. Besides, to initiate body motion in a desired direction, typically forward, external forces from the supporting surface have to be changed appropriately. To accomplish these mechanically necessitated goals, a rather stereotypical shift of the COP is observed prior to stepping (Figure 11.9). In the anterior–posterior direction, the COP shifts backwards. This allows a moment of the vertical ground reaction force to be generated, rotating the body forward. Simultaneously, the COP shifts in the medio-lateral direction, first towards the stepping leg and then towards the supporting leg, thus unloading the stepping leg. The COP shifts during step initiation are stabilized by multi-muscle mode synergies based on muscle modes that involve leg muscles and also muscles of the trunk.

11.2   Locomotion

Locomotion, by definition, is motor activity that leads to a change in location of the whole body in external space. There are numerous forms of locomotion used by animals, including crawling, hopping, flying, swimming, walking, and running. Many animals are able to use various forms of locomotion, for example to fly, to swim, and to walk. Lower animals do not locomote; as a result, their activity is limited to a small area in a close proximity to the body. The emergence of locomotion within the

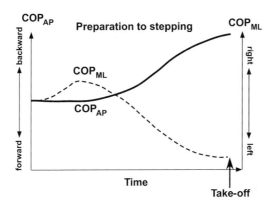

Figure 11.9 During preparation to stepping, the center of pressure (COP) is shifted backwards (COP$_{AP}$, solid line) and towards the supporting leg (COP$_{ML}$, dashed line) after a transient deviation towards the stepping leg.

evolutionary process led to the emergence of new motor and non-motor tasks and likely played a major role in the formation of the central nervous system of the contemporary higher animals, including humans.

Gaits

Within this chapter, the focus will be on the most common forms of locomotion used by humans, such as walking and running. Locomotor patterns are commonly described using sets of mechanical and electromyographic variables. These patterns demonstrate rhythmic, consistent changes during steady-state locomotion. For example, during walking, the angular joint trajectories within the right and left legs are nearly symmetrical. They show, however, a phase shift of about 180°. The relative phase of homologous joint trajectories across limbs is one of the main characteristics of locomotion that defines gait. Figure 11.10 illustrates the limb positions relative to the body when a quadrupedal animal walks, trots, and gallops. During walking, each of the right–left limb pairs shows out-of-phase movements (phase shift close to 180°); the forelimb–hindlimb pairs on each side also show out-of-phase movements. During *trotting*, the forelimb–hindlimb pairs move in phase, while the right–left pairs continue to move out of phase; in humans, this gait involves in-phase movements of the leg and arm on the same side of the body and looks rather awkward. During *galloping*, the situation is reversed: The right–left limb pairs move in phase, while the forelimb–hindlimb pairs move out of phase.

In humans, walking and running are associated with out-of-phase motion of the two legs and of the two arms, while the arm and leg on the same side of the body also move out of phase. The difference between walking and running is not in the relative phase of limb motion but in the presence or absence of the double-support phase, that is, the phase when both feet touch the ground (as in the left drawing in Figure 11.10).

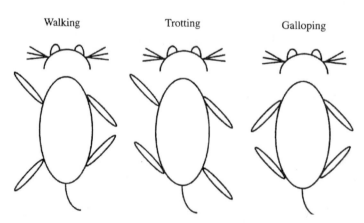

Walking   Trotting   Galloping

Figure 11.10 An illustration of gaits in quadrupeds: walk, trot, and gallop (left-to-right). Reproduced by permission from Latash, M. L. (2008). *Neurophysiological basis of movement*, 2nd edn. Urbana, IL: Human Kinetics.

Humans do not trot, unless they work in the infamous Ministry of Silly Walks immortalized by Monty Python, while galloping is possible—it is called hopping.

The purpose of the *accompanying arm movements* during walking is likely to minimize trunk rotation that would otherwise be produced by the asymmetrical leg motion and foot interaction with the ground. Minimizing trunk rotation, in turn, helps to stabilize head orientation in space and contributes to the relative stability of vestibular signals and constancy of visual perception. The lack of associated arm movements is a pathological sign that can be observed, for example, in patients with Parkinson's disease. It is a component of their bradykinesia (see Section 10.5).

Static and dynamic stability

Bipedal locomotion is a challenging task: It is performed on the background of the inherently unstable bipedal posture, plus it adds complicating factors such as transient changes in the decreased area of support and the reactive forces from the ground that show large transient peaks. However, as the reader can recall from his or her experience, walking is much easier than keeping balance while standing on one foot. This example illustrates the important difference between *static and dynamic stability*.

A mechanical system is considered to be in a *stable equilibrium state* if it returns to this state following a small transient perturbation. An equilibrium state is called *unstable* if a small perturbation leads to motion of the object away from the equilibrium. Figure 11.11 illustrates the notions of stable and unstable equilibrium using, as an example, a ball on a rigid surface.

For moving systems, the notion of stability is more complex. If the same ball rolls downhill along a semi-circular slide, a small perturbation would cause a change in the trajectory of the ball, but ultimately it will end up at the bottom of the slide, not too far from its central line. Similarly, if the ball is released several times at slightly different spots at the top of the slide, it will show somewhat different trajectories, but they will all lead to about the same location at the bottom of the slide. If the slide is not concave but flat or, even worse, convex, a small push will lead to a major change in the trajectory of the ball, and it will not return close to the expected location at the bottom. The two slides illustrated in Figure 11.12 would be called *dynamically stable* and *dynamically unstable*, respectively; a system is dynamically unstable if a small

(A)   **(B)**

Stable equilibrium   Unstable equilibrium

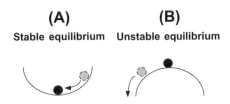

Figure 11.11 An illustration of stable (A) and unstable (B) static equilibrium. If the ball is pushed away from the equilibrium state (compare the gray and black circles), it tends to return to the equilibrium in A, but not in B.

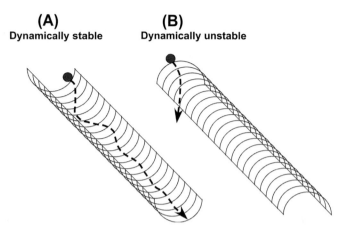

Figure 11.12 An illustration of the notion of dynamic stability. A ball released at different points of the concave slide (A) tends to return close to the center of the slide (assuming non-zero friction). A ball released at different points of the convex slide (B) drops off the slide.

change in the initial conditions or a small transient perturbation induces a deviation from a planned trajectory, and this deviation increases with time.

Bipedal locomotion can show dynamic stability. This has been demonstrated in studies of so-called *passive locomotion*. In those studies, inanimate bipedal objects looking like a crude doll with two legs and with only the "hip joint" per leg were placed on an inclined surface. The "feet" were shaped to allow a rolling motion, which lifted the contralateral leg. There were no motors, and energy for locomotion was provided by gravity. Such passive walkers were able to show stable locomotion without falling down within a range of slopes of the surface. Loss of stability most frequently happened in the medio-lateral direction, which could be remedied by adjusting the shape of the "feet."

Aspects of locomotion mechanics

The mechanical characteristics of locomotion differ across animals and depend strongly on the properties of muscles and tendons. Since locomotion involves cyclic loading and unloading of individual legs, the length-dependence of muscle and tendon forces is very important for storing energy during loading and recoiling it during unloading. The most famous example is hopping of kangaroos, whose very long, elastic tendons allow energy to be stored and recoiled during each hop with minimal energy losses. As a result, kangaroos do not have to produce large phasic changes in muscle activation levels, resulting in a very economic regime for traveling over large distances.

The mechanics of locomotion have been viewed as a combination of two pendular movements. On the one hand, the body may be viewed as an inverted pendulum swinging about the ankle joint of the supporting leg. On the other hand, the swing leg may be viewed as a pendulum swinging about the hip joint. Both models are very crude and fail to account for basic observations, such as energy generation and absorption and patterns of muscle activation during locomotion. These models have been made more sophisticated by adding springs acting at the suspension point of the pendulums. However, the relation of the model parameters to neurophysiology remains obscure.

Stepping and referent configuration hypothesis

Locomotion has been viewed as a particular example of voluntary motor action within the referent configuration hypothesis (see Section 8.4). Remember that within this hypothesis control of movements is produced by changing neurophysiological variables (levels of depolarization of neuronal pools) that translate into shifts of referent values for salient mechanical variables such as, for example, trajectories of important points on the body. Shifts of the referent configuration produce changes in the equilibrium state of the system "body + environment," and an action (movement and/ or force production) takes place towards the newly established equilibrium state. If the referent position of the body moves in such a way that it is always somewhat ahead of its current position (Figure 11.13), a whole-body motion will take place, and it will continue until the referent configuration stops, and the body rests in a new equilibrium state.

Spinal and supraspinal mechanisms of locomotion

In the 1960s, a series of studies on decerebrate cats by a team of Russian physiologists, Grigory Orlovsky, Feodor Severin, and Mark Shik, led to a major advance in the understanding of the spinal and supraspinal mechanisms of locomotion. *Decerebration*

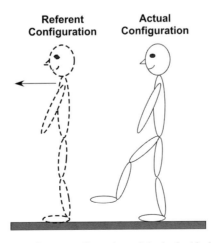

Figure 11.13 Motion of the referent configuration of the body (dashed) leads to whole-body motion.

involves a transection of the midbrain between the inferior and superior colliculi. As a result, no signals from the cortex can reach the spinal cord and affect movements. Such animals cannot maintain the typical standing posture on their own and have to be supported by a system of belts. If the paws of such an animal are placed on a treadmill, motion of the treadmill can produce rhythmic leg movements with corresponding phasic muscle activation patterns that resemble leg movements during natural loco-motion. The relative phase of motion of individual legs depends on the speed of the treadmill. At slow speeds, it is typical of the inter-limb coordination during walking. Speeding the treadmill up produces a switch to trot and then to gallop.

Using this preparation, the group of Orlovsky, Shik, and Severin explored the effects of electrical stimulation of different structures in the medulla and brainstem. They discovered an area in the reticular formation (an elongated structure that extends from the medulla into the midbrain, Figure 11.14) where electrical stimulation could produce locomotion patterns when the treadmill was in a passive mode, that is, the treadmill could be moved by the legs of the animal, but it was not powered. This area was termed the *mesencephalic locomotor region*. The frequency of the leg motion did not match the frequency of the electrical stimulation. Changing the strength (amplitude and/or frequency) of the stimulating current could produce a change in the gait patterns, from walking to trotting and to galloping. Later, similar effects were observed in response to stimulation within a particular zone in the upper cervical part of the spinal cord; this area was termed the *locomotor strip*.

These results suggested strongly that locomotion was produced by spinal struc-tures—*central pattern generators*—which received excitatory projections from supraspinal structures such as the mesencephalic locomotor region. To test this hypothesis, studies of so-called *fictive locomotion* were performed. In those studies, the cats were injected with *curare*, a chemical substance extracted from certain plants that had been used for centuries by hunters in South America. Curare blocks the neuromuscular transmission and paralyzes the animal. Curarized animals had to be placed on artificial ventilation because it paralyzes the muscles involved in breathing. Electrical stimulation of the mesencephalic locomotor area in such animals produced no motion; however, electrodes in the ventral horns of the spinal cord showed bursts of action potentials in the axons of alpha-motoneurons that innervated muscles involved in locomotion. These bursts showed the same phase relations as during actual locomotion in non-curarized cats.

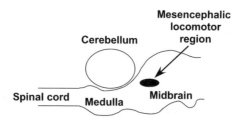

Figure 11.14 Location of the mesencephalic locomotor center is shown in this cartoon with respect to other structures of the central nervous system.

Taken together, these results show that the spinal cord contains neural structures able to generate patterned activity in response to peripheral information (as in the abovementioned experiments with treadmill motion) and to descending signals from structures within the brain. Changing the strength of the input (amplitude and/or frequency of the electrical stimulation or the speed to treadmill motion) can result in gait changes. Further studies showed that turning these locomotion central pattern generators (CPGs) on was also possible with the help of certain neurotransmitters injected into the spinal cord such as DOPA (a neuroactive substance, which is also known as a drug commonly used to treat Parkinson's disease).

Central pattern generators for locomotion

Spinal CPGs for locomotion have not been identified in mammals. Indirect evidence suggests that there are at least as many such CPGs as there are legs, and these individual leg-specific CPGs are coordinated by neural signals produced by a hierarchically higher neural structure, resulting in their relative phasing typical of quadrupedal gaits. Some studies even suggested the existence of joint-specific CPGs coordinated by neural signals from the corresponding leg-specific CPGs. In those studies electrical stimulation was applied directly to the lumbar enlargement of the spinal cord of patients with a *clinically complete spinal cord injury*. This means that the patients could not feel their legs (no feelings of touch, temperature, and motion) and could not produce visible muscle activation in the legs voluntarily. The patients were supine, and their legs were supported in the air by a system of belts. Stimulation of the lumbar enlargement could produce rhythmic muscle activation in the legs leading to leg motion that resembled running. The two legs could both be involved, moving in phase or out of phase, or the rhythmic activity could be limited to one leg and, sometimes, even to one joint. Since the frequency of the induced motion did not correspond to the frequency of the stimulation, it was concluded that the stimulation produced activation of leg CPGs, not direct activation of alpha-motoneurons.

The switching of gaits during locomotion with a change in the external stimulus resembles behavior of *dynamical systems*, which have been shown to switch to new relative phase values with a change in an input variable (see Section 9.3). Within the dynamical systems approach, the idea of CPGs is not very popular. Indeed, this approach considers the relative timing of motor patterns to be an emergent property of a complex system that involves the neural and peripheral structures of the body and the environmental mechanical and sensory variables. However, the existence of CPGs has received very strong experimental support in higher animals, and neural structures forming CPGs have been identified in lower animals such as the lamprey. Likely, the ideas of internal neural CPGs and dynamical systems (there is no argument that the body is a complex dynamical system) should be merged into a single coherent scheme.

Corrective stumbling reaction

Locomotion happens in an unpredictable environment. It is protected from unexpected perturbations by a system of *pre-programmed reactions* (also known as *long-latency reflexes*, see Section 3.4). In the case of locomotion, such reactions are called *corrective stumbling reactions*. Such reactions are seen in response to a sensory stimulus applied to the foot or lower leg; in humans, they have a latency of about 50–70 ms and appear in many muscles of the leg. When a stimulus (for example, a touch to the foot or an electrical stimulus applied to the sural nerve) occurs during the stance phase, a response is seen in the major extensor muscles leading to accelerated step (Figure 11.15). If a similar stimulus is applied in the swing phase, the response is seen in the major flexor muscles, and the leg "steps over" the invisible obstacle. The meaning of the responses becomes clear if one considers how such stimuli could occur in real life. When a person or an animal steps on a sharp object, it is impossible to withdraw the leg because it supports the weight of the body. Hence, accelerating the step minimizes the damage done to the foot by the object. When a foot hits an object (a stone or a branch) on its way during the swing phase, the flexor reaction lifts the foot and allows it to clear the obstacle.

Reflex reversals

Switching a reflex-like response to a standard stimulus from one muscle group to another is called *reflex reversal*. Reflex reversals were observed a long time ago in lower animals. In early studies, the choice between activation of one of the two opposing muscles (an agonist–antagonist pair) was defined by the relative muscle length: The longer muscle was more likely to respond. This rule was called the *Üexkull law*, after a German researcher who discovered it in studies of reflex responses in the starfish.

Reflex reversals have been documented in many animals, including humans. For example, high-frequency, low-amplitude vibration applied to the tendon of a major leg muscle produces an unusually high level of activation of muscle spindle endings which can lead to tonic muscle activation (*tonic vibration reflex*). The tonic vibration reflex is unusual in several aspects. First, it can be suppressed voluntarily by the

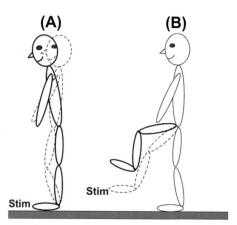

Figure 11.15 Corrective stumbling reaction. If a stimulus is applied to the sole of the foot at the beginning of the stance phase (A), extension in all major joints is observed and the step is accelerated. If a similar stimulus is applied during the swing phase (B), flexion of major joints is observed, and the leg "steps over" the invisible obstacle.

**Patterns of the
tonic vibration reflex**

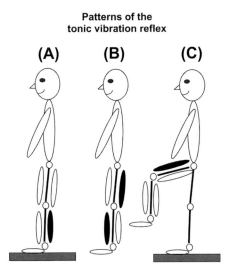

Figure 11.16 Patterns of the tonic vibration reflex (vibration can be applied to the Achilles and/or patellar tendon) when the person stands on the foot (A), when the person stands on the other foot only (B), and when the leg is flexed (C). The reflex activated muscles are shown with black ellipses. Note that the pattern of activation is similar to that observed during locomotion when the person moves through the illustrated phases.

subject. In other words, the subject may or may not allow muscle activation to happen. The reflex muscle activation is accompanied by strong presynaptic inhibition of Ia-afferent inputs into the alpha-motoneurons, resulting in suppression of monosynaptic reflexes (such as the H-reflex, see Section 3.4). In addition, reflex muscle activation can switch between the ankle flexors and extensors and between the knee flexors and extensors, depending on the leg posture and presence or absence of load applied to the foot. Typical patterns of muscle activation to vibration of the Achilles tendon (or the patellar tendon) in different postures are shown in Figure 11.16. They resemble muscle activation patterns observed when a person moves through the shown postures during walking. It seems possible, therefore, that the unusual afferent inflow produced by vibration projects on structures within the CPG and allows snap-shots of muscle activation that would be produced by the CPG during its natural activity to be observed. This interpretation has received support from recent studies demonstrating that muscle vibration can induce locomotor-like leg movements in healthy persons.

11.3   Reaching

Reaching arm movements represent building blocks for many everyday movements performed by humans. The purpose of such movements is to bring the end-effector (for example, the hand or a digit) into a certain point in space. Another common aspect of reaching movements is to ensure a proper orientation of the end-effector, for example during pointing at a remote object. Standing and locomotion rely on a variety of reflex-like mechanisms providing stability of those actions and commonly proceed without much conscious control. In contrast, reaching movements are produced to targets with different locations and orientations with respect to the body and the field of gravity. As a result, reaching movements involve conscious control to a much larger degree and offer a window into the organization of cortical and subcortical control of actions.

Typical features of reaching movements

The following common features have been described for multi-joint reaching (Figure 11.17). First, endpoint trajectories of point-to-point movements commonly follow a nearly *straight path*. This is not trivial given that individual joint rotations naturally produce curved endpoint trajectories; hence, to produce a straight-line path, joint rotations have to be coordinated. Such coordination is violated in patients after stroke, resulting in staggered involvement of joints and non-straight endpoint trajectories. Several approaches have been used to account for straight endpoint trajectories, including the *minimum-jerk optimization approach* (see Section 9.2).

Second, the tangential velocity of the endpoint typically shows a bell-shaped pattern and a double-peaked, not perfectly symmetrical acceleration. Note that individual joint trajectories do not necessarily show smooth bell-shaped profiles of angular velocities. In particular, for some tasks, some of the joints show a reversal of their motion. For example, if you extend your right arm all the way to the right at the shoulder level and then move the index finger to point at a distant object to the left, the elbow joint will produce a flexion–extension sequence (Figure 11.18).

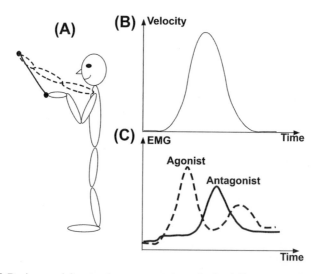

Figure 11.17 During a quick natural movement, the endpoint follows approximately a straight trajectory (A), the endpoint velocity time profile is bell-shaped (B), and many agonist—antagonist muscle pairs show tri-phasic patterns of muscle activation (C).

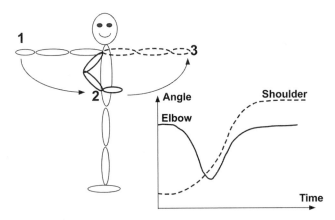

Figure 11.18 During a fast movement from posture-1 to posture-3 (via posture-2), the shoulder joint trajectory is monotonic while the elbow joint trajectory shows a sequence flexion–extension.

Third, agonist–antagonist muscle pairs acting at individual joints commonly show a tri-phasic pattern of muscle activation (EMG) that is particularly pronounced during fast actions (see Section 6.2). Sometimes, the EMG patterns show fewer than three or more than three bursts of muscle activation.

Finally, all movement characteristics during reaching movements show trial-to-trial variability. This variability is more pronounced at the individual-joint and individual-muscle levels and is typically the lowest for variables that characterize motion of the endpoint. Studies of motor variability have offered important insights into the control of multi-joint actions compatible with the ideas of multi-joint synergies (see Section 9.4) and the framework of the equilibrium-point (referent configuration) hypothesis (see Sections 8.3 and 8.4).

Joint coordination during reaching

Mechanical analyses of reaching movements have focused on the coordination of joint rotations and torques. At the kinematic level, it has been known since the classical studies of Bernstein on blacksmiths (see Section 2.6), that individual joint rotations co-vary to produce relatively invariant trajectories of the endpoint. More recently, such co-variation patterns—multi-joint synergies—have been studied quantitatively within the framework of the *uncontrolled manifold hypothesis* (see Section 9.4). These studies have shown that if in a particular trial one joint deviates from its preferred (average across trials) trajectory, other joints are likely to show deviations from their preferred trajectories that keep the endpoint trajectory relatively unchanged. Figure 11.19 shows an illustration of a three-joint system performing a two-dimensional reaching task. At each movement phase, there is a direction in the joint space that does not affect endpoint location. Joint variability across trials is mostly elongated along that direction (two configurations and two points are shown for selected phases in Figure 11.19). Certainly, this is possible only for kinematically redundant systems.

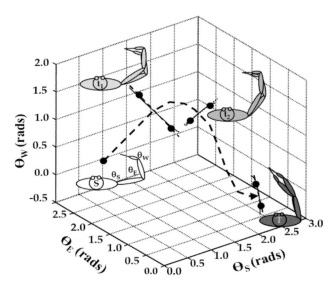

Figure 11.19 Trajectory of a reaching movement performed by a three-joint system in two dimensions is shown in the 3D joint angle space (dashed line). At each phase, the same endpoint location can be achieved with different joint configurations (two are illustrated for each of the three selected phases). All these configurations belong to the uncontrolled manifold (thin solid lines), which can be approximated linearly (thin dashed lines). Reproduced by permission from Latash, M. L., Scholz, J. P., & Schöner, G. (2007). Toward a new theory of motor synergies. *Motor Control, 11*, 276–308.

At the kinetic level, several hypotheses have been offered to account for the typical joint torque profiles observed during reaching movements. One of them, the *leading-joint hypothesis*, has been described in Section 5.2. To recap, this hypothesis assumes that control of movements of a multi-joint kinematic chain involves selecting a leading joint (commonly, the most proximal joint) that generates motion in all the joints of the chain with interaction torques. Other joints add muscle torques to the interaction torques in a task-specific way. Another hypothesis, the *linear torque synergy hypothesis*, was developed by Gerald Gottlieb and colleagues based on observations that, across many fast reaching tasks, individual joint torques scale linearly with each other. This hypothesis assumes that a single torque profile is used to produce a reaching movement by scaling the profile appropriately to produce individual joint torques. Unfortunately, this hypothesis cannot explain how movements are controlled when some joints follow a monotonic trajectory (for example, flexion), while other joints show a trajectory with a reversal (for example, the elbow joint in an example discussed earlier, Figure 11.18).

Muscle activation patterns during reaching

Muscle activation patterns during multi-joint movements show features related more to characteristics of the overall action than to characteristics of action at each individual joint. In particular, when a person performs a quick movement of the arm without a major rotation of the wrist joint, agonist–antagonist muscle pairs acting at the wrist show large-amplitude tri-phasic EMG patterns similar to those seen in the muscle pairs crossing more proximal joints that show large-amplitude rotations. The purpose of the phasic muscle activation at apparently postural joints is not to produce joint rotation but to avoid joint rotation that would otherwise occur under the action of interaction torques.

If an unexpected change in the external load happens during a one-joint movement, changes in the levels of muscle activation seen at a relatively short time delay (50–70 ms) follow a relatively simple rule: A muscle that is relatively stretched by the perturbation (as compared to unperturbed trials) will show additional activation, while its antagonist that is relatively shortened by the perturbation will show a decrease in its activation level. In Figure 11.20, two situations are illustrated—an unexpected increase (A) and a decrease (B) in the external load. When the load is increased, the agonist muscle shortens slower as compared with regular trials. As a result, its length is larger, and an additional activation is seen (shown with dashed lines). In those trials, the antagonist muscle stretched slower, and its EMG is decreased. Opposite EMG changes are seen when the load is suddenly decreased (B). If a similar perturbation is applied during a quick movement by a multi-joint limb, changes in the muscle activation levels at similar time delays may follow a different rule: They will be defined not by effects of the perturbation on individual joint trajectories but by those effects on the endpoint trajectory.

As already mentioned, the human arm is a multi-joint structure that possesses *redundancy* at both *kinematic* and *kinetic* levels. At the kinematic level, there are more degrees-of-freedom (joint rotations) than the number of constraints imposed by typical

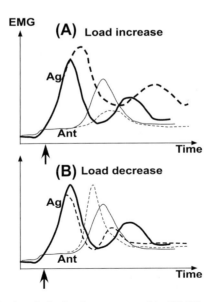

Figure 11.20 Changes in the tri-phasic electromyographic (EMG) pattern when the load is unexpectedly increased (A) and decreased (B). Regular trials are shown with solid lines (thick—agonist; thin—antagonist). Unexpectedly perturbed trials are shown with dashed lines.

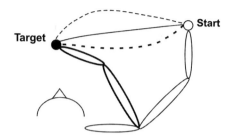

Figure 11.21 Even in the absence of kinematic redundancy, there is a possibility to use an infinite number of trajectories to move from a starting position to a target. Three such trajectories are shown for a two-joint system performing a movement in a two-dimensional space.

tasks. At the kinetic level, each joint is crossed by more muscles than necessary to produce joint torques about the individual axes of rotation. Studies not involving kinematic redundancy typically involve only two joints performing a planar task. As a result, for each endpoint location, there is only one possible combination of joint angles (Figure 11.21). However, there is motor redundancy at the level of joint trajectories since an infinite number of combinations of joint rotations can bring the limb from the initial to the final configuration. Three such trajectories are illustrated in Figure 11.21.

Reaching in unusual force fields. Internal models

A typical example of kinematically non-redundant reaching is the commonly used *center-out task*. This task has been used in studies of both monkeys and humans. Within this task, the subject grabs a handle that can be moved in a horizontal plane and places it into a comfortable initial position (since the task is non-redundant, the limb configuration is always the same). Then, the subject moves the handle to one of the targets distributed along a circle with the center in the initial position (Figure 11.22; the top figure). The handle may be linked to a programmable set of motors that can generate a force field, that is, a dependence of the external force vector (load) on kinematic variables associated with handle motion. Such setups have been used to study movement adaptation to different force fields.

One of the most common designs pioneered by the group of an Italian–American researcher Sandro Mussa-Ivaldi involved application of a force field with the external force proportional to the magnitude of the handle velocity vector and directed orthogonal to that vector (the insert on the top of Figure 11.22). The bottom four panels in Figure 11.22 illustrate typical trajectories produced by a subject in the absence of such a field (A) and after the field was turned on (B). Turning the field on produces major distortions in the shapes of the nearly straight trajectories observed without the field. The trajectories become curved in the direction of force. After some practice, the subjects adapt to the new environment, and the trajectories become nearly straight (C). If, following the adaptation, the field is turned off, an after-effect is observed: The trajectories become curved in the opposite direction as compared to the early effects of turning the field on (compare D and B).

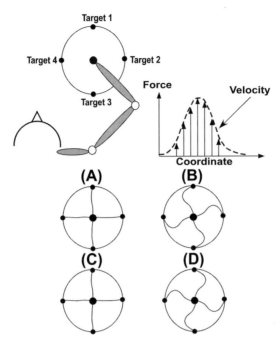

Figure 11.22 A person performs a center-out task illustrated in the top panel. An artificial force field can be produced by a programmable robot with the force orthogonal and proportional to the vector of velocity. Without the force field, the trajectories are nearly straight (A). After the force field has been turned on, the trajectories become curved (B). After some practice, the trajectories become straight again (C). When the force field is turned off, the trajectories become curved in the opposite direction (D).

These observations have been cited in support of the idea of a new *internal model* elaborated by the central nervous system in the process of practice. The new model has been assumed to take into account the artificially changed mechanical interactions between the body and the environment and to introduce corrections into the assumed computation of motor commands accordingly. After the force field was turned off, using the new, now inadequate, internal model resulted in the trajectories becoming curved again.

Adaptation of reaching to changes in visual information

Adaptation effects have also been observed during movements performed under visual control, when the visual information was distorted with prismatic glasses. For example, *prismatic glasses* can shift visual information by a certain angle. In such conditions, the first reaching movement deviates from the target by the distortion angle (Figure 11.23). If the subject repeats the movement again and again, the trajectories become accurate. If now the glasses are removed, *after-effects* of practice

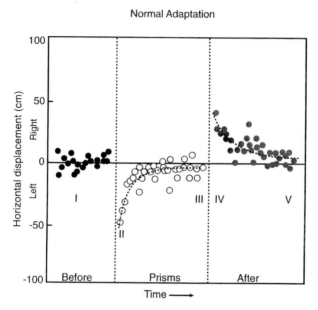

Figure 11.23 Adaptation of a reaching movement to prismatic glasses. When the glasses were put on, the first movement was to the perceived, not actual target location. After a few trials, the movement direction adapted. Taking the glasses off led to a directional error of the first movement in the opposite direction. Reproduced by permission from Martin, T. A., Keating, J. G., Goodkin, H. P., Bastian, A. J., & Thach, W. T. (1996). Throwing while looking through prisms. I. Focal olivocerebellar lesions impair adaptation. *Brain, 119*, 1183–1198. © 1996 Oxford University Press.

are observed: The first reaching movement shows an error in a direction opposite to that observed during the first movement after the glasses were put on. Adaptation and after-effects have been shown to be smaller or even disappear in patients with cerebellar disorders. These observations pointed to an important role of the cerebellum in adaptation to novel sensory and loading conditions.

Reaching with the dominant and non-dominant arm

Studies of adaptation of reaching movements to novel force fields revealed a qualitative difference between the dominant and non-dominant arm. The prevailing common sense view that every person has a "good arm" (*dominant*) and a "bad arm" (*non-dominant*) has been challenged. Each arm showed an advantage in specific aspects of movements after a novel force field was introduced similar to the one described earlier and illustrated in Figure 11.22. The dominant arm was better in achieving straight trajectories in the new force field. Following adaptation, the trajectories of the non-dominant arm were still rather curved, while this was not seen for the trajectories of the dominant arm. However, despite the curved trajectories, the non-dominant arm was more accurate in stopping at the target.

This and a few other experiments by the group led by Robert Sainburg have suggested a hypothesis (*dynamic-dominance hypothesis*) that the dominant arm was better equipped to deal with movement dynamics, particularly during fast actions, while the non-dominant arm was better suited for achieving a required equilibrium state. These conclusions are not completely unexpected. When you hammer a nail, you prefer to hold the nail with the non-dominant arm and hit it with the hammer held by the dominant arm. If you try to switch the arms, you will feel not only that the non-dominant arm is rather clumsy moving the hammer but also that the dominant arm is not as steady in holding the nail. So, we do not have a "good arm" and a "bad arm," but two good arms that are specialized for different aspects of everyday tasks.

Control of reaching within the equilibrium-point hypothesis

Most of the abovementioned studies used mechanical (and sometimes, electromyographic) variables to get insights into neural strategies of the control of reaching movements. As mentioned earlier (see Sections 5.1 and 5.3), it is highly unlikely that the neural structures operate with such variables or with their direct precursors. More likely, the central nervous system specifies neurophysiological signals that define parameters of equations that describe physical laws that govern the interactions among different parts of the body and between the body and the environment. All the abovementioned performance variables emerge given this paramerization and the actual (sometimes unpredicted) external force field. The only hypothesis that has tried to describe the control of reaching multi-joint movement using this approach is the equilibrium-point (referent configuration) hypothesis (see Sections 8.3 and 8.4).

This approach views multi-joint movement as controlled by a *hierarchical system* (Figure 11.24). At the upper level of the hierarchy, control signals related to referent values of salient task variables (for example, the coordinates of the endpoint of a multi-joint limb) are specified. For movement in three-dimensional space, these may involve referent values of the endpoint coordinates in three-dimensional space (a three-dimensional vector $\mathbf{R}$) and parameters that specify resistance of the endpoint to external forces that try to move it from the equilibrium state (in general, a six-component $\mathbf{C}$ command that specifies ellipsoid of apparent stiffness). In fact, several studies have shown that humans cannot voluntarily modify all six parameters related to $\mathbf{C}$, but only one or two of those. So, at the upper level of the hierarchy, there are likely about 4–5 parameters to be specified.

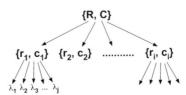

Figure 11.24 A control hierarchy. A pair of commands $\{\mathbf{R}, \mathbf{C}\}$ define referent configuration with respect to salient variables. They project on a redundant set of $\{r, c\}$ pairs—commands to joints. Each $\{r, c\}$ pair projects onto a redundant set of λ values—commands to muscles.

At the next level, signals related to referent values of joint-level variables are defined. These can be described as $\{r, c\}$ pairs for each axis of joint rotation (see Section 8.3). The human arm has at least seven potentially independent axes of joint rotation. This results in 14 variables specified at that level.

Finally, signals related to referent coordinates for individual muscles are produced. These correspond to λ values, thresholds of the tonic stretch reflex of the muscles. The redundancy of the human limbs at both joint and muscle level (see Section 3.5) suggests that transformation of signals at a higher level of the assumed hierarchy to the next, lower level is a few-to-many transformation. One can assume that such transformation involve multi-$\{r, c\}$ synergies at the joint level that specify the $\{\mathbf{R}, \mathbf{C}\}$ couple, and multi-$\{\lambda\}$ synergies at the muscle level that specify $\{r, c\}$ for the axis of rotation controlled by the muscles.

This account has been supported by many studies showing *equifinality* of multi-joint movements when an unexpected transient perturbation acted during the movement (see Section 4.5). Indeed, if the final state is defined by $\{\mathbf{R}, \mathbf{C}\}$ and the external field, any transient changes in the force field are not expected to lead to changes in the final equilibrium state. For example, in the described experiments with the artificial force field proportional to movement velocity, the novel force field acts only during the movement (when the velocity is non-zero); it becomes zero when the arm stops. So, despite the grossly distorted trajectories, equifinality of movement is expected, assuming that the subject is not trying to correct the ongoing movement. Note that the equifinality is expected to be violated if the subject of such an experiment tries to correct the movement in response to the perturbation.

This account offers an interpretation of the different performance of the dominant and non-dominant arms. The dominant arm has been trained to perform most fast everyday movements that are commonly produced in a not-perfectly-predictable external field. So, it learned to correct movements if a perturbation takes place. As a result of such corrections, its trajectories become much smoother and straighter. However, there is a by-product. It fails to take full advantage of the movement equifinality when changes in the force field are transient. The non-dominant arm, in contrast, has been trained to perform steady-state tasks (e.g. holding the nail). It is less likely to react to transient perturbations. As a result, its trajectories are much more curved, but it takes full advantage of the property of equifinality and reaches the endpoint final location more accurately, as compared to the dominant arm.

Violations of equifinality under Coriolis force

Violations of equifinality have been reported in a number of studies and are sometimes cited as evidence disproving the equilibrium-point hypothesis. Arguably the most famous experiment was that carried out by James Lackner and Paul DiZio. This involved reaching movements performed by subjects sitting in a rotating centrifuge (described in Section 4.5). The subject's body was aligned with the axis of rotation and he or she performed reaching movements to lit targets in otherwise complete darkness. When the centrifuge was stationary, the trajectories were nearly straight and rather accurate. Then the centrifuge was accelerated very slowly, so that the subject

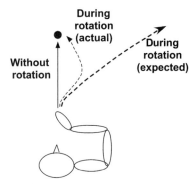

Figure 11.25 Natural reaching movements follow a nearly straight trajectory (solid line). During rotation in a centrifuge, Coriolis forces perturb reaching movements. However, the trajectory (thin dashed line) shows a tendency to come back to the same final position (with a residual error). If no joint torque corrections were introduced, the trajectory would not show the return phase (thick dashed line).

was unaware of the rotation. When the subject performed experiments while being rotated, the arm trajectory deviated from the straight line under the action of the *Coriolis force* (Figure 11.25). It then showed a return to the original trajectory but the return was incomplete, and there was a residual error: A violation of equifinality.

Note that the Coriolis force depends on the product of the linear velocity of the hand and the angular velocity (see Sections 4.5 and 5.1). As a result, it is high when the hand velocity is high, and it is zero when the hand stops. Figure 11.25 shows predicted deviations of the endpoint trajectory (thick dashed line) under the action of the Coriolis force if the controller applied the same force and moment-of-force time profiles during movements performed with and without rotation of the centrifuge. Obviously, the actual trajectory (dashed thin line) is very different. Deviations from the straight line are seen in the first half of the movement and then these deviations are reduced. Note that the Coriolis force does not change its direction during the second half of the movement, only its magnitude becomes smaller. So, why is the hand returning closer to the original trajectory?

There are two mutually non-exclusive explanations. First, there are involuntary mechanisms associated with equilibrium-point control that tend to bring the hand to its original equilibrium trajectory when the perturbation force is reduced. Second, despite the lack of conscious awareness of movement corrections, maybe the subjects' central nervous system did correct the $\{R, C\}$ time patterns. Likely, both processes took place and contributed to the early deviation of the observed trajectories from those expected under the action of added Coriolis forces and to the residual error in the final hand position.

Problems with studies of equilibrium trajectories

One of the major factors that has slowed down the development and acceptance of the equilibrium-point hypothesis is that it is notoriously hard to measure time profiles of the hypothetical control variables such as $\{\mathbf{R}, \mathbf{C}\}$, $\{r, c\}$ and λ. First, there is no place in the body where one could stick an electrode to measure those variables, even if participants of this hypothetical experiment gave permission for such procedures. So, researchers have to use indirect methods, that is, measure performance variables and compute hypothetical neural (control) variables. This has been done in a number of studies. However, this method requires the use of a model of the interactions within the body to link the performance variables with the control ones. Unfortunately, such models have been very crude, and estimates of their parameters have been quite unreliable. Typically, these have been *linear second-order models* with an inertial, a damping, and an elastic term. For a single-muscle system, a typical equation would be:

$$m\frac{d^2x}{dt^2} + b\frac{dx}{dt} + k(x - \lambda) = F_{EXT}, \tag{11.6}$$

where m is mass, b is damping coefficient, k is stiffness, and x is muscle length. For a single-joint system, a similar equation would be used adjusted for the fact that the action is rotation, not linear motion. Such models ignore important features of the actual system, such as its strong non-linearity, including threshold properties of the tonic stretch reflex loop, velocity dependence of λ (see Section 8.3), and the fact that some of the system's reactions come after time delays. As a result, such studies likely led to the reconstruction of distorted time profiles of the control variables.

N-shaped equilibrium trajectories

One of the results seems worth mentioning. During fast single-joint movements, reproducible non-monotonic (N-shaped) equilibrium trajectories have been reconstructed. Figure 11.26 shows an example of a quick movement ("actual trajectory," black dots) and a reconstructed N-shaped equilibrium trajectory (open dots). The shape could be distorted by the abovementioned simplifications of the underlying model. In another experiment, subjects performed a fast movement in one of the joints of the elbow–wrist two-joint system (Figure 11.27, left panel). As mentioned earlier, when one of the joints moves, the other joint experiences torques because of mechanical joint coupling. Hence, performing such an action requires control signals to be sent to both joints—the focal one (the one performing a fast movement), and the "postural" one (the one that is supposed not to move). Indeed, participants in such an experiment could easily move one joint (for example, the elbow) very fast while keeping the other joint nearly motionless. The reconstruction of the $\{r, c\}$ pairs to the two joints showed similarly timed, non-monotonic equilibrium trajectories that differed only in their final coordinate (Figure 11.27, right panels). For the moving joint, the final coordinate corresponded to the new position, while for the "postural" joint the final coordinate was very similar to the initial one. One can conclude that the control of such movements involves the generation of equilibrium trajectories to all the involved joints that are similarly timed but of different amplitudes. This allows compensation for the motion-dependent torques and achievement of a desired final joint configuration.

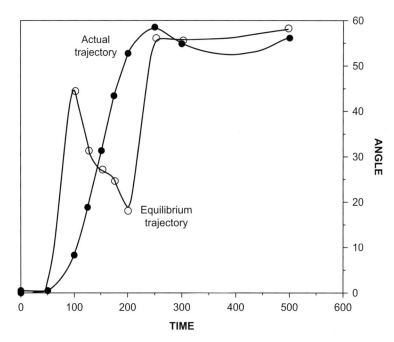

Figure 11.26 The actual trajectory during very fast elbow flexion movements (solid circles) and the reconstructed N-shaped equilibrium trajectory. Reproduced by permission from Latash, M. L., & Gottlieb, G. L. (1991). Reconstruction of elbow joint compliant characteristics during fast and slow voluntary movements. *Neuroscience, 43*, 697–712.

11.4   Prehension

The human hand possesses amazing dexterity and versatility. Despite impressive recent progress in engineering, most robotic grippers are clumsy and awkward in comparison with the human hand. This versatility is based on the mechanical design of the hand, its muscular apparatus, and sophisticated neurophysiological control. The motor function of the hand is closely linked to its sensory function: The hand is used to both explore objects by touch and manipulate them. The combined sensory–motor function of the grasping hand is called *prehension*.

Anatomy and mechanics of the hand

The hand is a complex anatomical structure. There are 27 bones in the human hand, wrist, and forearm; 14 phalangeal bones in fingers, five metacarpal bones in the palm area of the hand, and eight carpal bones in the wrist. These bones are connected by four major joint groups: The distal interphalangeal joints, the proximal interphalangeal joints, the metacarpophalangeal joints, and the carpometacarpal joints.

Most commonly, humans apply forces to hand-held objects with the fingertips. From the point of view of mechanics, the design of the hand combines both *serial* and

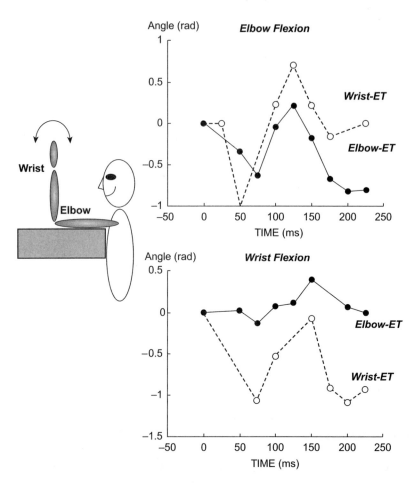

Figure 11.27 Equilibrium trajectories (ETs) for the elbow and the wrist reconstructed over series of one-joint fast flexion movements in a configuration illustrated to the left of the graphs. Note the large-amplitude non-monotonic ETs in both the moving joint and the "postural joint." Modified by permission from Latash, M. L., Aruin, A. S., & Zatsiorsky, V. M. (1999). The basis of a simple synergy: Reconstruction of joint equilibrium trajectories during unrestrained arm movements. *Human Movement Science, 18*, 3–30.

parallel chains (Figure 11.28). An individual digit can be viewed as a serial mechanism, with several joints connecting the fingertip to the wrist. Such mechanisms are *redundant* in kinematic tasks that typically have fewer task constraints than the number of the joints. However, if one wants to apply a certain force vector by the fingertip in isometric conditions, a serial mechanism becomes *over-constrained* because a vector of force ($\mathbf{F}$) at the endpoint defines unambiguously all the joint moments of force (a vector $\mathbf{M}$): $\mathbf{F} = \mathbf{J}^{\mathrm{T}}\mathbf{M}$, where $\mathbf{J}$ is the Jacobian of the system and T is the sign for transpose. In contrast, when several fingers press on a rigid object, they act in parallel. In this task, the fingers are over-constrained in kinematics, because

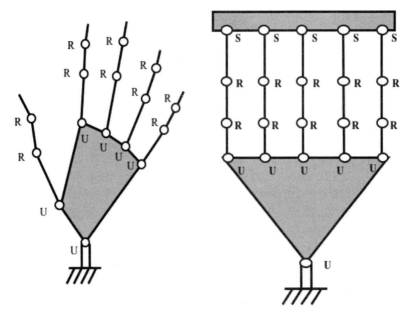

Figure 11.28 The human hand may be viewed as a combination of serial and parallel manipulators. U, universal joint; R, revolute joint; S, spherical joint. Reproduced by permission from Shim, J. K. (2005). Rotational equilibrium control in multi-digit human prehension. PhD dissertation. © 2005, J.K. Shim.

movement of one finger induces movement of all other fingers. However, such a parallel mechanism is redundant in isometric force production tasks because an infinite number of combinations of finger forces can produce a required total force.

Hand muscles

The hand is served by two major muscle groups, *intrinsic* and *extrinsic muscles* (Figure 11.29). The bellies of the intrinsic muscles lie within the hand (two are shown in the top panel of Figure 11.29). The *intrinsic flexor muscles* are digit-specific in their flexion and abduction–adduction action, that is, their distal tendons attach to proximal phalanges of one finger only. However, these muscles also attach to a tendinous structure that forms the so-called *extensor mechanism*, a network of passive elastic tissues that produce an extensor action in the distal finger joints (the bottom panel of Figure 11.29). As a result, activation of an intrinsic muscle produces a focal action in the corresponding metacarpophalangeal joint and also contributes to extension of the digit (and other digits) in the distal phalanges.

The bellies of the extrinsic muscles lie in the forearm. Each extrinsic muscle has several distal tendons that attach to individual fingers. For example, the *flexor digitorum superficialis* (FDS) sends four tendons to the four fingers of the hand. These tendons attach at the intermediate phalanges (dashed lines in the top panel of Figure 11.29). The other major flexor, *flexor digitorum profundis* (FDP) has four

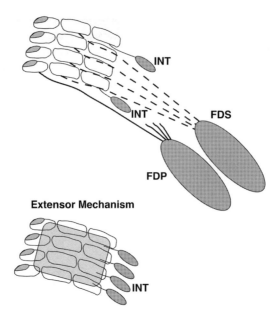

Figure 11.29 The action of extrinstic, multi-tendon muscles (FDP, flexor digitorum profundis; FDS, flexor digitorum superficialis) and intrinsic, digit-specific hand muscles (INT). INT also contribute to the extensor mechanism shown in the lower drawing.

tendons that attach to the distal phalanges of the four fingers (only one is shown in Figure 11.29). These muscles are sometimes viewed not as single physiological structures but as combinations of several *muscle compartments*. A compartment is a group of muscle fibers innervated by a subgroup of motor units from the pool innervating the whole muscle. Compartments produce forces transmitted primarily to one of the four tendons and lead to motor effects predominantly in one of the four fingers. This design of the muscular hand apparatus may be viewed as contributing to the interdependence of forces and movements produced by individual fingers. This interdependence is not absolutely obligatory; professional musicians, for example, learn to override it and produce much more independent finger actions.

Cortical maps of the hand

The human hand has a highly developed system of cortical control reflected in the large projections of the hand in different cortical areas, including the *primary motor cortex*. The primary motor cortex and the corticospinal tract are crucial for the proper functioning of the hand. In cases of stroke involving motor cortical areas, the clinical picture typically involves a major impairment of the hand function that is also notoriously hard to recover. In particular, patients following stroke become less able to move one finger at a time; rather, an attempt to move a finger leads to motion of all the fingers of the hand.

Studies using brain mapping techniques (reviewed in Sections 13.5 and 13.6) have shown major reorganizations of cortical maps following amputation of a digit or specialized training such as reading Braille, playing a musical instrument, or practicing an artificial laboratory task. This phenomenon called *neural plasticity* (see Section 12.5) is likely to mediate such processes as motor learning and motor rehabilitation.

Hierarchical control of the hand. Safety margin

During grasping tasks, control of the hand is frequently viewed as based on a two-level hierarchy (Figure 11.30). At the upper level, the task is shared between the actions of the thumb and the opposing virtual finger (VF). The latter term implies an imaginary digit with mechanical action equal to the combined action of the actual fingers involved in the task. More formally, VF produces a wrench equal to the sum of the wrenches produced by the fingers. At the lower level, the VF action is shared among the actual fingers. The two levels will be addressed as Task → {Th,VF} and VF → {I,M,R,L}. For example, imagine that the hand holds an object in the air using the so-called *prismatic grasp* with the contact points of all five digits in one plane, the *grasp plane* (Figure 11.31). For simplicity, assume also that external torque acts on the object in the same plane. Holding the objects requires that the following equations of statics are satisfied:

$$F_{VF}^n + F_{th}^n = 0$$

$$F_{VF}^t + F_{th}^t + L = 0 \tag{11.7}$$

$$Tq + \underbrace{F_{VF}^n d_{VF} + F_{VF}^t r_{VF}}_{\text{Moment of the VF} \equiv M_{VF}} + \underbrace{F_{th}^n d_{th} + F_{th}^t r_{th}}_{\text{Moment of the thumb} \equiv M_{th}} = 0$$

where the subscripts th and VF refer to the thumb and the virtual finger, respectively; the superscripts n and t stand for the normal and tangential force components, respectively; L is load (weight of the object), Tq is external torque, and coefficients d and r stand for the moment arms of the normal and tangential force with respect to a pre-selected center, respectively. In addition, to apply a certain tangential force to

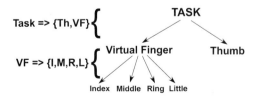

Figure 11.30 A two-level control hierarchy of the hand. At the upper level, the task is shared between the thumb and a virtual finger (VF). At the lower level, action of the VF is shared among the actual fingers.

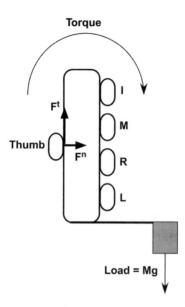

Figure 11.31 Prismatic grasp. All the points of digit contact are assumed to be in a plane (grasp plane). The external mass produces both a load and a torque. Each digit produces normal and tangential forces.

the object, the normal force should be large enough. Given a friction coefficient μ, the following inequality should be satisfied for each finger to avoid slippage: $F^n \geq F^t/\mu$. Typically, humans apply higher normal forces than necessary for the given friction conditions. This is quantified with an index called *safety margin* (SM): $SM = (\mu F^n - F^t)/F^t$. SM is a useful index that distinguishes different sub-populations, for example elderly persons have higher SM values than younger persons, while persons with Down syndrome have higher SM values than persons without Down syndrome.

Note that Equations 11.7 are redundant. This means that an infinite number of combinations of the thumb and VF forces and points of force application can solve these equations. If a person performs the task of holding an object statically many times, these variables show co-varied adjustments across trials. These adjustments reflect prehension synergies at the Task $\rightarrow$ {Th,VF} level.

The action of the VF is shared at the lower level among the actions by the individual fingers, i—index, m—middle, r—ring, and l—little:

$$F_{VF}^n = F_i^n + F_m^n + F_r^n + F_l^n$$

$$F_{VF}^t = F_i^t + F_m^t + F_r^t + F_l^t \tag{11.8}$$

$$M_{VF} = \underbrace{F_i^n d_i + F_m^n d_m + F_r^n d_r + F_l^n d_l}_{\text{Moment of the normal forces} \equiv M^n} + \underbrace{F_i^t r_i + F_m^t r_m + F_r^t r_r + F_l^t r_l}_{\text{Moment of the tangential forces} \equiv M^t}$$

This system of equations is also redundant. The equations allow an infinite number of solutions (sets of variables on the right hand sides), and different solutions are indeed realized in different trials for given actions of the VF (variables on the left hand sides of the equations). This means that prehension synergies can be studied at both Task $\rightarrow$ {Th,VF} and VF $\rightarrow$ {I,M,R,L} levels.

Finger interaction during pressing

Finger interaction at the VF $\rightarrow$ {I,M,R,L} level has been studied using multi-finger pressing tasks without thumb involvement. Performance of such tasks is characterized by the phenomena of *sharing, enslaving, force deficit*, and *synergic force adjustments*. Sharing implies that the total force (or another performance variable, for example the total moment of force) is shared among the four fingers in a certain way, and this sharing pattern is stable over a range of force magnitudes. Enslaving or lack of *finger individuation* can be seen when only one finger is instructed to produce force. In such tasks, other fingers show unintended force production, with the magnitude of the unintended force scaling proportionally with the magnitude of the task finger force. Force deficit reflects the fact that maximal voluntary force produced by a finger in a single-finger task is larger than the force of this finger in a maximal voluntary force production by several fingers pressing simultaneously.

The task of producing a constant, sub-maximal total force (or moment of force) with four fingers is redundant; it allows an infinite number of solutions. Analysis of finger force variance documented multi-finger force- and moment-of-force stabilizing synergies across a variety of pressing tasks. This means that in different trials participants of such studies used different finger force combinations to achieve required levels of total force with relatively high accuracy. Within the framework of the uncontrolled manifold hypothesis (see Section 9.4), this implies that most finger force variance was confined to the UCM.

Prehension synergies. Principle of superposition

In grasping tasks involving the thumb opposing the four fingers, synergies stabilizing such variables as total normal force, total tangential force, and total moment of force have been documented at both levels, Task $\rightarrow$ {VF,Th} and VF $\rightarrow$ {I,M,R,L}. Such co-varied adjustments of elemental variables that kept a value of a performance variable produced at the selected level have been referred to as *prehension synergies*.

Analysis of static prehension synergies revealed that not all possible combinations of elemental variables were used to satisfy the constraints. Typical tasks were performed as combinations of two sub-tasks: One of them was related to the production of *grasping force* (which is an example of an internal force) and *resultant force*, and the other to the production of *rotational action* (total moment of force). Correspondingly, there were two main synergies—force-stabilizing and moment-stabilizing. This organization complies with the *principle of superposition* introduced in robotics for the control of grippers. The principle states that skilled actions by a gripper can be decomposed into several elemental actions that are controlled independently by separate controllers. Such a decoupled control in robotics has been shown to reduce total computation time.

Feed-forward control of grip force

When the hand holds an object as shown in Figure 11.31, the digits have to produce net tangential forces that counterbalance the object's weight (as in Equation 11.7). If now the object is moved quickly to a target located above its initial position, the tangential digit forces have to show time modulation that corresponds to the modulation of inertial load:

$$F_{VF}^t + F_{th}^t + m[g - a(t)] = 0$$

where g is gravity acceleration and $a(t)$ is the time-varying object acceleration. In order to produce higher tangential forces that are required to accelerate the object, the normal forces have to be increased as well to prevent slippage and provide adequate safety margin. Several studies have shown that an increase in the normal forces takes place slightly before or simultaneously with the increase in the tangential forces associated with the movement initiation (Figure 11.32). Since there is no time lag in the normal force increase, it is viewed as being produced in a *feed-forward manner*.

The feed-forward adjustments of normal forces to expected changes in the external load that require modulation of tangential forces have been observed in a variety of conditions, such as manipulation of hand-held objects and whole-body movements performed with an object in the hand. Within the force-control ideas (see Section 5.1), these adjustments have been assumed to result from neural computations performed with the help of internal models reflecting the planned dynamics of the interaction between the hand and the hand-held object. A number of observations of impaired feed-forward adjustments in patients with cerebellar disorders have pointed to the cerebellum as a possible site where such internal models are created.

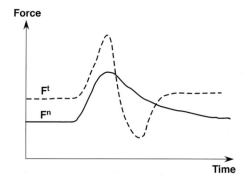

Figure 11.32 Typical changes in the tangential force (dashed line, F^t) and normal force (solid line, F^n) of the thumb during lifting quickly a hand-held object.

Voluntary movements of a hand-held object produce predictable modulations of the load. If the load changes unpredictably, signals from somatosensory receptors in the hand (and possibly more proximal segments) are used to produce quick adjustments of the normal (grip) force. For example, normal force adjustments are seen if a vertical force acts unexpectedly on a hand-held object, thus increasing the load in the vertical direction. Such adjustments are seen after very short time delays from the moment of load change, on the order of 50–70 ms. These delays are shorter than the simple reaction time; they suggest that the normal force adjustments in such conditions are of a reflex-type origin; possibly they belong to the group of *pre-programmed* or *triggered reactions* described in Section 3.4.

Hand control within the equilibrium-point hypothesis

An alternative view on the organization of force adjustments to planned actions is based on the equilibrium-point (referent configuration) hypothesis (see Section 8.4). To recap, this approach accepts the idea of predictive control but refutes the scheme of control signals based on computational processes within the central nervous system that model dynamic interactions within the body and between the body and the environment. According to the referent configuration hypothesis, the central nervous system uses neurophysiological signals that translate into changes in referent values of important kinematic variables.

In particular, at the Task $\rightarrow$ {Th,VF} level, changes in the grip force are assumed to be produced by centrally initiated changes in the referent value of the *grip aperture* (AP_{REF}), that is, the distance between the thumb and VF pads (Figure 11.33). A change in AP_{REF} leads to a change in the difference between the actual grip aperture (AP_{ACT}) and the referent one. This difference drives activation of muscles

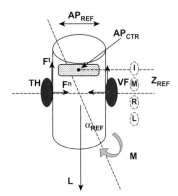

Figure 11.33 Illustration of three referent variables that form the referent configuration for the task of holding a grasped object: referent aperture (AP_{REF}), referent height (Z_{REF}), and referent tilt (α_{REF}). Reproduced by permission from Latash, M. L., Friedman, J., Kim, S. W., Feldman, A. G., & Zatsiorsky, V. M. (2010). Prehension synergies and control with referent hand configurations. *Experimental Brain Research, 202*, 213–229.

that try to bring AP_{ACT} closer to AP_{REF}. However, the rigid walls of the object do not allow AP_{ACT} to change. As a result, there is an increase in the normal force produced by both the thumb and VF.

Along similar lines, changes in the vertical position of the object may be described as produced by changes in the *referent vertical coordinate* (Z_{REF}). If there are changes in the external torque, adequate adjustments of digit force may be described as resulting from changes in the *referent orientation* of the object (α_{REF}). Taken together, for the task illustrated in Figure 11.33, specifying time profiles of referent values for three variables are sufficient to produce actions with a hand-held object.

Note that specifying a referent value of one of those variables, for example AP_{REF}, automatically satisfies one of the main equations of statics (or similar, appropriately modified equations that describe motion of the hand-held object). Indeed, for a given AP_{REF} and a fixed AP_{ACT}, there will be adjustments in both thumb and VF forces and also a possible adjustment in the location of the object in space until the two opposing normal forces balance each other. In different trials, this may involve different values of the normal forces and maybe different coordinates of the object in the external space resulting in prehension synergies at the Task $\rightarrow$ {Th,VF} level. So, synergies may result directly from the control with referent configurations without any additional computational action.

As described in Section 8.4, specifying a set of referent values at a higher level of a hierarchy may be expected to lead to the emergence of referent values for variables at a lower level. Referent values at the lower level may co-adjust across repetitive attempts at the same task to stabilize the referent value at the higher level. In other words, synergies may exist among referent values at the lower level stabilizing the referent values at the higher level. For prehensile tasks, the three referent values related to the task may be associated with AP_{REF}, Z_{REF}, and α_{REF} introduced earlier. These three values result in referent values for corresponding kinematic variables for the thumb and VF such as their coordinates. At the VF $\rightarrow$ {I,M,R,L} level, the referent values for the VF coordinates produce referent values for the corresponding coordinates for the individual fingers. At each such step, synergies may be expected that result in relatively high variability at the level of elements as compared to the relatively low variability at the level of their combined action.

Self-test questions

1. What mechanical factors complicate the neural control of vertical posture?
2. Define center of pressure.
3. What are the typical characteristics of postural sway?
4. What are the simplifications underlying the single-joint inverted pendulum model of vertical posture?
5. Can muscle fiber length changes be in the opposite direction to muscle + tendon length changes? Explain your answer.
6. Define rambling and trembling.
7. What is the relationship between the notion of rambling and the equilibrium-point hypothesis?

8. Define eigenmovement.

9. Formulate the posture–movement paradox for vertical standing.

10. What are the main lines of defense of vertical posture against perturbations?

11. What main factors define the characteristics of anticipatory postural adjustments?

12. How do anticipatory postural adjustments change in conditions of increased and decreased postural stability?

13. How can preflexes be used to stabilize posture against perturbations?

14. What are the main differences between pre-programmed reactions and polysynaptic reflexes such as the tonic stretch reflex?

15. What are the ankle strategy and the hip strategy? In what conditions are they typically observed?

16. What mechanical variables are the vestibular receptors sensitive to?

17. What are the main effects of light touch on vertical posture?

18. What is sensory reweighting?

19. How can multi-muscle synergies be defined for postural tasks?

20. What postural adjustments happen during preparation prior to making a step?

21. What is the difference between walk, trot, and gallop?

22. Define dynamic stability. Define unstable equilibrium.

23. How is locomotion viewed within the referent configuration hypothesis?

24. Can a deafferented spinal cord produce rhythmic patterns related to locomotion?

25. Stimulation of what supraspinal structures can induce locomotion in the decerebrated cat?

26. What is corrective stumbling reaction?

27. Present a few examples of reflex reversals.

28. What are the typical features of reaching movements?

29. Define multi-joint synergy for a reaching movement.

30. What data on reaching in unusual force fields support the idea of internal models?

31. What are the main differences in reaching movements by the dominant and non-dominant hands?

32. Describe hierarchical control of reaching within the equilibrium-point hypothesis.

33. Explain violations of equifinality under the action of Coriolis force.

34. What are the main complicating factors in studying equilibrium trajectories?

35. Describe the main differences in the extrinsic and intrinsic hand muscles.

36. What are the specific features of hand representation in the primary motor cortex?

37. Describe the two-level hierarchical control of the hand?

38. Define safety margin.

39. Define principle of superposition for prehensile tasks.

40. Describe grip force adjustments during manipulations of a hand-held object.

41. What variables are used for the control of the hand according to the equilibrium-point hypothesis?

Essential references and recommended further readings

Alexandrov, A. V., Frolov, A. A., & Massion, J. (2001). Biomechanical analysis of movement strategies in human forward trunk bending. I. Modeling. *Biological Cybernetics, 84,* 425–434.

Arbib, M. A., Iberall, T., & Lyons, D. (1985). Coordinated control programs for movements of the hand. In A. W. Goodwin, & I. Darian-Smith (Eds.), *Hand Function and the Neocortex* (pp. 111–129). Berlin: Springer Verlag.

Arimoto, S., Tahara, K., Yamaguchi, M., Nguyen, P. T. A., & Han, H. Y. (2001). Principles of superposition for controlling pinch motions by means of robot fingers with soft tips. *Robotica, 19*, 21–28.

Baud-Bovy, G., & Soechting, J. F. (2001). Two virtual fingers in the control of the tripod grasp. *Journal of Neurophysiology, 86*, 604–615.

Berkinblit, M. B., Feldman, A. G., & Fukson, O. I. (1986). Adaptability of innate motor patterns and motor control mechanisms. *Behavioral and Brain Science, 9*, 585–638.

Berkinblit, M. B., Gelfand, I. M., & Feldman, A. G. (1986). A model for the control of multijoint movements. *Biofizika, 31*, 128–138.

Birbaumer, N., & Cohen, L. G. (2007). Brain-computer interfaces: communication and restoration of movement in paralysis. *Journal of Physiology, 579*, 621–636.

Bizzi, E., Accornero, N., Chapple, W., & Hogan, N. (1982). Arm trajectory formation in monkeys. *Experimental Brain Research, 46*, 139–143.

Bongaardt, R. (2001). How Bernstein conquered movement. In M. L. Latash, & V. M. Zatsiorsky (Eds.), *Classics in Movement Science* (pp. 59–84). Urbana, IL: Human Kinetics.

Cole, K. J. (1991). Grasp force control in older adults. *Journal of Motor Behavior, 23*, 251–258.

Cordo, P. J., & Nashner, L. M. (1982). *Properties of postural adjustments associated with rapid arm movements Journal of Neurophysiology, 47*, 287–302.

Flash, T. (1987). The control of hand equilibrium trajectories in multi-joint arm movements. *Biological Cybernetics, 57*, 257–274.

Forssberg, H. (1979). Stumbling corrective reaction: A phase dependent compensatory reaction during locomotion. *Journal of Neurophysiology, 42*, 936–953.

Gorniak, S. L., Zatsiorsky, V. M., & Latash, M. L. (2009). Hierarchical control of static prehension: I. Biomechanics. *Experimental Brain Research, 193*, 615–631.

Gorniak, S. L., Zatsiorsky, V. M., & Latash, M. L. (2009). Hierarchical control of static prehension: II. Multi-digit synergies. *Experimental Brain Research, 194*, 1–15.

Grillner, S. (1975). Locomotion in vertebrates: central mechanisms and reflex interaction. *Physiological Reviews, 55*, 247–304.

Jeka, J. J., & Lackner, J. R. (1994). Fingertip contact influences human postural control. *Experimental Brain Research, 100*, 495–502.

Kiemel, T., Oie, K. S., & Jeka, J. J. (2002). Multisensory fusion and the stochastic structure of postural sway. *Biological Cybernetics, 87*, 262–277.

Latash, M. L., Aruin, A. S., & Shapiro, M. B. (1995). The relation between posture and movement: A study of a simple synergy in a two-joint task. *Human Movement Science, 14*, 79–107.

Li, Z. M., Latash, M. L., & Zatsiorsky, V. M. (1998). Force sharing among fingers as a model of the redundancy problem. *Experimental Brain Research 119*, 276–286.

Massion, J. (1992). Movement, posture and equilibrium–interaction and coordination. *Progress in Neurobiology, 38*, 35–56.

Morasso, P. (1983). Three-dimensional arm trajectories. *Biological Cybernetics, 48*, 187–194.

Nashner, L. M. (1979). Organization and programming of motor activity during posture control. *Progress in Brain Research 50*, 177–184.

Orlovsky, G. N., Deliagina, T. G., & Grillner, S. (1999). *Neuronal control of locomotion. From Mollusc to Man*. New York: Oxford University Press.

Santello, M., & Soechting, J. F. (2000). Force synergies for multifingered grasping. *Experimental Brain Research 133*, 457–467.

Schieber, M. H., & Santello, M. (2004). Hand function: peripheral and central constraints on performance. *Journal of Applied Physiology, 96*, 2293–2300.

Soechting, J. F., & Lacquaniti, F. (1981). Invariant characteristics of a pointing movement in man. *Journal of Neuroscience, 1*, 710–720.

Stuart, D. G., Pierce, P. A., Callister, R. J., Brichta, A. M., & McDonagh, J. C. (2001). Sir Charles S. Sherrington: Humanist, mentor, and movement neuroscientist. In M. L. Latash, & V. M. Zatsiorsky (Eds.), *Classics in Movement Science* (pp. 317–374). Urbana, IL: Human Kinetics.

Zatsiorsky, V. M., & Duarte, M. (2000). Rambling and trembling in quiet standing. *Motor Control, 4*, 185–200.

Zatsiorsky, V. M., Latash, M. L., Gao, F., & Shim, J. K. (2004). The principle of superposition in human prehension. *Robotica, 22*, 231–234.

Westling, G., & Johansson, R. S. (1984). Factors influencing the force control during precision grip. *Experimental Brain Research, 53*, 277–284.

Winter, D. A., Prince, F., Frank, J. S., Powell, C., & Zabjek, K. F. (1996). Unified theory regarding A/P and M/L balance in quiet stance. *Journal of Neurophysiology, 75*, 2334–2343.

12 Effects of practice and adaptation

Chapter Outline

12.1   Introduction

Motor learning is a field of its own with numerous books and textbooks. This field is loosely related to motor control, but the emphasis of motor learning has traditionally been on applied aspects of movement studies, such as the effects of different practice schedules, retention of the effects of learning, transfer of learning across tasks, external conditions and effectors, etc. In this chapter I focus on a few issues that are traditionally covered in textbooks on motor learning. These issues have been selected for the lessons they teach relevant to issues of motor control. As a reminder, motor control is an area of natural science that tries to discover laws of nature that govern interactions within the body and between the body and the environment, leading to coordinated movements. So, in this chapter issues relevant to hypotheses on motor

Fundamentals of Motor Control. DOI: 10.1016/B978-0-12-415956-3.00012-9

control and coordination are discussed, while with respect to other issues, which may be of higher practical importance but not so obvious theoretical implications, readers are directed to traditional textbooks on motor learning.

Many years ago, Nikolai Bernstein coined the expression "repetition without repetition." He meant the following: When a person tries to perform the same motor task more than once in identical conditions (note that "same" and "identical" are practically impossible to achieve during actual motor performance by humans), he or she demonstrates different patterns of mechanical and neural variables in different attempts. The notion of "repetition without repetition" was crucial in the arguments of Bernstein against the then dominant theory of Ivan Pavlov. According to Pavlov's theory, performing a movement many times led to strengthening of neural connections in the involved neural pathways, resulting in movement automation. According to Bernstein, since every time the involved pathways were different from each other, no such "beating a path" through the central nervous system was possible.

So, what is repeated when a person executes the same task again and again? It seems that the only answer is: Solving the problems posed by the task again and again. The *redundancy* of transformations at different levels of the neuromotor system and the inherent variability of both neural and motor variables leave no room for repeated patterns of any single variable at any level of analysis. Learning to improve behavior in an ever-changing environment may be viewed as a major requirement for survival in the process of evolution.

Depending on the duration and intensity of practice, its effects may involve different structures within the neuromotor system. For example, strength-training exercises typically require substantial muscle forces and weeks of practice to lead to visible results. The effects of such practice can be seen at the level of muscle anatomy and physiology as well as within the central nervous system. Practicing highly specialized skills such as playing musical instruments, reading Braille, juggling, and certain sports (for example, gymnastics and figure skating) may require a very long time (10 000 hours to achieve expert performance according to some estimates) with significant changes seen at all levels of the neuromotor hierarchy.

Here, we will focus primarily on effects of relatively short practice sessions, commonly limited to one day or even one hour. The effects of such short-term practice on the muscle anatomy and physiology are commonly assumed to be small and not permanent. So, all the effects on performance may be attributed to changes within the central nervous system.

Explicit and implicit task components

While analyzing the effects of practice, it is useful to consider separately the explicit and implicit components of typical tasks. For example, a person may be asked to make a quick hand movement to a visual target in an unusual force field or in conditions of unusually distorted visual signals. The *explicit* task component is to reach the target, and a participant of this experiment is expected to pay attention primarily to this task component. However, natural reaching movements typically follow nearly straight trajectories (see Section 11.3). While moving along a nearly straight trajectory may not be an explicit task component, practice in unusual conditions may result in the trajectories becoming less and less curved. This is an example of an *implicit* task component, a component that is not prescribed by the task formulation but is self-imposed by the central nervous system of the participant.

Other examples of implicit task components are those related to safety and comfort. Any task performed by a standing person implies not falling down, even if this is not explicitly spelled out in the instruction. Transporting a hand-held object implies that it should be neither crushed nor dropped. If the object is a mug filled with coffee, it is implied that coffee should not be spilled. Earlier, the notion of a *safety margin* was discussed as a measure of extra gripping force above the minimum required to avoid slippage (see Section 11.4). This notion can be introduced for various other tasks, and keeping a safety margin at a certain value may be viewed as a common implicit task component.

12.2   Learning to be quick and accurate: Speed–accuracy and speed–difficulty trade-offs

Speed–difficulty trade-off, Fitts' law

Being able to perform a task quickly and accurately is a common goal of practice in athletics (consider, for example, throwing a baseball or fencing), professional movements (from butchers to violin virtuosi) and laboratory experiments. From everyday experience, we know that speeding-up commonly leads to diminished accuracy. This common knowledge has been studied experimentally since the nineteenth century. In the middle of the twentieth century, an equation was proposed to describe the trade-off between task difficulty and speed. This equation describes what is known as *Fitts' law*.

The formulation of Fitts' law is very simple. If a person is asked to move "as quickly and accurately as possible" to targets of different size placed at different distances from the initial position (Figure 12.1), movement time (MT) scales as a logarithmic function of the ratio of movement distance (D) to target width (W):

$$MT = a + b \cdot \log_2(2D/W), \tag{12.1}$$

where a and b are constants. This equation has been shown to be valid for discrete and rhythmic movement, movements performed by young and elderly persons, in different loading conditions, by different effectors, and in different environments. A change in the experimental conditions only leads to an adjustment in the coefficients a and b while the functional form of Fitts' law remains unchanged.

Scaling of MT with D is not surprising, for example because of purely mechanical reasons: It takes longer to move an inertial object over a larger distance. It is less obvious, however, that MT scales linearly with $\log(D)$. Scaling of MT with W is far from being trivial: Why would one slow down to land in a smaller target? To account for this effect, one has to make assumptions with respect to processes residing within

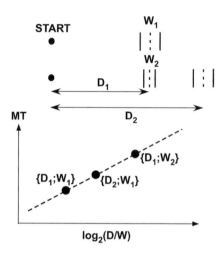

Figure 12.1 If a person is asked to move "as fast and accurately as possible" to a target, movement time (MT) is a linear function of log-transformed ratio of target distance (D) to target width (W). Making the target smaller has the same relative effect on MT as increasing the distance.

the central nervous system. Finally, it is rather unexpected that changing distance, for example increasing it by a factor of two, leads to the same effect on movement time as decreasing target width by the same factor of two.

Hypotheses on the origins of Fitts' law

Originally, Fitts came up with this formulation based on the classical *information theory*. In further studies, Fitts' law has been discussed as originating at both *movement planning* and *movement execution* levels. One of the hypotheses assumed that Fitts' law resulted from a series of corrective *sub-movements* used by a person to land in a small and distant target (Figure 12.2). It assumes that each sub-movement is performed at the highest possible speed and leads to an error in the distance traveled proportional to the distance. So, if one faces a small and distant target, the first sub-movement is likely to land somewhere in the target vicinity but outside the target. Then, a second sub-movement is used to bring the end-effector even closer to the target. And so on, until the target is reached. The sub-movements are not expected to come to a complete stop before the next sub-movement is initiated. Rather, their existence is revealed in inflections of trajectories and sequences of acceleration–deceleration pairs (as in the bottom panel of Figure 12.2).

Another idea is that human motor actions are associated with an irreducible "noise," which is *signal-dependent*. This implies, in particular, that typical errors in force (quantified as standard deviation across several trials) are proportional to force magnitude. So, using high forces and moments of force that are needed for fast movements is expected to lead to proportionally large errors in those variables, resulting in larger movement amplitude errors. The idea of signal-dependent noise, therefore, suggests that in order to land in a small target, one has to slow down.

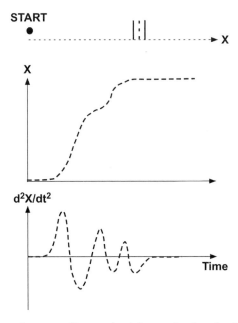

Figure 12.2 Movements into a small target (top) frequently show hesitations (middle) corresponding to multiple acceleration–deceleration cycles (bottom).

The dependence of force variability on force level has been studied extensively, in particular by the group of Karl Newell. These studies have shown that force standard deviation increases with force level in a nearly linear fashion within a broad range of forces. This, however, is true only for single-effector tasks, for example in tasks that require force to be produced by pressing with a single digit or producing torque in a single joint. When a redundant system is involved in force production, for example several fingers pressing in parallel, variance of total force shows little dependence on force level. This is illustrated in the left panel of Figure 12.3, which shows the data for young and elderly persons who performed slow ramps of total force increase while pressing with the fingertips (distal) or with the proximal phalanges (proximal). In contrast, each finger's force shows an increase in its variance (and standard deviation) with an increase in the force level; this is illustrated in the right panel of Figure 12.3, which shows the sum of the force variances of the four fingers. But most of this variance is channeled into *good variance* (variance within the *uncontrolled manifold*, see Section 9.4), while only a small fraction results in bad variance and affects performance (variance of the total force). Since most natural actions involve redundant sets of effectors, it is not obvious that the dependence of force variability on force level has to lead to slowing down when a smaller target is presented.

Besides, several studies have shown that Fitts' law can be observed in postural adjustments prior to movement initiation (for example, *in anticipatory postural adjustments*, APAs, described in Section 11.1). These observations speak against the idea of sub-movements as the origin of Fitts' law; otherwise, one would have to

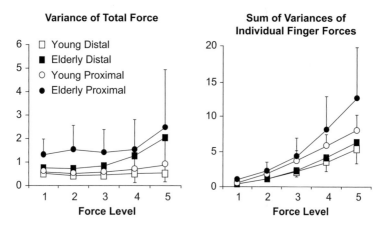

Figure 12.3 Force variance typically increases with force level. However, when several effectors act in parallel, the sum of variances of individual effectors (fingers) increases with force level (right panel) while variance of total force is nearly immune to force level variation (left panel). Data for young and elderly persons are shown who produced force while pressing with distal phalanges and while pressing with proximal phalanges. Averages across participants are shown with standard error bars. Reproduced by permission from Shinohara, M., Scholz, J. P., Zatsiorsky, V. M., & Latash, M. L. (2004). Finger interaction during accurate multi-finger force production tasks in young and elderly persons. *Experimental Brain Research, 156,* 282–292.

assume that the central nervous system predicts the number of sub-movements before the initiation of the very first sub-movement. Also, since no forces related to the explicit task are generated during the APAs, these observations also speak against the idea of signal-dependent noise as the origin of Fitts' law. These and other observations have resulted in a view that Fitts' law originates at the level of movement planning. Simply put, humans are scared of moving to small and distant targets and, as a result, they slow down.

Within the *equilibrium-point hypothesis*, a quick movement into a target may be associated with changing neural variables, such as λ (see Section 8.3), to new values. These new values define a new equilibrium position of the system where it will come to rest (Figure 12.4). If the external loading conditions do not change, accuracy in landing within the target is defined exclusively by accuracy of specifying the final value of λ (λ_{FIN}). There is no obvious reason to expect variability of λ_{FIN} to show a strong dependence on the initial value of λ (λ_{INIT}) that corresponds to the initial position of the effector(s). Note that movement distance is defined by $\Delta\lambda = (\lambda_{FIN} - \lambda_{INIT})$. Compare the distances D_1 and D_2 in Figure 12.4 corresponding to movements from two different starting positions (defined by the load and the initial values λ_1 and λ_2) into the same final position corresponding to the equilibrium point EP_{FIN}. This implies that accuracy in reaching λ_{FIN} is not expected to depend on movement distance, in contradiction to Fitts' law. Indeed, if a subject is told to ignore the target size and always move as fast as possible while aiming at the center of the target, after a bit of practice Fitts' law starts to disintegrate as predicted by the equilibrium-point hypothesis.

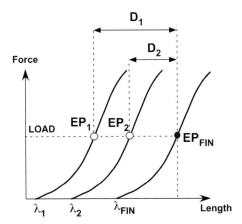

Figure 12.4 Within the equilibrium-point hypothesis, movements to the same final position from different initial positions (over distances D_1 and D_2) in isotonic conditions corresponds to shifts of the threshold (λ) of the tonic stretch reflex (three force–length characteristics are shown with curved lines) from different initial values (λ_1 and λ_2) to the same final value (λ_{FIN}).

Traditionally, Fitts' law is described using the expression *speed–accuracy trade-off*. This expression is imprecise, because no measure of accuracy of actual performance is included into the formulation of Fitts' law, only parameters of the task and movement time (which correlates with average speed for obvious mechanical reasons). Since task parameters define the difficulty of the task, not accuracy in its performance, it seems more appropriate to call it a *speed–difficulty trade-off*. In contrast, there is a relation between movement time and an index of variability of the final position, which deserves the name speed–accuracy trade-off.

Speed–accuracy trade-off

While Fitts' law links movement time to parameters of the task, there is a speed–accuracy trade-off that links movement time to parameters of actual performance. If a person is asked to produce a series of movements to a very small target quickly and accurately, movements will show some variability in the final position about some average location, which may not correspond to the center of the target (Figure 12.5). Let us assume that the person moved over a distance D_{ACT} and showed a scatter of final positions that can be characterized by a standard deviation SD_{ACT} about some average final position. Richard Schmidt and his colleagues introduced a notion of effective target width (W_E) with the size of $\pm 2SD_{ACT}$; then, about 95% of trials are expected to fall within W_E. It has been shown that W_E demonstrates a linear increase with the average movement speed:

$$W_E = c + d \cdot (D_{ACT}/MT), \tag{12.2}$$

where c and d are constants. Note that, in contrast to Fitts' law, this equation links MT to parameters characterizing actual performance such as W_E and D_{ACT}, and the

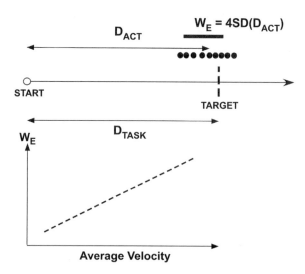

Figure 12.5 During movements to a very small target, average movement velocity scales linearly with standard deviation of actual movement distance, SD(D_{ACT}). A hypothetical distribution of final positions is shown with filled circles. Note that D_{ACT} may differ from the task distance (D_{TASK}).

relationship is linear rather than logarithmic. This speed–accuracy trade-off gets contribution from all the levels involved in the production of a fast movement, from motor planning to movement mechanics.

Methodological issues in studies of speed–accuracy trade-offs

The experimental procedures used to study the speed–accuracy and speed–difficulty trade-offs are somewhat controversial. First, the typical instruction "be as fast and accurate as possible" is ambiguous. It requires the subject to decide which is more important—speed or accuracy. In typical Fitts' experiments with an explicitly set target width, commonly the subjects are told that they can land outside the target in not more than, for example, 10–20% of trials. So, the subjects are expected to speed-up until they cannot satisfy this requirement and then slow down just a bit to be within the allowed error range. However, some subjects try to play it safe and slow down even more to make sure that they always land within the target. So, this instruction allows freedom for interpretation by the subjects. The consistency of Fitts' law suggests that, as long as a person sticks to a certain interpretation of the instruction (that is, what the relative importance of speed and accuracy is), the law holds.

In typical experiments with a very small target (sometimes just a point), there is even more freedom for the subject to decide what accuracy is acceptable. Since it is virtually impossible to land exactly on the target, the participant has to self-impose a criterion of acceptable accuracy, which may be very subjective. But once again, as long as this criterion is kept unchanged over the duration of the experiment, the speed–accuracy trade-off illustrated by Equation 12.2 holds.

The mechanical properties of the muscles and tendons and the length- and velocity-sensitive reflexes (see Sections 3.1 and 3.4) contribute to the behavior of human limbs that is sometimes imprecisely referred to as "viscoelastic." This term implies the following. Imagine that a limb is in equilibrium against an external load applied to its endpoint (for example, a heavy object in the hand). If a small change in the external load takes place, the endpoint will move away from the equilibrium. The limb will generate force against the perturbation, and the magnitude of this force will be approximately proportional both to the magnitude of the deviation and to its velocity. The term *viscoelastic* is not recommended because it implies that the object (the limb) possesses classical physical properties of viscosity and elasticity (stiffness). As explained in earlier chapters (see Section 5.1), this is not true. Unfortunately, there is no other established term in the field.

As a result of the described property of human limbs, fast movements typically show oscillations about the final position. This is the source of yet another problem for studies of the accuracy of fast movements: What if a subject in a typical Fitts' experiment lands inside the target while the terminal trajectory oscillations land outside the target? Is this a hit or a miss? Sometimes, a certain value of *dwell time* within the target is required to count a movement as a hit. Obviously, subject behavior will depend on whether the experimenter counts or does not count terminal oscillations outside the target as errors. So, there is a lot of arbitrariness and imprecision in performing such experiments. It is even more amazing that the two trade-offs are very robust at describing the observations.

Effects of practice on the speed–accuracy and speed–difficulty trade-offs

Practice does not change the form of Equations 12.1 and 12.2 but it can change the coefficients in those equations. According to Equation 12.2, speeding the movement up is expected to lead to larger W_E, that is, to larger variability of the final coordinate. Practice, however, allows this effect to be overcome and leads to an increase in both movement speed (D_{ACT}/MT) and accuracy (lower W_E) in a seeming violation of Equation 12.2.

The same is true with respect to Fitts' law. With practice, subjects show shorter movement times (higher average speed) when moving to targets characterized by the same ratio D/W. There are different interpretations for these findings within the two main hypotheses on motor control.

Learning internal models

Improvement of motor performance with practice has been associated with the elaboration of better (more adequate) internal models within the central nervous system. Most studies using the language of internal models studied the effects of practice on movements performed in artificially changed force fields or under distortion of visual feedback. A common manipulation has been to apply an artificial force field with the external force magnitude proportional to movement speed and the vector of force acting orthogonally to the speed vector. Movement trajectories and their changes with practice in such a field were illustrated earlier (see Figure 5.16 in

Section 5.1 and Figure 11.22 in Section 11.3). Before practice and without an artificial force field, the trajectories were straight. The application of the force field distorted the shape of the trajectories, which became rather curved. After some practice, the trajectories became nearly straight again, similar to their shape without force application. Finally, when the force field was turned off, there was an after-effect on the trajectories, which became curved in the opposite direction compared to their shape during the first trials after the force field was turned on.

Similar effects were observed when the subjects performed pointing arm movement to a visual target and visual feedback was distorted, for example with prismatic glasses that rotated the visual field by a fixed angular deviation (see Figure 11.23 in Section 11.3). During the first trials with the glasses on, participants pointed not at the target but at a place where they perceived it to be. After a few trials, however, the pointing movements became accurate. After the glasses were taken off, a few initial trials showed directional errors in the opposite direction.

The observations of the after-effects suggest that the central nervous system learns to take into consideration the artificially distorted sensory information and/or the artificial force field. In particular, it generates neural signals that lead to the generation of muscle forces and joint torques that differ from those prior to practice and are adequate to produce desired trajectories in the presence of an artificial sensory or motor manipulation.

One feature of movements in artificial force fields does not fit well with the idea of new internal models elaborated during practice: There is very limited transfer of the effects of practice to movements performed in another work space. For example, if the center-out task illustrated in Figure 5.16 is practiced only within a small range of endpoint directions, for example only using movements performed within a $\pm 20°$ range, movements within that range adapt well and show after-effects similar to those described earlier. However, movements in directions that are far away from the practiced range do not. They remain curved as if no practice happened. There are also no after-effects on such movements after the force field has been turned off. The trajectories remain straight. These observations question the usefulness of the term "internal model," which implies a computational operation that is applicable to both practiced and unpracticed directions.

Learning equilibrium trajectories

Within the equilibrium-point hypothesis, changes in neural commands that happen with practice are described in terms of control trajectories, such as the time changes in the tonic stretch reflex threshold, $\lambda(t)$ for a single muscle or changes in the threshold for activation of higher order neuronal pools that produce $\{r(t), c(t)\}$ for a joint, and $\{R(t); C(t)\}$ for a multi-joint system (see Sections 8.3, 8.4, and 11.3). Currently, rules that result in adjustments of control trajectories during practice are unknown. A simple and elegant solution has been offered by the Canadian researchers David Ostry and Paul Gribble. This solution takes advantage of the fact that equilibrium trajectories are expressed in actual kinematic variables. If a deviation of an actual trajectory happens from a desired trajectory (top panel of Figure 12.6), the referent (equilibrium) trajectory

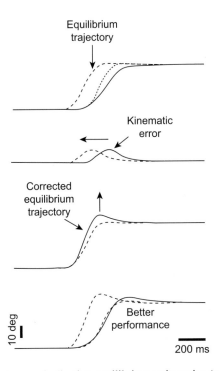

Figure 12.6 A simple scheme of adjusting equilibrium trajectories (top) based on kinematic errors (second set of lines) can lead to quick adaptation to novel conditions of movement execution (bottom lines). Reproduced by permission from Gribble, P. L., & Ostry, D. J. (2000). Compensation for loads during arm movements using equilibrium-point control. *Experimental Brain Research, 135*, 474–482.

(shown as dashed lines in Figure 12.6) is adjusted in the next trial following a simple rule. The kinematic difference between the actual and desired trajectories (second panel in Figure 12.6) is added to the previous equilibrium trajectory (the third panel of Figure 12.6). This simple rule has been shown to lead to a very quick adaptation to novel conditions taking 2–3 trials. It also leads to after-effects, that is, trajectories curved into the opposite direction, after the force field has been turned off unexpectedly for the subject. Note that, unlike the ideas of internal model adjustment, this simple rule does not involve any computations related to the complex transformations of neural and mechanical variables involved in producing the task mechanics.

12.3   Learning motor synergies

Most tasks are performed in conditions of *motor redundancy*, that is, the number of elements is higher than the number of task constraints. As a result, there are an infinite number of solutions available to solve the task (see Section 3.5). According to the idea of *synergies* and the *uncontrolled manifold hypothesis* (see Section 9.4), such tasks

are performed using families of solutions that reduce variance of important performance variables. Variance in the space of elemental variables can be viewed as
consisting of two components—*good variance* and *bad variance*. By definition, only
bad variance has an effect on variance of the important performance variable, while
good variance does not. It is natural to expect bad variance to drop with practice;
otherwise, accuracy of performance would not improve. It is much less obvious,
however, what could happen with good variance.

Let us use the same, simple example as in Section 9.4—two elements that try to
produce an accurate magnitude of their summed output. So, the task may be
formulated as $E_1 + E_2 = C$, where E_1 and E_2 are the outputs of the elements, and C is
a desired constant value. Let us assume that prior to practice there was a degree of co-
variation between E_1 and E_2 such that the good variance (V_{GOOD}) was larger than the
bad variance (V_{BAD}). With practice, V_{BAD} drops. What will happen to V_{GOOD}?

There are three scenarios illustrated in Figure 12.7. First, V_{BAD} drops, while V_{GOOD}
stays unchanged (or decreases less, or even increases) leading to a larger proportion of
the total variance accounted for by V_{GOOD}. This may be interpreted as the synergy
becoming stronger (panel B). Second, V_{GOOD} decreases in proportion to V_{BAD}. This
implies more accurate performance without a change in the synergy strength, only
due to the fact that each element's output became less variable (panel C). Third,
V_{GOOD} may drop more than V_{BAD}, leading to a more spherical data distribution
illustrated in panel D. Although the last scenario may look counterintuitive, data
compatible with all three scenarios have been reported.

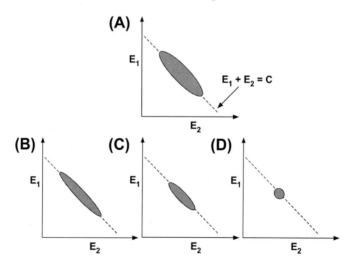

Figure 12.7 Three scenarios of changes in synergy with practice. (A) Prior to practicing a task
of constant common output production with two effectors (E_1 and E_2), a synergy is seen
reflecting a data distribution across trials elongated along the line $E_1 + E_2 = C$. After practice,
variance orthogonal to that line ("bad variance") is expected to be reduced. Variance along that
line may (B) remain unchanged, (C) decrease proportionally, or (D) decrease more than "bad
variance". In other words, improved accuracy of performance may correspond to a stronger
synergy (B), similar synergy (C), or weaker synergy (D).

Within the equilibrium-point hypothesis, practice may be expected to lead to more accurate specification of control variables at the highest level of the control hierarchy related to the production of the most relevant performance variable. This is expected to lead to a drop in V_{BAD} without a comparable change in V_{GOOD} (as in panel B of Figure 12.7). A drop in V_{GOOD} suggests that the controller cares not only about producing accurate values of the task variable (a drop in V_{GOOD} does not help accurate performance) but also about other factors. These may be summarized as performing the task in an optimal way with respect to some cost function such as, for example, minimal fatigue or minimal effort (see Sections 7.3 and 9.2). This would require combining control at the highest hierarchical level with control at lower levels that favors some combinations of elemental variables over others, despite the fact that they lead to the same values of the important performance variable.

Studies of the effects of practice in unusual force fields have typically been performed using non-redundant systems such as pointing at targets in a two-dimensional workspace by a two-joint (shoulder–elbow) effector. When similar studies are performed using a kinematically redundant system, a three-joint limb performing a planar task, adaptation to the novel force field results in higher V_{GOOD} even after the movements adapt fully and show straight trajectories. Figure 12.8

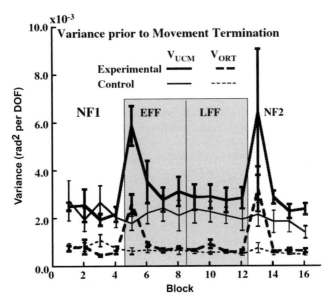

Figure 12.8 Practicing movements by a kinematically redundant effector in a destabilizing force field leads to higher variance within the uncontrolled manifold (UCM) even after seemingly perfect adaptation (variance that affects performance, V_{ORT} is as low as without the force field). Data are shown averaged across subjects in the null-field (no artificial force) before (NF1) and after (NF2) adaptation, early after the force field was turned on (EFF) and after much practice (LFF). Reproduced by permission from Yang, J.-F., Scholz, J. P., & Latash, M. L. (2007). The role of kinematic redundancy in adaptation of reaching. *Experimental Brain Research, 176,* 54–69.

illustrates the changes in the two variance components, within the UCM (V_{UCM}; same as V_{GOOD}) and orthogonal to the UCM (V_{ORT}; same as V_{BAD}) quantified during adaptation to the novel force field (EFF—early effects of force field, LFF—late effects of force field). Note the elevated level of V_{UCM} (thick solid line) as compared to no force field (NF1) while V_{ORT} (thick dashed line) is reduced to the original level. This observation suggests that there is more to adaptation to new force fields than learning new internal models. Indeed, there is no reason for a new, optimal internal model to lead to more variable joint trajectories across repetitive trials.

12.4   Stages in motor learning

Bernstein's three-stage scheme

Bernstein suggested a three-stage scheme of processes associated with motor learning. He viewed the typical redundant design of the motor apparatus as a computational problem that required *elimination of redundant degrees-of-freedom* to make the system controllable. So, the first stage was assumed to be associated with elimination of or *freezing degrees-of-freedom*. During the second stage, the controller is assumed to become comfortable with the task and start *releasing degrees-of-freedom* to achieve flexibility of performance in the changing environment and its stability in cases of unexpected perturbations. The third stage was assumed to lead to an *optimal interaction with external forces* such that only those external forces that hurt performance are counteracted, while those that help performance are not.

This three-stage scheme has become classical despite the imprecise expressions "freezing degrees-of-freedom" and "releasing degrees-of-freedom." Indeed, what does it mean that a degree-of-freedom has become frozen? In practice, this means that the peak-to-peak amplitude of change in that particular degree-of-freedom dropped below a certain arbitrarily selected threshold. For example, in a multi-joint fast movement, frozen degrees-of-freedom are associated with joint rotations that are small according to some criterion. This is assumed to simplify the control of the multi-joint limb. The last statement is not at all obvious: To avoid motion in a joint of a multi-joint limb during a fast movement requires precisely timed non-trivial control of muscles crossing that joint (see Sections 5.2 and 11.3). A study of the equilibrium trajectories during fast movement of one joint in a two-joint (elbow–wrist) system has shown large-amplitude changes in the control variables to the apparently postural joint (see Figure 11.27 in Section 11.3). So, trying to freeze a joint does not automatically make the task simpler.

There may be another reason for reducing the amplitude of some degrees-of-freedom. It is well established that standard deviation of a variable (for example, force) increases nearly linearly with the magnitude of change of that variable. So, if a redundant set of elemental variables contribute to a common task, and there is no neural mechanism in place to arrange co-variation of the variables, minimizing the amplitude of a subset of degrees-of-freedom (freezing them) is a sensible mechanism to reduce variance of the combined output. After a synergy has been developed stabilizing the salient performance variable, the previously frozen degrees-of-freedom can be released. This will be accompanied by more flexible and adaptive performance.

Two stages in learning motor synergies

Recent studies of multi-element actions produced by redundant systems showed that the polar strategies illustrated in Figure 12.7B and D typically follow each other in a certain order. Namely, when a person practices a novel task, synergies (that may be absent before practice) emerge and strengthen. This is associated with a drop in bad variance without a comparable drop in good variance. After some time, the subject reaches a level of performance that is close to perfection so that no further drop in bad variance is possible. If the subject of this mental experiment continues to practice, the goal of practice changes from improving accuracy of performance (since it cannot be improved any more) to performing the task better according to other criteria. During this second stage of practice, bad variance stays nearly unchanged (it cannot drop more), so all further improvement is achieved by modifying good variance. This naturally leads to a drop in the synergy index as illustrated in Figure 12.7D.

Figure 12.9 illustrates what happens with data distributions during these two stages of practice using the example of the task: $E_1 + E_2 = C$. During the first stage, a relatively fat ellipse of data observed before practice becomes thinner and thinner until bad variance reaches the smallest value it can possibly reach. Further, the large range of good variance, which is apparently irrelevant to performance of the explicit task, starts to shrink corresponding to search for more optimal solutions with respect to a new, secondary criterion. For example, the element that produces E_1 may fatigue more

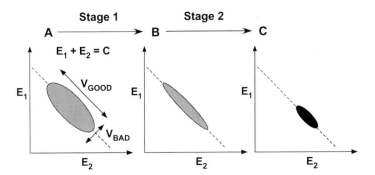

Figure 12.9 Two hypothetical stages of learning a synergy in the same task as in Figure 12.7: Constant output production with two effectors, E_1 and E_2. During the first stage, "bad variance" (V_{BAD}) drops while "good variance" (V_{GOOD}) stays nearly unchanged. So, the synergy becomes stronger. During the second stage, V_{BAD} cannot drop any more. An optimal working range is selected (the black ellipse in the rightmost graph) corresponding to smaller V_{GOOD}. The synergy weakens.

quickly, and so the controller may prefer to use a narrow range of solutions corresponding to a smaller contribution of E_1 to C (the small black ellipse in Figure 12.9C).

Is there a third stage corresponding to the Bernstein utilization of external forces? Maybe there is, but this stage is yet to be defined in terms of changes in control variables.

12.5   Neural maps and their changes with practice

Topographic organization is typical of the neural pathways within the central nervous system. This feature means that neighboring receptor cells commonly project to neighboring neurons in relay nuclei, which end up projecting to neighboring neurons in the corresponding cortical sensory area (see Figure 10.13 in Section 10.3). The same is true for descending (motor) pathways: Those pathways that originate from neighboring neurons of a brain area (cortical or not), the origin of a descending pathway, project onto interneurons, and further to motoneurons that induce muscle contractions resulting in movements of neighboring body segments. As a result, there are many *motor maps* and *sensory maps* within the central nervous system that look like distorted drawings of the whole body or of body parts.

Early cortical maps were drawn as distorted pictures of the body with unchanged relative location of body parts. Those maps were based on classical studies with direct electrical stimulation of cortical areas during brain surgery by a Canadian neurosurgeon Wilder Penfield. More recently, however, the development of new methods such as transcranial magnetic stimulation (see Section 13.5) has resulted in findings of much less somatotopically organized, mosaic neuronal representations. Stimulation of neurons in relatively remote brain areas could induce muscle contractions in similar body parts, while stimulation of neighboring neurons could produce contractions leading to movements of different effectors. Those phenomena have been called *convergence* and *divergence* (Figure 10.16 in Section 10.4).

Changes in cortical projections following injury

For a long time it was assumed that changes in the wiring within the central nervous system occur only during early childhood, and then few or no changes occur. This view was challenged by the pioneering works of an American neuroscientist Michael Merzenich and his group, who showed that cortical maps in monkeys could change dramatically and rather quickly following amputation of a digit (Figure 12.10). The cortical area dedicated to the amputated digit was quickly taken over by representations of the neighboring digits, and the whole hand representation changed. Later, similar results were observed after suturing two digits together such that they could not act independently.

Plastic changes within the central nervous system are not limited to those involving supraspinal structures. For example, classical studies by the group of Jonathan Wolpaw demonstrated changes in the excitability within the spinal, monosynaptic H-reflex loop during prolonged *operant conditioning* in monkeys. In such studies, the animal is allowed to explore the environment and it gets a reward (typically, a drop of juice) for certain types of action. It took many days and tens of thousands of repetitions to

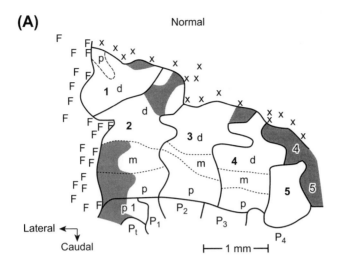

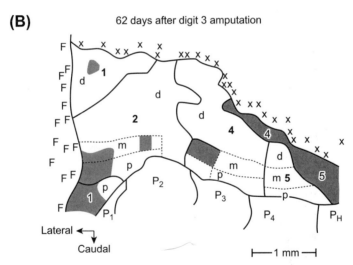

Figure 12.10 Amputation of the third digit of a monkey leads to a reorganization of the cortical projections: The areas previously occupied by the third digit become occupied by the neighboring digits. Projections corresponding to the distal (d), medial (m), and proximal (p) phalanges are shown for the digits 1–5. Reproduced by permission from Merzenich, M. M., Nelson, R. J., Stryker, M. S., Cynader, M. S., Schoppman, A., & Zook, J. M. (1984). Somatosensory cortical map changes following digit amputation in adult monkeys. *Journal of Comparative Neurology, 224*, 591–605.

produce changes in the H-reflex magnitude, but ultimately these changes took place showing that spinal reflex loops can show plasticity just like supraspinal structures.

Most dramatic changes in the cortical projections in humans have been reported following amputation of a part of the body. Commonly, projections of the amputated body part were taken up by another part of the body leading to phantom limb sensations, for example sensation of the missing hand could migrate to more proximal arm segments after lower arm amputation. Migration of hand sensation to other body parts, such as the face, has also been described (Figure 12.11).

Plastic changes within the central nervous system have also been documented following a neurological injury, for example stroke. Unilateral stroke affecting the corticospinal tract commonly leads to complete or partial loss of voluntary muscle control in the contralateral extremities. Remember that the corticospinal tract has a substantial proportion of uncrossed fibers that, in a healthy person, mostly participate in the control of axial trunk muscles. Can plastic changes lead to a functionally important increase in the role of ipsilateral projections in the control of more distal muscles? There are observations suggesting that the answer to this question is yes.

Symmetrical cortical motor areas are connected by inhibitory pathways. After stroke, the balance of the pathways is violated and there is an increase in interhemispheric inhibitory projections from the non-affected hemisphere to the affected hemisphere. These changes may interfere with recovery of the residual function of the body parts controlled by the affected hemisphere. Several strategies have been suggested to deal with this problem by inducing plastic changes within the central nervous

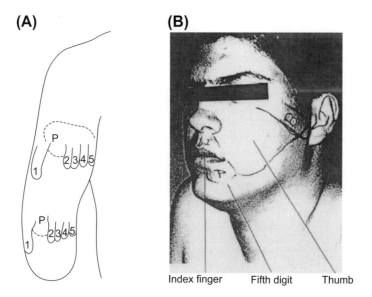

Figure 12.11 Amputation of the lower arm can lead to reorganization of the cortical projections with the amputated body part taken over by another part of the body leading to phantom sensations. As a result, sensation of the missing hand could migrate to more proximal arm segments (A) or to other body parts, such as the face (B). Projections of the palm (p) and digits 1–5 are shown. Reproduced by permission from Cohen, L. G., Bandinelli, S., Findley, T. W., & Hallett, M. (1991). Motor reorganization after upper limb amputation in humans: a study with focal magnetic stimulation. *Brain, 114*, 615–627.

system, in particular by using transcranial magnetic stimulation (and, more recently, other means of cortical stimulation using direct electrical current) with different parameters.

Changes in cortical projections following specialized practice

A number of studies have shown that plastic changes happen within the central nervous system of a healthy adult in the absence of any injury. Such changes have been commonly documented using transcranial magnetic stimulation (TMS) and observing changes in the area from which a motor response could be produced, in the threshold for inducing a response, and in the size of the response. Most such studies reported an increase in the cortical area, a decrease in the threshold, and an increase in the response amplitude with training involving that particular body part. In particular, such changes have been reported in people who learned how to read Braille or to play a musical instrument.

Several studies have shown that plastic changes within the central nervous system could occur within a very short time limited to a single experimental session (1–1.5 hours). In one such study (Figure 12.12), the subjects received single TMS stimuli over the thumb projection in the primary motor cortex. Each stimulus produced an involuntary jerky thumb motion in a particular direction (top panel of Figure 12.12).

Further, the subjects practiced thumb motion in a direction different from the one produced by the TMS (middle panel of Figure 12.12). After about 30 min of practice, the TMS stimuli of the same amplitude and applied over the same cortical area produced thumb motion in a direction shifted from the original one towards the practiced one. This effect slowly disappeared with time (bottom panel of Figure 12.12).

In another study, single TMS stimuli were applied during the execution of a task that required accurate force production by three fingers of the dominant hand pressing on force sensors. The task also imposed a constraint on the total moment of force the fingers produced since the frame with the sensors rested on a very narrow pivot (Figure 12.13). In this study, the unexpected TMS-induced responses were detrimental for performance since they produced irregular, unexpected jerky changes in the finger force. After about an hour of practice in such conditions, the amplitude of the force response to the TMS decreased. So, practice can lead not only to an increase in the excitability of neural structures involved in the task but also to a decrease in their excitability if this helps perform the task better.

The latter study provided evidence for the two stages of practice as suggested in Section 12.4. The three-dimensional space of finger forces was redundant with respect to the two constraints related to the required total force and moment of force. Figure 12.14 illustrates the UCM for a certain value of the total force (UCM_F, the dotted triangle) and for a certain (close to zero) value of the total moment of force (UCM_M, the gray triangle). The intersection of the two (the thick line) corresponds to the sub-space of good variance with respect to both total force and total moment of force. During the first 100 trials of practice, finger force variance related to total force dropped. The same

Pretraining (TMS-evoked movements)

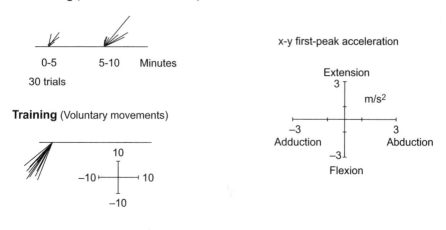

0-5   5-10   Minutes

30 trials

x-y first-peak acceleration

Extension
3
m/s²
−3   3
Adduction   Abduction
−3
Flexion

Training (Voluntary movements)

10
−10   10
−10

Posttraining (TMS-evoked movements)

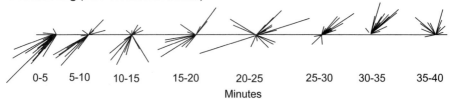

0-5   5-10   10-15   15-20   20-25   25-30   30-35   35-40
Minutes

Figure 12.12 Training can lead to changes in short-latency movements produced by a standard transcranial magnetic stimulus (TMS) applied over the contralateral primary motor area of the cortex. Top: Typical movement directions prior to practice. Second row: Movement directions during practice. Third row: Movement directions after practice are shifted towards the practiced directions. Reproduced by permission from Classen, J., Liepert, J., Wise, S. P., Hallett, M., & Cohen, L. G. (1998). Rapid plasticity of human cortical movement representation induced by practice. *Journal of Neurophysiology, 79*, 1117–1123.

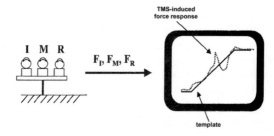

Figure 12.13 Illustration of a task of ramp force production by three fingers, index (I), middle (M), and ring (R), pressing in parallel. The fingers had to keep balance about a pivot placed under the M finger. Unexpectedly, a transcranial magnetic stimulus (TMS) was applied over the contralateral primary motor cortex and produced both force and moment of force perturbations. Modified by permission from Latash, M. L., Yarrow, K., & Rothwell, J. C. (2003). Changes in finger coordination and responses to single pulse TMS of motor cortex during practice of a multi-finger force production task. *Experimental Brain Research, 151*, 60–71.

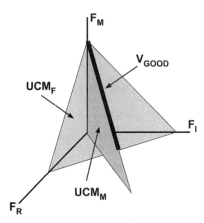

Figure 12.14 In the three-dimensional space of finger forces, two sub-spaces are shown corresponding to a constant value of total force (the dotted plane, UCM_F) and to a zero value of the total moment of force (the gray plane, UCM_M). Their intersection (the thick line) is the space of "good variance" (V_{GOOD}) for both force and moment of force.

was true for finger force variance related to moment of force. There were no major changes in the third variance component, which led to changes in neither total force nor total moment of force (good variance). During the next 100 trials, however, good variance showed a significant drop while the two other variance components remained largely unchanged. Within the two-stage scheme suggested in Section 12.4, these observations correspond to the stage of development of synergies (the first 100 trials), and to optimizing performance with respect to other factors, likely trying to cope with the perturbations produced by the TMS (the second 100 trials).

Self-test questions

1. Explain Bernstein's expression "repetition without repetition."
2. What was Pavlov's idea on effects of practice for motor skill learning?
3. Present examples of typical implicit task components.
4. Formulate Fitts' law.
5. Suggest at least three hypotheses on the origin of Fitts' law.
6. How does force variability (standard deviation) depend on force level?
7. Can Fitts' law be observed prior to movement initiation?
8. What is a major difference in the dependence of force variability on force level for a multi-element system?
9. What happens with variability in the final position when the same task is performed faster? Formulate the speed–accuracy trade-off.
10. What are the main methodological problems in studies of speed–accuracy trade-offs?
11. What happens with characteristics of the speed–accuracy trade-off with practice?
12. How much transfer to unpracticed directions is observed after practicing movements in an artificial force field?

13. How does the equilibrium-point hypothesis handle effects of practice in unusual force fields?
14. What can happen with indices of synergies during practice?
15. Explain why sometimes indices of synergies drop with practice.
16. Describe Bernstein's three-stage scheme of motor learning.
17. What stages can be identified in changes of motor synergies with practice?
18. What can happens with cortical maps following an injury to a part of the body?
19. What can happen with responses to standard transcranial magnetic stimuli applied over the primary motor cortex following practice?

Essential references and recommended further readings

Bhushan, N., & Shadmehr, R. (1999). Computational nature of human adaptive control during learning of reaching movements in force fields. *Biological Cybernetics, 81*, 39–60.

Birbaumer, N., & Cohen, L. G. (2007). Brain–computer interfaces: communication and restoration of movement in paralysis. *Journal of Physiology, 579*, 621–636.

Celnik, P. A., & Cohen, L. G. (2004). Modulation of motor function and cortical plasticity in health and disease. *Restorative Neurology and Neuroscience, 22*, 261–268.

Classen, J., Liepert, J., Wise, S. P., Hallett, M., & Cohen, L. G. (1998). Rapid plasticity of human cortical movement representation induced by practice. *Journal of Neurophysiology, 79*, 1117–1123.

Cohen, L. G., Bandinelli, S., Findley, T. W., & Hallett, M. (1991). Motor reorganization after upper limb amputation in humans: a study with focal magnetic stimulation. *Brain, 114*, 615–627.

Crossman, E. R. F. W., & Goodeve, P. J. (1983). Feedback control of hand-movement and Fitts' law. *Quarterly Journal of Experimental Psychology, 35A*, 251–278.

Domkin, D., Laczko, J., Jaric, S., Johansson, H., & Latash, M. L. (2002). Structure of joint variability in bimanual pointing tasks. *Experimental Brain Research, 143*, 11–23.

Fitts, P. M. (1954). The information capacity of the human motor system in controlling the amplitude of movement. *Journal of Experimental Psychology, 47*, 381–391.

Fitts, P. M., & Peterson, J. R. (1964). Information capacity of discrete motor responses. *Journal of Experimental Psychology, 67*, 103–112.

Graybiel, A. M. (2005). The basal ganglia: learning new tricks and loving it. *Current Opinions in Neurobiology, 15*, 638–644.

Gribble, P. L., & Ostry, D. J. (2000). Compensation for loads during arm movements using equilibrium-point control. *Experimental Brain Research, 135*, 474–482.

Hallett, M. (2001). Plasticity of the human motor cortex and recovery from stroke. *Brain Research Reviews, 36*, 169–174.

Latash, M. L. (2010). Stages in learning motor synergies: A view based on the equilibrium-point hypothesis. *Human Movement Science, 29*, 642–654.

Latash, M. L., Yarrow, K., & Rothwell, J. C. (2003). Changes in finger coordination and responses to single pulse TMS of motor cortex during practice of a multi-finger force production task. *Experimental Brain Research, 151*, 60–71.

Malfait, N., Gribble, P. L., & Ostry, D. J. (2005). Generalization of motor learning based on multiple field exposures and local adaptation. *Journal of Neurophysiology, 93*, 3327–3338.

Merzenich, M. M., Nelson, R. J., Stryker, M. S., Cynader, M. S., Schoppman, A., & Zook, J. M. (1984). Somatosensory cortical map changes following digit amputation in adult monkeys. *Journal of Comparative Neurology, 224*, 591–605.

Newell, K. M. (1991). Motor skill acquisition. *Annual Reviews in Psychology, 42,* 213–237.

Nudo, R. J., Plautz, E. J., & Frost, S. B. (2001). Role of adaptive plasticity in recovery of function after damage to motor cortex. *Muscle and Nerve, 24,* 1000–1019.

Pascual-Leone, A. (2001). The brain that plays music and is changed by it. *Annals of the New York Academy of Science, 930,* 315–329.

Schwartz, A. B. (2004). Cortical neural prosthetics. *Annual Reviews in Neuroscience, 27,* 487–507.

Thach, W. T. (1998). A role for the cerebellum in learning movement coordination. *Neurobiology of Learning and Memory, 70,* 177–188.

Vereijken, B., van Emmerick, R. E. A., Whiting, H. T. A., & Newell, K. M. (1992). Free(z)ing degrees of freedom in skill acquisition. *Journal of Motor Behavior, 24,* 133–142.

Wolpaw, J. R. (1987). Operant conditioning of primate spinal reflexes: the H-reflex. *Journal of Neurophysiology, 57,* 443–459.

13 Methods in motor control studies

Chapter Outline

13.1   General methodological issues

Experimental methods in motor control form three large groups that focus on *mechanical, electrical,* and *metabolic* variables. Patterns of mechanical variables are obviously more closely related to success of movements and the interactions between the body and the environment. On the other hand, electrical variables reflect processes within the body, within muscles—*electromyography* (EMG) and within the brain—*electroencephalography* (EEG). Many indices used in brain imaging studies such as *magnetic resonance imaging* (MRI) and *positron emission tomography* (PET) are

Fundamentals of Motor Control. DOI: **10.1016/B978-0-12-415956-3.00013-0** reflections of metabolic processes that are expected to correlate with synaptic activity in the corresponding areas.

Quite commonly, methods from two or three groups are used simultaneously. In such cases, one has to keep in mind that electrical signals propagate and are being recorded by instruments nearly instantaneously, while mechanical signals typically have to reach a particular threshold to be identified. For example, if one measures muscle activation level and a mechanical variable produced by the muscle, a delay is expected between detectable changes in the former and in the latter. This delay, known as *electromechanical delay*, reflects methods of measurement and accuracy of equipment to a larger extent than physiological processes within the muscle. Different methods of measurement result in values of electromechanical delay varying from under 10 ms to over 100 ms. Metabolic signals show changes at an even larger time delay following the neural processes they reflect. As a result, the time resolution of such methods is rather poor.

Studies of biological motion typically involve observation with or without applying perturbations. Observations of unperturbed motor behavior in various tasks and under various instructions allow more or less natural patterns of variables of interest to be quantified and later interpreted. A researcher may be interested in average across repeated trials patterns and/or in trial-to-trial variability of such patterns over repeated attempts.

Application of controlled perturbations is potentially a powerful method that has been developed in engineering to identify characteristics of systems with unknown parameters. It may lead, however, to major problems when applied to biological systems. In non-living systems, it is typically assumed that the properties (parameters) of the system do not change while it responds to a perturbation. As a result, comparing the system's states prior to and after the perturbation allows the values of its important parameters to be computed. This assumption is commonly violated in biological systems: Their responses to perturbations almost always involve a change in the parameters the method is trying to identify.

Consider the following very simple example. Imagine that you are trying to identify the gain in a reflex loop that involves a few synapses (Loop 1 in Figure 13.1). Prior to the perturbation, the system is in a steady-state characterized by states of all the involved neurons that define a value of the gain. If a perturbation is applied providing an adequate stimulus for the sensory receptors (for example, muscle stretch providing a stimulus for spindle sensory endings), the reflex response will depend on the state of the neurons in the loop. It is possible, however, that the same stimulus changes the states of some of the neurons at a time delay that is shorter than the one involved in signal transmission along the loop of interest (compare Loops 1 and 2 in Figure 13.1). So, when the signal produced by the stimulus arrives at those neurons via the longer loop, their response differs from what would have been given the pre-perturbation state. As a result, the overall response to the perturbation will change and reflect not the steady-state parameters but a potentially complex pattern of their time changes.

This ability of biological systems to change their parameters when subjected even to a subtle perturbation makes defining even such basic parameters as muscle

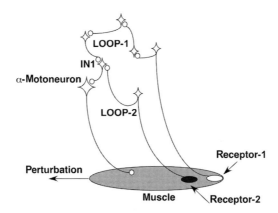

Figure 13.1 If a perturbation is used to study a reflex loop originating from a certain group of receptors (Loop-1 from Receptor-1), it is possible that the state of one of the interneurons (IN1) will be changed via a different loop (Loop-2) that originates from a different group of receptors (Receptor-2), also sensitive to the perturbation.

apparent stiffness (length dependence of muscle force) problematic. Note that the reaction of a muscle to perturbation depends on the muscle's peripheral mechanics, on short latency reflex responses, on longer latency polysynaptic reflex responses, and on other reactions that come after varying time delays and may be modified by the state of the subject of this mental experiment (see Section 3.4 and Figure 13.2). If a measurement is performed a very short time after a perturbation, not giving the system time to change its parameters via reflex loops, it may provide information about the state of peripheral structures. Such a measurement, however, is obviously unable to provide information on the state of any loops that involve elements within the central nervous system since these loops have not been given enough time to transmit action potentials.

Another approach commonly used in studies of animals is to introduce controlled lesions to structures involved in movement production. Then, observation of movement deficits may provide information on the role of the structure with the lesion in the intact body. One has to be very careful drawing such conclusions. First, an injured neural system shows remarkably quick and powerful plasticity (see Section 12.4), and its wiring after the injury may show changes in places that are far away from the injury site. Second, an injury may lead to dramatic differences in a behavior due to reasons that are not directly related to a function the researcher is interested in.

Consider the following well-known (to some) story: "A group of very smart researchers have decided to study where the organ of hearing in the cockroach is. First, they induced in a cockroach a conditioned reflex to a sound signal (a bell). In a few days, the cockroach learned to run to a corner in the cage where it expected to get a morsel of food after the bell rang. Then, the smartest of the researchers took all the legs off the poor cockroach. Then, the researcher rang the bell, and the cockroach did not run to the corner. So, the conclusion is that the organ of hearing in cockroaches is in the legs." It is useful to keep this rather stupid story in mind when reading reports with

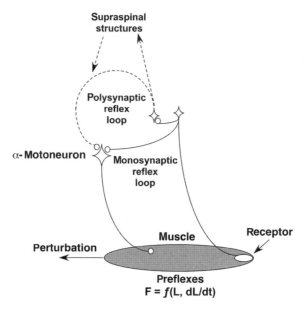

Figure 13.2 Muscle response to an external perturbation gets a contribution from different mechanisms with different characteristic time delays, such as instantaneous muscle reaction to stretch (preflexes) defined by the dependence of muscle force on length and velocity, which is a function of muscle activation level. The activation level will depend on the action of monosynaptic reflexes, long-loop polysynaptic reflexes, and reactions mediated by supraspinal structures.

conclusions on a function of different brain areas based on observations of animals with an injury to that area or of patients with a documented disorder of that area.

13.2   Mechanical analysis

Studies of mechanical variables during biological movement date back a few hundred years (see Chapter 2). In the nineteenth century, photographic methods were developed specifically for analysis of natural movements. These methods obviously could provide information only on movement *kinematics*, while *kinetic variables* (such as forces and moments of force) had to be computed based on kinematic variables and estimated mechanical (in particular, mass-inertial) properties of the body segments. The problem of linking body kinematics to muscle forces remains one of the central issues. Typically, during natural movements, only forces of interaction with the environment can be recorded more or less reliably, while forces and moments within the body (in particular, muscle forces) have to be computed based on certain assumptions and not very accurate estimations of essential mechanical parameters of the body. Even basic parameters such as mass of a body segment may change during movements, for example with changes in the blood flow distribution.

Methods of kinematic analysis

Most commonly, mechanical analysis of movement involves measurement and/or computation of coordinates, velocities, and acceleration of specific points on the body (for example, the tip of the index finger during pointing). These variables are most directly related to success or failure in motor tasks. Since skeletal muscles produce joint rotations, another group of intrinsic kinematic variables is frequently measured and/or computed, such as joint angles, rotational velocities, and rotational accelerations.

For each group of variables, commonly, only one of the variables from the group is measured while the other two are computed. For example, one of the commonly used methods to study individual joint kinematics involves *goniometers*, devices that produce electrical signals related to joint angle (Figure 13.3A). Historically, early goniometers used potentiometers (devices with variable resistance) attached to two straight planks that were strapped to two adjacent body segments. The resistance of the potentiometer changed when one of the planks rotated with respect to the other plank. Some of these goniometers showed high accuracy and linearity. Their main problem was that they assumed rotation of the two segments about a single axis whose orientation did not change during the movement. It is well established today that this assumption is violated during many human movements. Another problem was that the accuracy of measurement depended on accuracy of placement of the goniometer with respect to the joint.

More advanced goniometers measure rotations about two axes simultaneously. They are sometimes based on measuring the forces at the ends of a thin flexible piece of metal created by its deformation during movement (Figure 13.3B). The rigid end-pieces of such goniometers are attached to adjacent body segments, and the flexible metal pieces are connected in the end-pieces to force transducers. This construction does not require a specific part of the goniometer to be placed over an assumed center of joint rotation. Hence, no assumption on the location and orientation of the joint axis

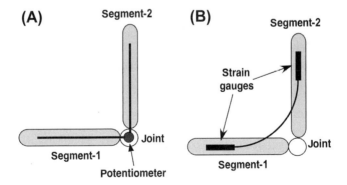

Figure 13.3 Two commonly used types of potentiometers. (A) Potentiometer is placed over the joint of interest, and two rigid planks are fixed to the two segments. (B) Two rigid end-pieces are attached to two adjacent body segments. They are connected with a flexible piece that produces forces at its ends that are functions of the joint angle.

of rotation is made. The goniometer measures the angles between the two segments viewed as two rigid bodies.

In each of the two methods illustrated in Figure 13.3, only joint angle (α) is measured. Other kinematic variables, such as *rotational velocity* (ω) and *acceleration* (*A*) have to be computed: $\omega = d\alpha/dt$; $A = d^2\alpha/dt^2$. As of now, there are no goniometers that would record three angles between two body segments; this naturally limits the applicability of this method to movements in three dimensions.

Two main groups of methods are commonly used to measure variables that characterize body kinematics with respect to the external space. The first group— jointly referred to as *optoelectronic methods*—is based on recording the coordinates of markers placed on segments of interest. (Alternatively a movement can be filmed without markers, and specific points on the body identified at each time sample— digitized—using special software under the supervision of an experienced researcher.) The second group uses distortions of an artificially created electromag- netic field by sensors attached to the body segments to compute both coordinates and orientations of the sensors in the external space. The second group provides more directly measured variables. Its drawbacks are, however, significant. In particular, it does not tolerate the presence of certain metal objects, particularly moving ones, in the space of analysis.

There are two main types of optoelectronic systems, with *active markers* and with *passive* (reflective) *markers*. The former use light-emitting diodes (LEDs) connected to the data-acquisition computer by wires. The coordinates of the LEDs are measured by a pre-calibrated system of cameras, and each marker is always unambiguously identified. The main advantage of such systems is that they by-pass the frequently tedious process of tracking inherent to systems with passive markers. The main drawback is the wires that connect the person to the system and naturally constrain movements.

Systems with passive markers are more versatile but, potentially, require more time for extracting the trajectories of individual markers. Although software is able to identify markers and track them in most situations, sometimes the images of the markers overlap in some of the camera views, and then marker switch can happen. This can only be resolved by rather tedious, manual identification of the markers.

Two main characteristics of all systems that measure body kinematics in external space are *frequency* of data acquisition and *accuracy*. Obviously, higher frequency systems are needed to study fast movements, particularly if accurate computation of velocities and accelerations is needed. Typical frequencies of data acquisition for systems with passive markers are between 60 (slow) and 240 (fast) Hz. In systems with active markers and systems that use magnetic sensors, frequency of data acquisition may depend on the number of sensors; it may be very fast (hundreds of hertz) for a few sensors but drops proportionally with an increase in the number of sensors.

It is very hard to estimate accuracy of systems that use markers placed on the skin. Specifications supplied by the manufacturers mention error values on the order of a fraction of a millimeter. Unfortunately, these values are not realistic with respect to typical variables of interest. Even if the coordinates of the individual markers are detected with such a high accuracy, this does not mean that important kinematic variables are also measured with a comparable accuracy. The main problem is that the markers, for obvious reasons, cannot be attached to the bones. They are typically placed on the body surface. During movements, unavoidable skin motion takes place, in particular due to bulging of activated muscles. This changes the geometry of the body segments and affects the relative location of the markers. Such marker displacements may be on the order of a few millimeters.

Another source of problems in estimating joint angles based on measured coordinates of markers placed on adjacent body segments is that axes of joint rotation can migrate during movements. Some body segments do not only rotate but also translate with respect to an adjacent segment. All these factors make typically used simplified geometric models of body segments (see Figures 13.4 and 13.5) valid only within relatively small ranges of changes in body configuration.

Despite all the complicating factors, body movements are usually viewed as combinations of rotations of body segments with respect to each other, with each segment considered as an elongated (commonly, one-dimensional) *rigid body*. In three-dimensional space, location and orientation of a rigid body can be described with six variables, a six-component vector (Figure 13.4).

Defining the location of a selected point on a rigid body (point *a* in Figure 13.4) is relatively simple: One has to define the origin of a coordinate system, the directions of its axes, and unit vectors, and then find projections of a vector connecting the origin of coordinates and point *a* on the axes x_a, y_a, and z_a. There are several methods of defining rigid body orientation. One of the common methods uses direction angles of the three vectors forming the local system of coordinates linked to the rigid body with respect to the axes of the global reference frame. Figure 13.4 illustrates the angles for one such vector aligned with the longest dimension of the rigid body (vector **V** in Figure 13.4).

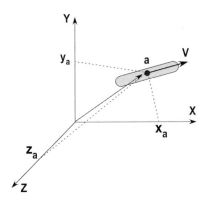

Figure 13.4 Location of a rigid body in the three-dimensional space is defined by its three coordinates (x_a, y_a, and z_a), while its orientation can be described with angles formed by the three vectors of the local system of coordinates linked to the rigid body with the axes of the global reference frame (a total of nine angles). One of such vectors (**V**) in the local coordinate system is shown.

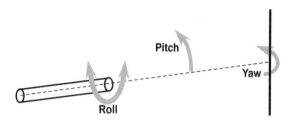

Figure 13.5 Yaw, pitch and roll angles are commonly used to describe rotation of an elongated object in the external three-dimensional space.

Defining a change in the rigid body orientation in space is less trivial. The problem is that rotations are *non-commutative*. This means that the outcome of performing a sequence of rotations about orthogonal axes depends on the order in which the rotations are performed. Therefore, rotations are commonly described using *Euler's angles*, which are successive angles of rotation about pre-defined axes. Frequently, yaw, pitch, and roll are used. For an elongated object (such as the one shown in Figure 13.5), these angles are defined as successive rotations about the vertical axis of the global reference frame, rotation about a horizontal axis of the moving reference frame orthogonal to the longer dimension of the rigid body, and rotation in the local reference frame about the longer axis of the rigid body.

Having three markers per segment is an absolute minimum to define orientation of a rigid body representing the segment in space. Typically, more markers are used and an orientation is computed that is best compatible with the recorded coordinates of the markers. Sometimes, additional constraints have to be introduced on results of such computations to make them compatible with anatomical integrity of the body: Due to the abovementioned factors, such as skin motion, computation may result in an apparent motion of the rigid bodies that corresponds to segments of the body moving away from each other in impossible ways.

If a researcher is interested in defining joint angles and their changes during movements, rigid body orientations recorded in the external system of coordinates have to be transformed into joint angle values. For computational details on such transformations, please see the book *Kinematics of Human Motion* (Zatsiorsky 1998).

Another commonly used type of kinematic sensor are those sensitive to linear acceleration—*accelerometers*. These sensors measure forces associated with an accelerating small mass placed inside the accelerometer. There are miniature accelerometers that can be attached to the body with adhesive tape. Some of them measure acceleration in one direction only—along the axis of sensitivity of the accelerometer. Others measure acceleration along two or three directions simultaneously. Typically, accelerometers are very sensitive and provide better estimates of acceleration than those computed with double differentiation of a position-related signal. Their signals can be used for computation of angular acceleration and kinetic variables (see below). Accelerometers are also frequently used to identify the moment of movement initiation because their signals show abrupt changes during posture-to-movement transitions.

There are certain problems associated with using accelerometers. Due to their design, accelerometers measure the gravity acceleration when the sensor is motionless. On the other hand, if the sensor is in a free-fall state towards the center of the Earth, it will produce no signal. Since accelerometers are sensitive to gravity, changes in their orientation with respect to the gravity line lead to changes in their output. Even in static conditions, muscle activation may lead to changes in the geometry of the body surface. This may lead to changes in the orientation of the axes of sensitivity of accelerometers placed on the body surface, resulting in acceleration-related signals while no body motion takes place.

The use of measured acceleration-related signals to compute other kinematic variables, such as velocities and coordinates, is also prone to errors. This requires the acceleration signals to be integrated, which only allows a change in velocity to be computed, not its magnitude. Velocity magnitude also depends on the initial velocity when the acceleration signal started to be recorded; in general, the initial velocity is unknown. Double-integration to compute coordinate involves two unknown constants of integration (initial velocity and initial coordinate).

There are also sensors that measure velocity—linear and/or rotational. They are based on a variety of physical principles and methods, including magnetic induction, piezoelectric phenomena, gyroscopes, and fiber optics. The measured velocity signals can be differentiated to compute acceleration and integrated to compute coordinate. Such systems are reported to achieve high precision, for example up to 0.01 deg/s for rotational velocity. Note, however, that, as with any other sensors placed on the body surface, the signal will also reflect changes in the body surface geometry with muscle activation.

Overall, direct measurement of a physical variable always has an advantage compared to its computation based on other variables that have been measured. Some systems for analysis of movement kinematics combine various sensors sensitive to different variables to improve accuracy of measurement.

Computation of kinetic variables from kinematic recordings

Measuring kinetic variables, such as muscle forces and joint torques, during natural human movements is very difficult. There are sensors that generate electrical signals proportional to the components of the force and moment of force vectors acting on the sensor, but placing them inside the body (implanting them) is associated with obvious medical and ethical problems (although this has been done by volunteers in some laboratories, for example in the laboratory of Professor Paavo Komi in Finland). Placing the sensors on the body surface is easy, but then they measure other forces such as contact forces with the environment and inertial forces, not forces between anatomical structures within the body.

Most commonly, joint moments of force during movements are computed based on measured and/or computed kinematic signals and equations of motion (for example, see Section 5.1). The equations contain a number of parameters related to the geometry of the moving body and to its mass–inertial characteristics such as masses of the segments, their moments of inertia, and corresponding center-of-mass coordinates.

These parameters differ between people. While the length of a segment can be measured more or less accurately, the mass–inertial characteristics cannot be measured and have to be estimated. Such estimates are typically based on earlier studies on cadavers or indirect measurements in groups of persons (for example, using gamma-rays to estimate tissue density). Those studies produced regression models that allow mass–inertial characteristics to be computed based on a set of readily accessible measures such as height, body mass, segment length, segment circumference, etc. Unfortunately, the natural differences in the body proportions and composition among people introduce errors into such estimates on the order of about 10%. Besides, during movements, migration of the axes of joint rotation, changes in the blood flow, and muscle bulging result in changes in the parameters in typical equations of motion.

There have been attempts to estimate muscle forces based on muscle activation signals (electromyogram, EMG) combined with estimated values of muscle physio-logical cross-sectional area, length and velocity; the latter are based on measured joint kinematics. The EMG signal depends on placement of the electrodes, orientation of the muscle fibers, and skin resistance (see Section 13.3). Some of these factors may change during movements, making this method of muscle force estimation potentially rather inaccurate. Besides, parameters of the transformation of electrical muscle signals into forces cannot be measured directly and have to be assumed.

Force platforms

It is relatively easy to measure forces and moments of force between the body and the environment. Force sensors are relatively accurate and inexpensive. The simplest ones measure only one variable, the force vector component orthogonal to the sensor surface. More sophisticated sensors measure six variables representing three components of the force vector and three components of the moment of force vector in the local reference frame of the sensor (Figure 13.6). Historically, the first six-component sensors were rather large and used to measure the forces and moments of

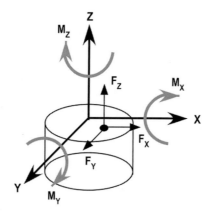

Figure 13.6 A six-component force sensor measures three components of the force vector (F_X, F_Y, and F_Z) and three components of the moment-of-force vector (M_X, M_Y, and M_Z).

force during standing between the person and the supporting surface. These have been called *force platforms*. Force platforms remain one of the most commonly used tools in studies of whole-body actions such as posture and stepping.

When a person stands on a force platform, he or she generates a normal force (during absolutely quiet standing it corresponds to the weight of the person), a two-dimensional vector of shear force, and moments of force about the three platform axes. Note that moments of force are measured with respect to axes passing through a pre-defined center of the platform, which sometimes is located deep inside the platform (Figure 13.7).

Commonly used variables in postural studies are coordinates of the center of pressure (COP, Figure 13.7). The COP is, by definition, the point of application of the resultant vertical force acting on the body. The coordinates of this point in the platform reference frame can be computed from the measured forces and moments of force:

$$\mathrm{COP}_X = \frac{-M_Y + (F_X * dz)}{F_Z}; \mathrm{COP}_Y = \frac{-M_X + (F_Y * dz)}{F_Z}, \tag{13.1}$$

where F stands for force, M for moment of force, and dz stands for the moment arm of the shear forces with respect to the center of the coordinate system. In some

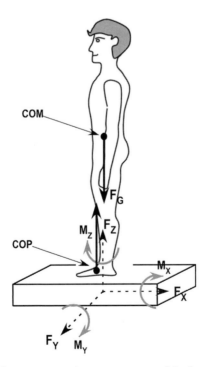

Figure 13.7 A force platform measures three components of the force vector (F_X, F_Y, and F_Z) and three components of the moment-of-force vector (M_X, M_Y, and M_Z). These can be used to compute the coordinates of the center of pressure (COP). Estimating coordinates of the center of mass (COM) during quiet standing may be a complicated procedure.

platforms, $dz = 0$, while in others it is on the order of a few centimeters. Since in most studies the subject does not stand exactly over the origin of the coordinate system, shifts of the COP are of interest rather than its absolute coordinates.

Relatively recently, miniature force platforms have been built to study the contact forces between digits and environment. Overall, they function exactly as the larger force platforms. Components of the force and moment of force vectors, as well as COP coordinates, are most commonly used variables to describe the contact between the digit and the environment.

When a person stands on a force platform, the signals can be used to estimate the motion of the center of mass (COM) projection on a horizontal plane. According to Newton's second law, $F_{X,Y} = m \cdot A_{X,Y}$, where F stands for force, A for acceleration, and m for mass. The mass of the person can be estimated from the measured vertical force component: $F_Z = m \cdot g$, where g is gravity acceleration. So, acceleration of the COM is relatively easy to compute from the platform signals. However, as mentioned earlier, estimation of the coordinates of the COM projection on the horizontal surface of the platform from acceleration is non-trivial because this procedure requires the initial COM coordinates and velocity to be known.

If the person stands quietly and then performs a fast action (for example, quickly sways the body forward), the initial conditions may be assumed to be $COM_{X,Y} = COP_{X,Y}$, and $dCOM_{X,Y}/dt = 0$. Since COP coordinates can be measured (see Equation 13.1), the initial conditions for the COM become known. However, if the person stands quietly for a long time, and the task is to compute migration of the COM over time, the assumption on the initial conditions is no longer valid.

Several methods have been suggested for estimating COM trajectory. One of them is based on the fact that when shear force along a coordinate is zero (for example, $F_X = 0$ at t_0), coordinates of the COP and COM projection may be assumed to coincide. This makes the COM coordinate known at selected times. Further, COM velocity may be assumed to be zero at t_0, and COM coordinates computed until the next time when $F_X = 0$. Comparing the computed and actual coordinates allows the error in the initial COM velocity to be estimated. This procedure results in estimating the magnitudes of both variables, COM_X and $dCOM_X/dt$ at t_0.

If only COM shifts are of interest, not absolute coordinates, another method may be used. It assumes the initial COM position along a coordinate to be zero, $COM_X(t_0) = 0$. Assuming (wrongly) $dCOM_X/dt = 0$ at t_0 leads to a drift of the computed $COM_X(t)$ from the actual one. This drift will lead to a trend in the $COM_X(t)$ trajectory, moving it beyond the limits of a reasonable area, for example the area of support. The trend can be estimated quantitatively, and the initial value of $dCOM_X/dt$ can be corrected to eliminate the trend.

13.3   Electromyography

Recording of muscle activation patterns is usually performed using one of the two main methods. Within the first method, a thin wire is inserted into the muscle of interest (or, more precisely, into an area of interest of the muscle of interest) and the electrical potential recorded by the tip of the wire with respect to a remote (indifferent) electrode is measured. Within the second method, two electrodes are placed on top of the muscle of interest, and the difference in the potentials at the two electrodes in measured. These two methods are commonly referred to as *intramuscular electromyography* and *surface electromyography*. In both cases, the measurements reflect electrical processes inside the muscle without a time delay.

Even when using intramuscular electromyography, one can only record extracellular electrical potentials since the tip of the wire does not pierce the muscle cell membrane. As a result, typical electromyographic (EMG) signals are much smaller than the typical action potential peak-to-peak amplitude (which may be about 100–120 mV, see Section 3.1). Typical magnitudes of signals recorded by intramuscular electromyography are about 1 mV, while typical signals recorded from the muscle surface are an order of magnitude smaller. Such small signals have to be amplified before recording; they may also be corrupted by extraneous electromagnetic fields. The most common source of noise is the 60 Hz power supply. Sometimes, activation of other muscles generates large-amplitude extraneous signals, for example signals from the heart muscle commonly affect recordings made from trunk muscles.

The main advantage of intramuscular electromyography is that it allows the patterns of activity of individual motor units to be recorded. Note that each motor unit contains many muscle fibers, which are all innervated by short terminal branches of a single axon of an alpha-motoneuron and, therefore, they generate action potentials nearly synchronously. As a result, the changes in the electrical field produced by those individual action potentials sum up and result in a signal that has a specific, reproducible pattern. If relative location of a recording electrode with respect to the muscle fibers does not change, it may be expected to record a specific "signature" pattern for the compound action potential of each motor unit in its vicinity. Typically, a thin wire electrode is able to record the electrical activity of a few motor units whose muscle fibers happen to be in close proximity to the electrode. The differences in the "signature" patterns of individual motor units make it possible to record several motor units with one intramuscular electrode and identify their compound action potentials using specially designed pattern recognition software.

There are several pitfalls of this method. First, it allows activation of only a portion of the muscle, close to the tip of the wire, to be recorded. As a result, this method is more commonly used to study activation of small muscles, for example intrinsic hand muscles (see Section 11.4) or compartments of larger muscles, for example extrinsic hand muscles. Second, even a small shift in the location of the tip of the electrode with respect to the muscle fibers may corrupt the recordings by distorting individual motor unit action potentials. Since muscle contractions always lead to changes in the muscle fiber geometry, in particular, during production of large forces, intramuscular electromyography is commonly used only during small to moderate force production tasks.

The other method, surface electromyography, is frequently used in studies of movements that involve large muscles with the bellies close to the surface of the body. Typically, two electrodes are attached to the skin over the muscle belly, and the difference of potentials between the electrodes is measured. Researchers select the size of electrodes used in surface electromyography based on their particular goals. The electrodes may be from 1 mm to 20 mm in diameter; the distance between the centers of the electrodes may vary from 5 mm to 100 mm. Most commonly, the purpose of this method is not to focus on individual motor unit firing patterns but to obtain a measure of overall muscle activation. One has to note that surface electrodes with very small contact areas have been developed to be able to identify individual motor unit compound action potentials. This method, however, is plagued with the same problems as intramuscular electromyography. In particular, during muscle contractions, there may be major changes in the location of muscle fibers with respect to the skin as well as changes in skin resistance. So, electrodes fixed on the skin surface are likely to record signals from different motor units when the muscle contracts, and the magnitude of these signals can change.

Another potential problem with using large electrodes attached to the skin is that they may pick up signals from other muscles that happen to be not far from the recording site, particularly if those muscles show large changes in their activation levels. For example, surface electrodes placed over wrist flexors may record signals during activation of wrist extensors. This phenomenon, referred to as "cross-talk," has to be controlled for. There are standard methods that allow the magnitude of signals recorded by an electrode whose origin is in a different muscle to be quantified. One such method involves large voluntary contraction of a suspected "wrong muscle" and recording signals with two sets of electrodes, one placed over that muscle and the other placed over the original muscle of interest. If the two recorded signals show large cross-correlation, cross-talk may be suspected.

There is no single method for recording and processing electromyograms. In each project, methods have to be adjusted to the goals of the project. The following data-processing operations are frequently used in the analysis of electromyograms.

One of the most common and least standardized operations is *filtering*. Recall that individual action potentials are very brief events with typical times of potential changes on the order of a few milliseconds. Since limb movements are much slower, researchers sometimes use high-pass filters, which get rid of possible movement artifacts, that is, signals produced by motion that changes the relative location of the recording electrodes with respect to muscle fibers. To get rid of the abovementioned 60 Hz noise, notch filters are used, for example from 59 Hz to 61 Hz that effectively remove all signals with the frequency within the window with minimal effects on signals outside that window. If a complex signal has to be removed, for example one produced by rhythmic heart contractions, *wavelet filtering* is used. Wavelets are standard time patterns that may be used to construct a complex signal by time and amplitude scaling. If an extraneous "noise" signal is identified (for example, when the muscle is completely relaxed), its pattern can be quantified by software and in further recordings it can be removed from the signal at each of its occurrences.

Another common data-processing technique is *rectification*. Since recorded EMG signals have nearly symmetrical potential deviations into positive and negative values, integrating such a signal over a time interval will likely produce a number very close to zero. Since researchers are frequently interested in the amount of muscle activation over a certain time interval, before integrating the signal, one has to make sure that all the potential deviations have the same sign (conventionally, they are assumed to be positive). Most commonly, full-wave rectification is used. This procedure converts all negative values of the recorded potentials into positive ones with the same absolute magnitude. Figure 13.8 illustrates an EMG signal before and after full-wave rectification. While full-wave rectification allows the signal to be integrated and a measure of its overall magnitude obtained, it corrupts the frequency content of the signal. Indeed, when the original signal crosses the zero line (Figure 13.8, circled area), smooth changes in the signal are substituted with an abrupt change in its derivative. So, if a researcher is interested in the frequency content of an EMG time series, analysis of non-rectified signals provides a more reliable result.

Frequently, researchers record EMG signals to quantify involvement of muscles and muscle groups in a particular task. At this step, rectified EMG signals are used. To get a signal reflecting the overall shape of the electromyogram, frequently an *EMG envelope* is calculated. This procedure involves either low-pass filtering or integration of the original signal within a particular time window, then shifting the center of the window by one time sample, repeating the procedure, and so on until the end of the time series (called *moving window average*). The size of the window is selected by researchers depending on the characteristic times of the EMG signal changes that are of interest. Moving window average can be computed using a window of a few milliseconds to a few hundred milliseconds. If specific time windows can be defined (for example, based on changes in the movement mechanics and/or timing), within which changes in the EMG signal are of particular interest, the rectified signal can be integrated over those windows.

Electromyographic signals depend on many factors, including the number of recruited motor units, their size, the frequency of their firing, the orientation of their fibers with respect to the recording electrodes, the distance from the electrodes to the muscle fibers, and the skin resistance. All these factors differ from one person to another and from one muscle to another within the same person. Moreover, some of the factors may change even when activation of a single muscle within a single person is studied. For example, this may happen if the person starts to sweat during the experiment, thus leading to a change in the skin resistance. There are also unavoidable changes in the relative location and orientation of the muscle fibers with respect to recording electrodes placed on the skin when the muscle contracts and changes its geometry. As a result, absolute magnitudes of an EMG signal frequently carry little meaning if one wants to perform comparisons across different persons within a population, across different muscles, or across populations (for example, between healthy persons and patients with a movement disorder).

To make such comparisons possible, a procedure termed *normalization* is used. The purpose of this procedure is to record an EMG signal during a standard action ($EMG_{ST.ACT}$), rectify and integrate it over a time window of the same size as the time windows of interest during the main part of the study, and then divide the recorded, rectified and integrated EMG signal ($\int EMG_{DATA}$) by that magnitude. It is assumed that differences in the magnitudes of $\int EMG_{ST.ACT}$ (across persons and muscles) reflect all the factors that contribute to the differences in the conditions of signal

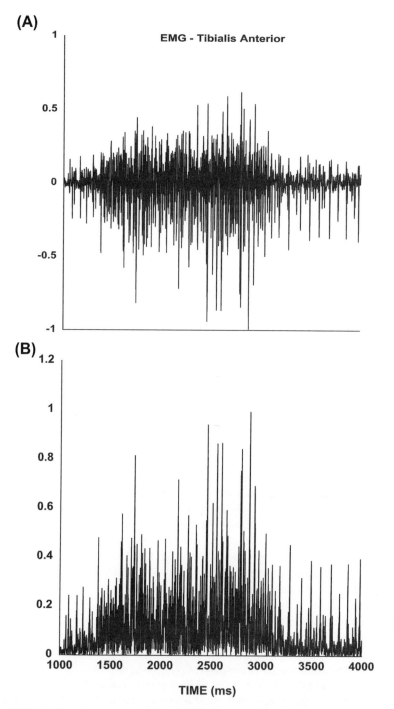

Figure 13.8 (A) Raw electromyographic (EMG) signal recorded from tibialis anterior during voluntary sway by a standing person. (B) The same signal after full-wave rectification.

recording. Dividing the signals of interest by corresponding $\int EMG_{ST.ACT}$ makes them comparable: $EMG_{NORM} = \int EMG_{DATA} / \int EMG_{ST.ACT}$.

The normalization procedures are very subjective and are selected by researchers based on their experience and intuition. The main problem is in selecting an appropriate "standard action." Commonly, this action represents *maximal voluntary contraction* (MVC) of each of the muscles of interest. There are several problems with this method. First, during MVC the unavoidable changes in the muscle geometry are maximal. As a result, signals recorded by surface electrodes are likely to be distorted maximally as compared with relatively weak contractions (that are more common during everyday tasks). Second, people differ in their ability to show truly maximal muscle contractions. Since such tasks are typically performed when the body segments are prevented from moving (in isometric conditions), some people are not even sure what kind of action produces maximal contraction of a specific muscle group. This may be particularly true for older persons, patients with neurological disorders, and atypically developing people. Third, sometimes it is impossible or painful to fix the body segments that are moved by the muscle during its maximal

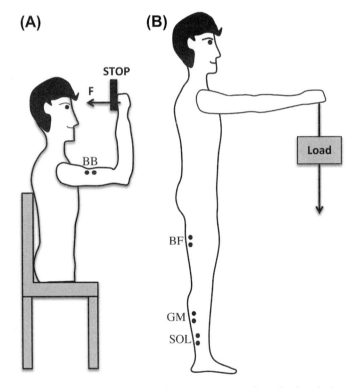

Figure 13.9 EMG normalization is done with respect to muscle activation during maximal voluntary contraction (MVC) or with respect to a standard task. (A) MVC task can be performed in isometric conditions (pressing against a stop "as strongly as possible"). (B) Holding a load in extended arms can be used as a standard test involving naturally dorsal leg muscles.

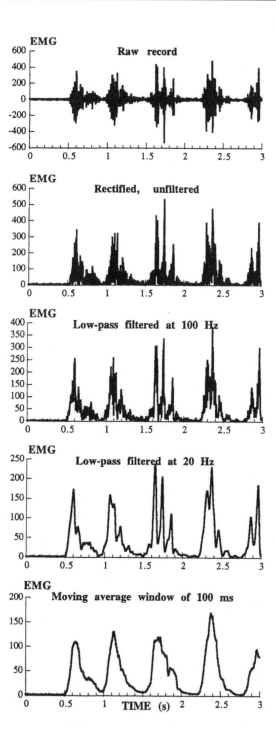

contraction. Consider, for example, muscles that move the human eye, facial muscles, or abdominal muscles.

Another method of normalization involves using muscle activity at a steady state prior to action as $EMG_{ST.ACT}$. On the one hand, this method is most immune to possible changes in the conditions of signal recording over time. On the other hand, many muscles in such steady-states show activation levels close to zero. Dividing a signal of interest by a very small number that may be primarily defined by noise is obviously not a good idea.

An alternative method has become more popular recently. It involves asking a participant to perform a standard task that naturally involves the muscles of interest to a substantial, but not very high, degree. For example, a person may be asked to stand quietly with the arms extended and produce a standard force against an external load (Figure 13.9). This force will require all the postural leg and trunk muscles to be activated to keep balance. Integrating such rectified EMG signals is associated with changes in the muscle geometry expected during natural tasks that the researcher may wish to explore and yields $EMG_{ST.ACT}$ of a reasonable magnitude.

Figure 13.10 illustrates the effects of some of the described procedures on an EMG signal recorded from the author's left biceps brachii muscle. The upper trace is the unprocessed EMG signal that was amplified and sampled at 1000 Hz by a computer. The panel below shows a full-wave rectified signal without any additional filtering. The next two panels show the effects of low-pass filtering (with a commonly used bi-directional fourth-order Butterworth filter—if you are interested, look into a textbook on signal processing) at the frequencies of 100 Hz and 20 Hz. The lowest panel shows the same signal processed with a moving average window of 100 ms (an EMG envelope). Obviously, the time series in different panels have both similarities and differences. Depending on particular research questions, different data processing techniques may be selected.

Until now, all the steps have been described for processing of EMG data recorded from individual muscles. In Section 6.4 a few methods for processing EMG signals recorded over large sets of muscles were mentioned. The purpose of those methods is to identify groups of muscles with close to parallel scaling of their activation levels. The methods use rectified EMG signals that may also be filtered and normalized. If absolute levels of muscle activation are analyzed, the *non-negative matrix factorization* method may be preferred because it takes into consideration that muscle activation can never be below zero. If deviations of muscle activation from a certain level are analyzed (these can be both positive and negative), *principal component analysis* with factor extraction may be used.

There are many other research questions that can be addressed using electromyographic techniques. For example, correlation methods may be used to quantify

Figure 13.10 Effects of different processing steps on the raw EMG signal (top). The signal was rectified (second panel), low-pass filtered at 100 Hz (middle panel), low-pass filtered at 20 Hz (fourth panel), and processed with moving average window of 100 ms (bottom panel). Reproduced by permission from Latash, M. L. (2008). *The neurophysiological basis of movement*, 2nd edn. Urbana, IL: Human Kinetics.

the amount of common neural drive received by alpha-motoneuronal pools innervating different muscles or different muscle compartments. Complex analysis of both
electromyographic and electroencephalographic signals has been used to identify
sources in the brain of changes in muscle activity. These issues are beyond the scope
of this book.

13.4   Electroencephalography and magnetoencephalography

Electroencephalography

Electroencephalography (EEG) is a method of non-invasive recording of the combined
activity of large groups of neurons. It has certain similarities with surface
electromyography. Both methods use electrodes placed on the surface of the body
close to the anatomical site of interest. While surface electromyography typically
records the difference of potentials between pairs of electrodes placed close to each
other over the muscle belly, EEG more commonly records electrical potentials at
single electrodes with respect to an *indifferent electrode*, commonly placed on the
person's earlobe. There is a large difference in the magnitudes of the recorded signals.
Surface EMG signals are typically on the order of a few hundred microvolts. Typical
EEG signals are two orders of magnitude smaller, about 1 μV. In part, this is due to the
larger distance between the electrodes and the neurons, which are separated by the soft
tissues, skull and meninges. As a result, EEG recordings have usually been performed
in specialized rooms isolated from extraneous electromagnetic fields. Modern
amplifiers and signal conditioners are able to identify and reject external noise automatically, which allows recording EEG in a variety of environments.

   Another source of extraneous signals that may corrupt EEG signals is the activity
of cranial and facial muscles. For example, if a person moves the eyes, the relatively
large-amplitude signals from eye muscles frequently overpower EEG signals and
make them undecipherable. This obviously requires a degree of cooperation by the
subject.

   The dominant source of the EEG signals are currents that move along dendrites
and bodies of the neurons. Detectable deviations of the signals reflect processes that
happen simultaneously in large neuronal populations. As a result, the overall EEG
signal depends on the geometrical organization of groups of neurons, their connections with other neurons, and properties of their electrical fields. The main source of
EEG signals that can be recorded from the scalp is cortical pyramidal cells.

EEG rhythms

Although commonly EEG signals look rather noisy, their patterns allow for identification of rhythms that result from synchronized activation of large groups of
neurons. The accepted classification of the main EEG rhythms is: 2–4 Hz—*delta
rhythm*; 4–8 Hz—*theta rhythm*; 8–13 Hz—*alpha rhythm*; 13–30 Hz—*beta rhythm*;
and anything with a frequency over 30 Hz is a *gamma rhythm* (Figure 13.11). Most of

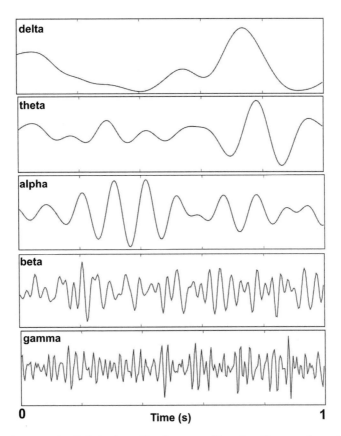

Figure 13.11 The main EEG rhythms. The data were filtered to illustrate the main rhythms from a recording at one of the standard recording sites on the midline on the top of the head, OZ. Created by Hugo Gambo, Reproduced from Wikipedia Commons under the GNU Free Documentation License.

the rhythms are represented throughout many brain structures. The alpha rhythm was the first one described by the pioneers of electroencephalography in the 1920s. It is seen in many persons during relaxed wakefulness in the absence of distracting stimuli, for example while lying relaxed in a quiet room with eyes closed. The low-frequency delta and theta waves typically have the biggest amplitude; these rhythms are commonly seen during certain phases of sleep.

Typical electrode placement covers all the areas of the skull over the main cortical lobes, frontal, temporal, parietal, and occipital (Figure 13.12). The number of recording electrodes varies within a broad range, from about 20 to over 200. The purpose of increasing the number of electrodes is to improve the notoriously *poor spatial resolution* of EEG signals and to be able to relate these signals to specific areas of the brain.

In a healthy awake person, EEG produces a low-amplitude signal with waves covering a broad spectrum of frequencies. Large-amplitude, synchronized waves may

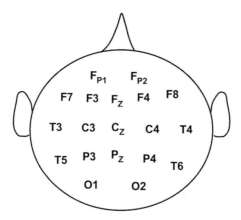

Figure 13.12 A typical scheme of electrode placement over the skull during electroenceph-alographic (EEG) recording.

be a sign of pathology. For example, such waves are commonly seen in recordings over large areas of the brain during epileptic seizures.

Methods of EEG analysis

Early methods of EEG analysis did not go far beyond classification of the signal according to its most pronounced rhythms and measuring their amplitudes. Later, spectral analysis became widely used as a method of automatic identification of the main waves and the relative amounts of power of the signal within different frequency windows. Spectral analysis involves representation of a signal as the sum of sine waves of different frequencies and with different amplitudes.

More recently, more advanced methods of processing EEG signals have been developed that allow the strength of connections between pairs of brain areas to be estimated based on measures of coherence. *Coherence* is a measure of stability of phase shifts between pairs of signals (independently of the amplitude), which is computed for each frequency separately. This measure is typically high for adjacent pairs of electrodes, and it drops dramatically for pairs of electrodes that are far from each other. Sometimes, however, coherence between signals recorded over two distant areas is unexpectedly high, suggesting interactions between these areas, possibly reflecting their common involvement in a functional activity. It is also possible to quantify coherence between an EEG signal and an EMG signal recorded in a muscle involved in a functional task. Such analysis yields information relevant to direct projections from the brain to alpha-motoneurons and to common supraspinal drives to groups of muscles.

EEG has many advantages over other methods of brain study. First, it has very high temporal resolution. Indeed, it records electrical signals that propagate nearly instantaneously and can be sampled at any rate, even from a millisecond to a milli-second. It is relatively cheap and simple to use compared with methods such as magnetic resonance imaging (MRI) and positron emission tomography (PET) (see Section 13.6). It directly reflects electrical processes in the brain, while MRI and PET reflect metabolic processes that are only indirect consequences of the electrical brain activity.

Event-related potentials

Frequently, researchers have to extract a useful biological signal from a recording that has a high level of noise (reflecting signals other than the signal of interest). This is common in studies of changes in the background brain activity produced by a sensory stimulus (in such cases another term is frequently used, *evoked potentials*) or associated with a self-generated action. The idea of the method is rather straightforward. It assumes that there is an identifiable event, which happens at a fixed time interval with respect to the event-related potential. In studies of sensory evoked potentials, the event is commonly the moment of stimulus application. It is assumed that transmission of the stimulus-produced neural activity to the recording site takes a fixed time such that the potential of interest is time-locked to the stimulus. In studies of brain potentials associated with motor actions, the event is frequently the first change in the electromyogram of a muscle that is supposed to initiate the action. Note that this is not a trivial assumption that may be violated sometimes.

Brain event-related potentials are commonly studied using electroencephalographic techniques. The noisy EEG signal is recorded several times, individual recording are aligned by the time of stimulus presentation or action initiation, and then the recordings are averaged for each data sample. This procedure produces an averaged time series, where noise is reduced (assuming that it is not synchronized with the stimulus or action) while the event-related potential is expected to be relatively unaffected. The procedure leads to an increase in the ratio of the amplitude of the useful signal to the amplitude of the noise, the *signal-to-noise ratio*. The amplitude of typical event-related potentials is very low, and this requires a large number of trials to be averaged, sometimes hundreds of trials, to make the potential visible on the background of the relatively large-amplitude brain waves. If the shape of the potential can be predicted, filtering may also be used to increase the signal-to-noise ratio.

Event-related potentials may also be recorded in peripheral structures in response to brain stimulation. A typical example would be changes in muscle activation produced by a pulse of *transcranial magnetic stimulation* (TMS, see Section 13.5).

The shape, size, and timing of evoked potentials may differ across subjects, types of sensory stimulation, and sites of recording. Since a stimulus can lead to several responses in the brain via different pathways, event-related potentials are frequently complex, representing sequences of positive and negative deviations of the baseline brain potential. To characterize the potentials, such indices as latencies, amplitudes, and durations of their identifiable components are commonly used. Figure 13.13 illustrates five single trials and the average of 45 trials for a simulated response on the background of a noisy signal. Note that the response can hardly be seen in the individual trials, and it becomes clearly visible after the averaging.

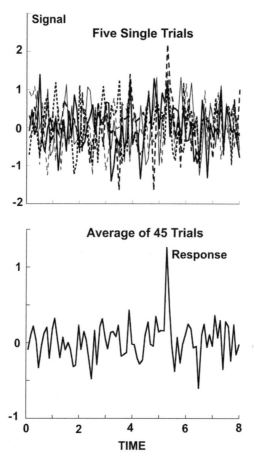

Figure 13.13 Five single trials (top panel) and the average of 45 trials (bottom panel). In each trial, a response is present, time locked to the beginning of the time scale. The response can hardly be seen in the single trials, while it is clearly seen in the averaged time series.

Movement-related potentials represent a complex sequence of changes in the brain potential that may be recorded over large areas of the scalp, in particular over the *supplementary motor area* and *primary motor area* of the cortex (see also Section 10.4). Changes in the brain potential may start as early as 1 s prior to action initiation (or even earlier) representing a slow drift of the potential, typically into more negative values. This phase is addressed as *readiness potential* or, using the original term in German, *Bereitschaftpotential*. The readiness potential is followed by a *pre-motor potential* (100–200 ms prior to action initiation) followed by the *motor potential* (about 50 ms prior to action initiation). If an action is performed as quickly as possible to an unpredictable sensory signal (simple reaction time), the early brain potentials shorten in duration or even disappear, while the motor potential is unaffected. This suggests that the early potentials represent processes related to movement preparation (which may be not necessary if the action is known in advance), while the motor potential reflects a neural volley to the spinal cord that ultimately initiates the action.

Magnetoencephalography

A relatively recent method combines the high temporal resolution of EEG with a much higher spatial resolution. This method is called *magnetoencephalography* (MEG). MEG is based on the fact that electrical current is accompanied by a magnetic field. So, electrical currents in cortical neural cells produce magnetic fields that can be recorded non-invasively. A huge problem is that those magnetic fields are extremely weak (0.01–1 pT, picotesla), 8–10 orders of magnitude smaller than the earth magnetic field and several orders of magnitude smaller than magnetic fields produced by equipment in a typical laboratory. MEG is recorded in special chambers using highly sensitive sensors called SQUIDs (superconducting quantum interference devices) that convert magnetic field into voltage. The ambient noise is measured by special dedicated sensors and further subtracted from the signal to produce signals related to brain activity.

MEG shares some of the abovementioned advantages of EEG. It reflects electrical phenomena in the brain and has very high temporal resolution. Its spatial resolution is comparable to that of PET and MRI (on the order of a few millimeters). There are a few disadvantages. In particular, MEG does not reflect well currents that run orthogonal to the scalp surface; such currents are likely to occur in cortical gyri where the cortex surface is tangential to the skull. Note that EEG can record such currents. MEG loses its high spatial resolution for sources that are deep in the brain (unlike MRI and PET). The last, but for many researchers not the least, important drawback is that MEG equipment is prohibitively expensive for most laboratories.

13.5   Transcranial magnetic stimulation

Electrical stimulation of brain structures has been a powerful tool for the study of connections among different parts of the central nervous system and their roles in movement production. Attempts to use electrical stimulation of the brain in humans have been marginally successful. One of the problems is that, for obvious ethical reasons, researchers cannot penetrate the skull and the meninges and apply stimulation directly to the neural tissue for purely scientific purposes. Direct brain stimulation was done during surgeries on the open brain by the famous Canadian neurosurgeon Wilder Graves Penfield (1891–1976), and the results of his experiments led to the idea of brain representations of the human body in different parts of the brain in the shape of a distorted human figure, the *homunculus*.

In order to stimulate an excitable biological tissue (neural or muscle cells) with pulses of electrical current applied to the surface of the body, one has to use rather large stimulation currents. This is due to dissipation of the currents in tissues that separate the object of stimulation and the stimulation site. It is relatively easy to stimulate a muscle on the surface of the body through electrodes placed on the skin directly over the muscle belly because the distance between the skin surface and muscle fibers may be small, on the order of a few millimeters. Brain tissues are separated from the skin surface by soft tissues, the skull, and meninges. As a result, much higher stimulation currents have to be applied to induce activation of brain neurons. This is possible to achieve but only with rather unpleasant side effects, such as quick, strong contractions of nearby muscles and pain.

The problem of non-invasive brain stimulation has been partly solved with the invention of *transcranial magnetic stimulation* (TMS). This method has its limitations but it allows brain neurons in areas close to the surface of the body to be stimulated without significant unpleasant side effects.

Physical foundations of TMS

The idea of TMS is based on the phenomenon of electromagnetic induction. An electric current produces a magnetic field (Figure 13.14) which can penetrate tissues and is not perceived by humans. If the current magnitude changes quickly, this leads to comparably quick changes in the strength of the magnetic field. Changing magnetic field produces so-called *eddy currents* (also known as *Foucault currents*) in conducting structures. Since biological tissues are good conductors of electric currents, sufficiently strong eddy currents can be produced in them by a sufficiently quickly changing magnetic field.

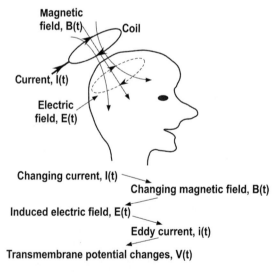

Figure 13.14 Transcranial magnetic stimulation (TMS) uses a coil placed close to the surface of the skull. The strong pulse of current in the coil, $I(t)$, produces changing magnetic field, $B(t)$, which induces electric field in the brain tissue under the coil, $E(t)$, resulting in eddy currents, $i(t)$, and changes in the transmembrane potential in neurons.

So, the sequence of physical events during TMS is as follows (Figure 13.14): A very short pulse of a rather strong electric current is generated. It travels along the stimulating coil that is positioned close to the skull of the subject over the area of interest (without touching the skin). The pulse produces a very quickly changing, strong magnetic field **B**. The field **B** produces eddy currents in the brain tissue (electric field **E**). The field **E** affects the transmembrane potential in nearby neurons, which can lead to the generation of action potentials. The action potentials may have many effects depending on their targets—sensory, cognitive, motor, or none.

By its very nature, TMS cannot be focused precisely on a very small brain area. Indeed the currents (**E**) spread in all directions and are likely to affect large numbers of neurons. There are different coil designs that allow focusing the stimulation. The simplest design is a circular coil (bagel-shaped). When electric current runs along such a coil, it generates the strongest magnetic field **B** on a line passing through its center and orthogonal to the plane of the coil. Even better focused **B** can be obtained using figure-of-eight coils (Figure 13.15) with the current running in opposite directions along the wires that run close to each other in the center of the coil. Sometimes, figure-of-eight coils are used with the two coils oriented at an angle to each other. Overall, selecting the right shape and size of stimulating coils is part of the art of TMS.

Motor effects of TMS applied to M1

When a single pulse of TMS is applied over the primary motor area of the cortex (M1), there is a sequence of events in the body. First, there are direct effects of the stimulation upon neuronal elements, dendrites, axons, and somas. These excited

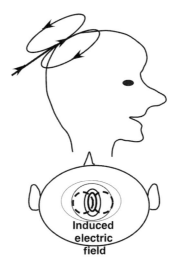

Figure 13.15 A figure-of-eight coil allows focusing the stimulation better as compared to circular coils. It produces a strong field under the central part of the coil (bottom drawing), which becomes weaker with the distance away from the central area.

elements activate other cells (in particular, pyramidal neurons) *trans-synaptically.* Most short-latency motor effects of TMS are commonly assumed to be produced by such secondary trans-synaptic activation of neurons whose axons form the *cortico-spinal tract.* Since a single pyramidal neuron receives tens of thousands of synaptic inputs and produces outputs to thousands of other cells, the effects of a single TMS pulse may be rather complex.

A single TMS pulse produces two types of responses that can be observed in axons that form the corticospinal tract—*direct (D)* and *indirect (I).* The D-response results from action potentials sent along the corticospinal tract by cortical neurons that are the first to be activated by the TMS. These neurons also send action potentials to other cortical neurons that also contribute to the activity along the corticospinal tract (I-response) and continue to affect activation of their neighbors in the cortex. As a result, a single TMS pulse can produce a single D-response and a sequence of I-responses (also known as *I-waves*). The D-response occurs at the shortest latency, while the I-waves occur at variable latencies that are longer than the one of the D-response. Amplitude of the waves scales with the strength of the stimulation (Figure 13.16).

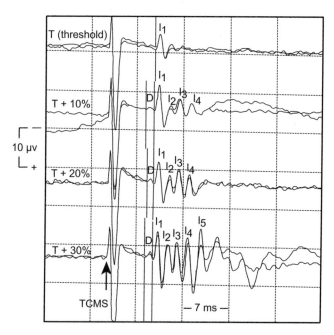

Figure 13.16 D- and I-waves recorded in a human subject at the T8 level of the spinal cord in response to transcranial magnetic stimulus (TMS) applied at the location for optimal stimulation of the left tibialis anterior. Note the increase in the wave magnitude with the stimulation magnitude above the threshold (*T*). Two trials are superimposed in each trace. Reproduced by permission from Houlden, D. A., Schwartz, M. L., Tator, C. H., Ashby, P., & MacKay, W. A. (1999). Spinal cord-evoked potentials and muscle responses evoked by transcranial magnetic stimulation in 10 awake human subjects. *Journal of Neuroscience, 19,* 1855–1862.

Muscle responses to a single pulse of TMS applied over the corresponding M1 area occur when the strength of the stimulation exceeds a certain threshold. The *latency* of the earliest muscle response (*motor evoked potential*, MEP) depends on the target muscle and anatomy of the subject. In arm muscles, typical latency values are about 20 ms (Figure 13.17). Since TMS stimulus is not very precise and usually activates neurons within large cortical areas, MEPs to a single stimulus are commonly seen in several muscles within the same anatomical region of the body. The earliest quick phasic response (a twitch contraction) is a direct consequence of the D-response in the corticospinal tract. It is commonly followed by a relatively long *silent period*, which is frequently interrupted in the middle by a short-lasting *rebound*; both the silent period and the rebound can be seen in Figure 13.17. Different phases of the silent period are likely to represent the different mechanisms such as cortical inhibition, the action of Renshaw cells, and inhibitory reflex effects from cutaneous afferents.

Factors that affect MEP characteristics

MEP magnitude depends on a variety of factors including the background level of activation of the target muscle(s). In general, higher levels of voluntary muscle activation are associated with larger MEPs to a standard TMS stimulus. This phenomenon reflects an increase in the excitability of cortical cells during voluntary muscle activation. Voluntary activation can also change TMS-induced responses in symmetrical contralateral muscles; both *facilitation* and *inhibition* of the MEPs in contralateral muscles have been described.

MEPs are affected by such factors as fatigue, specialized practice, injury, and rehabilitation. Fatigue typically leads to smaller MEPs. In contrast, specialized practice (for example, learning how to read Braille or how to play a musical instrument) typically leads to lower thresholds to TMS, larger MEPs, and larger areas from which TMS-induced responses can be evoked. Effects of practice on MEPs can be

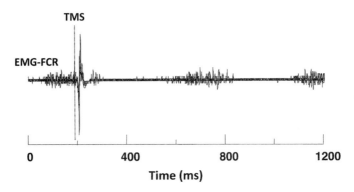

Figure 13.17 Five superimposed trials show the response of flexor carpi radialis to single-pulse transcranial magnetic stimulus (TMS) over the contralateral primary motor cortex. Note the large short-latency response followed by a silent period interrupted by a rebound.

very fast; some studies described such effects after only one hour of practice (see Section 12.5).

TMS can be used to study the functioning of *intra-hemispheric* and *inter-hemispheric* loops. If a subthreshold stimulus is applied over a cortical area followed by a supra-threshold stimulus, the response to the second stimulus (MEP) is inhibited, if the two stimuli follow each other at a short delay (a few milliseconds). This phenomenon is referred to as *short-interval intracortical inhibition* (SICI). To study inter-hemispheric effects, two stimulation coils are used. One of them produces a conditioning stimulus, while the other one—applied over the other hemisphere—produces a motor response (MEP). When the conditioning stimulus is applied about 10 ms prior to the MEP-producing stimulus, the latter is reduced in amplitude. This phenomenon reflects signal transmission via the corpus callosum; it is called *inter-hemispheric inhibition* (IHI). Both SICI and IHI change with practice. These changes can contribute to motor impairments following a neurological injury (such as stroke) and motor recovery during rehabilitation.

13.6 Brain imaging

Radiography (X-rays)

X-radiation (also called *Röntgen radiation* after Wilhelm Conrad Röntgen, 1845–1923) represents electromagnetic radiation with the frequencies outside the visible range; the range of frequencies of X-rays is rather wide, between 10^{16} and 10^{19} Hz. The X-rays at relatively low frequencies are called *soft X-rays*, while those at high frequencies are *hard X-rays*. Radiography is a method of creating visual images of objects and their parts with different abilities to absorb X-rays. Since most biological objects studied with the X-ray methods are much larger in size compared with the typical wavelength of the X-rays, these rays may be viewed as particles rather than waves. Most commonly, X-rays have been used to make images of bones because of their much larger absorption of X-rays as compared to soft tissues. Other traditional medical applications include identification of lung diseases, intestinal obstructions, gallstones etc. Traditional X-ray methods are less useful in imaging soft tissues such as the brain or muscles.

A widely used variation of conventional radiography uses contrast agents with an ability to absorb X-rays injected into the bloodstream. When the agent is distributed throughout the circulatory system, it makes X-ray images of blood vessels visible. This method, called *angiography*, is commonly used to identify changes in the structure of the blood supply to different body organs, including the brain. If several X-ray images are taken in a quick succession (a few per second), this method allows blood flow through the vessels of interest to be visualized. Although angiography is an invasive method, it has important advantages in visualizing the circulatory system with high precision. It is commonly used to determine aneurysms (balloon-like bulges filled with blood in the wall of a blood vessel), malformations in blood vessels, and strokes.

Computerized tomography

Computerized tomography (CT) is a method that combines radiography with computer processing that allows three-dimensional images to be created based on a sequence of two-dimensional X-ray images. The object of interest (for example, the head of a person) is placed between an emitter of X-rays and a receiver. Then, a sequence of images is made while rotating the system around a single axis of rotation that allows the object to be looked at from different sides (Figure 13.18). The method has several important advantages over conventional X-ray methods. First, it allows the object of interest to be looked at from different viewpoints. Second, CT eliminates the superimposition of images of structures outside the area of interest. This is particularly important in studies of brain tissues because of the high degree of absorption of X-rays by the skull. Third, it increases contrast between tissues with relatively small differences in their ability to absorb X-rays. In particular, it allows the gray and white matter of the brain to be visualized.

Taken together, methods based on using X-rays have an important advantage of creating images with very high spatial resolution (fractions of a millimeter). Potentially, one can achieve high temporal resolution as well but this would require making numerous images at short time intervals. Such an excessive exposure to radiation would present a significant health risk, and therefore it is not used.

Positron emission tomography

Positron emission tomography (PET) is an imaging technique that produces a three-dimensional image of a part of the body reflecting functional processes within the area

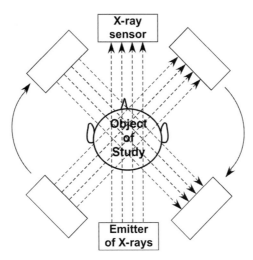

Figure 13.18 Computer tomography uses an emitter of X-rays and a sensor. The object is placed in-between the emitter and the sensor. Further, the orientation of the emitter–sensor with respect to the object is changed resulting in a series of two-dimensional images that allow reconstructing a three-dimensional image of the object.

of interest. A radioactive isotope (tracer) with short half-life is incorporated into a molecule that participates in biological processes within the body and injected into the bloodstream. For example, an analogue of a molecule of glucose can be used with radioactive ^{18}F (fluorine) substituting for the normal hydroxyl group. As the radio-isotope decays, it emits positrons, anti-particles to electrons. Since there are numerous electrons within the body, all positrons meet electrons quickly and anni-hilate. This process results in the birth of two gamma-particles that fly in opposite directions and can be detected by an array of gamma-ray detectors (Figure 13.19). Further, methods similar to computer tomography can be used to reconstruct three-dimensional images of the area of interest, and the images will reflect the density of metabolized glucose-like molecules. This signal may be interpreted as reflecting the intensity of biological processes within the area.

Studies of brain activity with PET are based on an assumption that areas of high density of gamma particles reflect increased brain activity. What is actually measured (indirectly) is the flow of blood to different parts of the brain, which does correlate with intensity of neural activity, but this correlation is far from perfect. PET has been proven useful in diagnosing brain tumors, strokes, and neurodegenerative diseases such as Alzheimer's disease.

There are a few limitations of the PET method. First, as mentioned earlier, it provides only indirect information on neural brain processes. Second, because the radioactivity decays rapidly, the method can only be used to monitor short tasks. On the other hand, temporal resolution of the method is limited because it is based on transport of the tracer with the blood flow, which is a slow processes compared to typical neurophysiological processes (for example, typical times of the generation of a motor action). A major advantage of the PET method is its very high spatial resolution (on the order of a fraction of 1 mm).

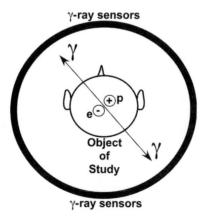

Figure 13.19 Positron emission tomography uses radioactive substances that emit positrons. A positron (p) meets an electron (e). The result is the annihilation of both, which produces two gamma quants. The gamma quants are detected by an array of gamma-ray sensors.

Magnetic resonance imaging

Magnetic resonance imaging (MRI) is an imaging technique that is particularly effective in providing contrast between different soft tissues. As a result, it is commonly used to create images of neural tissues and muscles (including the heart). MRI machines use a powerful magnetic field to align the spin axes of the nuclei of certain elements, in particular the protons of hydrogen atoms. Furthermore, a brief pulse of the electromagnetic field at a radiofrequency is used to perturb the orientation of the spin axes. After the pulse is over, the spin axes return to their original orientation and release photons during this process. Characteristics of the photons (electromagnetic waves) are measured and analyzed. The frequency of the waves and the time it takes the nuclei to return to the original state depend on both the type of atom and its physical environment.

Since the human body is largely composed of water molecules, the nuclei of the hydrogen atoms of those molecules are most commonly used as the targets of MRI methods. The photons of the perturbing electromagnetic field have just the right energy (the resonance frequency) to be absorbed and flip the spin of the protons in the body to a higher energy state. Furthermore, the spin returns to the original lower energy orientation, and this process is accompanied by the release of electromagnetic waves. Several variables are used to characterize the released electromagnetic waves. Changing the settings on the scanner can be used to distinguish between different tissues within the body as well as between different states of a tissue.

A major advantage of the MRI method is that it is harmless to humans. It uses strong magnetic fields and non-ionizing radiation in the radiofrequency range, unlike traditional X-rays and CT, which both use ionizing radiation. Compared with other methods, MRI provides *superb spatial resolution* (fractions of a millimeter) and *great contrast* between different soft tissues, for example between a healthy tissue and a tumor.

There are a few disadvantages. Scanning is associated with loud noise, and the method does not tolerate metal objects (including implants and dentures). In addition, the person in the scanner has to be motionless during the examination, and persons with claustrophobia may not tolerate it. The biggest disadvantage perhaps, however, is that scanning takes time, which limits the *temporal resolution* of the method to a few seconds, which is rather long compared with many neural processes.

Recently, a method has been developed called *real-time MRI*. This term refers to the continuous monitoring ("filming") of moving objects in real time. The real-time MRI technique can produce a temporal resolution of 20–30 ms for images with spatial resolution of 1.5–2.0 mm.

There are a few modifications of the method that, in particular, can be used to track neural connections among brain areas. Water molecules in biological tissues diffuse non-randomly because of the constraints imposed by the cellular membranes. In particular, they tend to diffuse along axons. This phenomenon is used in *diffusion MRI* and *diffusion tensor imaging* (DTI, a more sophisticated analysis that takes into account diffusion rates in different directions in different mini-volumes—voxels—of the brain). These methods have been found to be sensitive to the changes that occur in areas of brain lesion (for example, following stroke).

Functional magnetic resonance imaging

Functional MRI (fMRI) has been widely used in studies of brain processes associated with a variety of motor and cognitive actions in both healthy persons and patients with different disorders. The idea is to perform two MRI examinations, before and after an action, and to quantify differences between the results of the two brain scans. These differences are assumed to reflect task-specific changes in the neuronal activity in various brain structures. Since MRI reflects neuronal activity only indirectly, conclusions on the involvement of different brain structures in various actions should be drawn with a pinch of salt, preferably with additional confirmation from more direct methods, for example EEG or MEG.

Because neurons do not store glucose and oxygen, their activity requires energy delivered by the blood. Differences in the relative amount of oxyhemoglobin and deoxyhemoglobin are detected by MRI because the former is a *diamagnet* (an object which creates a magnetic field in opposition to an externally applied magnetic field, thus causing a repulsive effect) while the latter is a *paramagnet* (an object which is attracted when in the presence of an externally applied magnetic field). These differences produce a BOLD ("blood oxygen level dependent") signal, which is the most common response studied with fMRI. Changes in the BOLD signal within a particular brain area correlate with local neuronal activity, but this correlation is usually not very strong. Different studies have linked the BOLD signal to action potential generation by neurons, local field potentials, and the presence of neuro-transmitters. Another complication in interpreting the BOLD signal is that it differs depending on the blood perfusion of different brain areas. Strong magnetic fields are required to detect action-related changes in this signal in smaller blood vessels such as arterioles, venules, and capillaries. On the other hand, larger blood vessels that collect blood from many smaller vessels are more likely to reflect neural processes that occur within larger brain volumes. This obviously decreases the spatial resolution of the method.

The method of fMRI requires a very high degree of cooperation by the subject. Even small movements of the head may corrupt the results. Another problem is the relatively long examination time. Actions have to be given time to affect the meta-bolic processes in the brain tissues, and these processes typically take a few seconds. And, as mentioned earlier, the BOLD signal is only an indirect reflection of neural processes in the brain.

Nevertheless, fMRI offers a range of advantages that make it a commonly used method in studies of brain activity. The method is non-invasive and is not associated with health risk. Its spatial resolution is high (on the order of 1–3 mm) compared to methods that study electrical brain activity, and it can produce information about deep brain structures that may not be directly accessible to such methods as EEG. And— very importantly!—the method produces beautiful colorful pictures of the brain.

As of now, there is no single perfect method that allows the combination of high temporal resolution, high spatial resolution, low cost, lack of health hazards, and ease of use. In many clinical cases, detection of violations of the structural integrity of brain tissues is most important, while accurate detection of time changes in the brain activity may not be as crucial. Then, methods that offer the highest spatial resolution (such as MRI and PET) with no associated health hazard may be preferred. On the other hand, if the main purpose of an examination is to detect rapid changes in neuronal activity, EEG and MEG are the best tools.

Self-test questions

1. What variables are typically measured in motor control studies?
2. Why is it hard to measure such parameters as joint apparent stiffness and damping?
3. Define electromechanical delay. What properties of the neuromuscular system are reflected in electromechanical delay?
4. What conclusion can be drawn from an observation that lesion in a particular brain structure leads to a particular functional impairment?
5. What kinematic variables are measured by goniometers? What variables can be computed based on those original variables?
6. What are the advantages and drawbacks of motion analysis systems with passive markers as compared to systems with active markers?
7. What factors are the main contributors to errors in kinematic variables measured using motion analysis systems?
8. What does the expression "large-amplitude rotations are non-commutative" mean?
9. What is the minimal number of markers per body segment that allow rigid-body analysis to be performed?
10. What kinematic variables are measured in accelerometers?
11. What are the main sources of errors in inverse dynamic computations?
12. What variables are measured by force platforms?
13. What are the main problems in computing the center of mass trajectory during quiet stance based on force platform signals?
14. What are the advantages and disadvantages of intramuscular electromyography compared with surface electromyography?
15. Why is it hard to use intramuscular electromyography to measure muscle activation during very strong contractions?
16. What is the purpose of rectification?
17. What are the commonly used methods of normalization of electromyographic signals?
18. What is a notch filter? Present an example when using this filter may be needed.
19. What are the main brain waves that can be recorded with electroencephalographic methods?
20. What are the main advantages and disadvantages of EEG compared with brain imaging methods such as PET and MRI?
21. Define evoked potential. What is the purpose of averaging many responses in avoked potential studies?
22. What is coherence?
23. What are the technical difficulties of magnetoencephalography? What are the advantages and disadvantages of this method compared with EEG?
24. Define eddy current. Why do these currents emerge during transcranial magnetic stimulation?
25. What are D-waves and I-waves? Why is there only one D-wave but several I-waves in response to a single TMS stimulus?

26. How can TMS be used to study interactions within a hemisphere and between hemispheres?
27. What factors contribute to the silent period after the muscle response to a TMS pulse?
28. What are X-rays? Why are X-rays useful for imaging of internal body organs?
29. What is computer tomography? What are its main advantages and disadvantages compared with other imaging methods such as PET and MRI?
30. What is the physical principle of PET?
31. What objects cannot be used during MRI scanning?
32. What is functional MRI? What are the main difficulties in interpreting its results?

Essential references and recommended further readings

Asanuma, H. (1973). Cerebral cortical control of movements. *Physiologist, 16*, 143–166.

Burgess, R. C. (2011). Evaluation of brain connectivity: the role of magnetoencephalography. *Epilepsia, 52. Supplement, 4*, 28–31.

Cheng, K. (2011). Recent progress in high-resolution functional MRI. *Current Opinions in Neurology, 24*, 401–408.

Crivello, F., & Mazoyer, B. (1999). Positron emission tomography of the human brain. In U. Windhorst, & H. Johansson (Eds.), *Modern techniques in neuroscience research* (pp. 1083–1098). Berlin: Springer-Verlag.

Diekmann, V., Erne, S. N., & Becker, W. (1999). Magnetoencephalography. In U. Windhorst, & H. Johansson (Eds.), *Modern techniques in neuroscience research* (pp. 1025–1054). Berlin: Springer-Verlag.

Evarts, E. V. (1968). Relation of pyramidal tract activity to force exerted during voluntary movement. *Journal of Neurophysiology, 31*, 14–27.

Fink, G. R. (2004). Functional MR imaging: from the BOLD effect to higher motor cognition. *Supplement to Clinical Neurophysiology, 57*, 458–468.

Fortin, C., Feldman, D. E., Cheriet, F., & Labelle, H. (2011). Clinical methods for quantifying body segment posture: a literature review. *Disability and Rehabilitation, 33*, 367–383.

Frahm, J., Fransson, P., & Krüger, G. (1999). Magnetic resonance imaging of the human brain function. In U. Windhorst, & H. Johansson (Eds.), *Modern techniques in neuroscience research* (pp. 1055–1082). Berlin: Springer-Verlag.

Houlden, D. A., Schwartz, M. L., Tator, C. H., Ashby, P., & MacKay, W. A. (1999). Spinal cord-evoked potentials and muscle responses evoked by transcranial magnetic stimulation in 10 awake human subjects. *Journal of Neuroscience, 19*, 1855–1862.

Ivanitsky, A. M., Nikolaev, A. R., & Ivanitsky, G. A. (1999). Electroencephalography. In U. Windhorst, & H. Johansson (Eds.), *Modern techniques in neuroscience research* (pp. 971–998). Berlin: Springer-Verlag.

Krasnow, D., Wilmerding, M. V., Stecyk, S., Wyon, M., & Koutedakis, Y. (2011). Biomechanical research in dance: a literature review. *Medical Problems in Performing Art, 26*, 3–23.

Langheim, F. J., Leuthold, A. C., & Georgopoulos, A. P. (2006). Synchronous dynamic brain networks revealed by magnetoencephalography. *Proceedings of the National Academy of Sciences, USA, 103*, 455–459.

Lange, D. H., & Inbar, G. F. (1999). Modern techniques in ERP research. In U. Windhorst, & H. Johansson (Eds.), *Modern techniques in neuroscience research* (pp. 997–1024). Berlin: Springer-Verlag.

Makeig, S., Gramann, K., Jung, T. P., Sejnowski, T. J., & Poizner, H. (2009). Linking brain, mind and behavior. *International Journal of Psychophysiology, 73*, 95–100.

Martin, N., Grafton, S., Vinuela, F., Dion, J., Duckwiler, G., Mazziotta, J., Lufkin, R., & Becker, D. (1992). Imaging techniques for cortical functional localization. *Clinical Neurosurgery, 38*, 132–165.

Rossini, P. M., & Pauri, F. (2000). Neuromagnetic integrated methods tracking human brain mechanisms of sensorimotor areas 'plastic' reorganisation. *Brain Research Reviews, 33*, 131–154.

Turner, R. (2000). fMRI: methodology—sensorimotor function mapping. *Advances in Neurology, 83*, 213–220.

Walsh, V., & Pascual-Leone, A. (2003). *Transcranial magnetic stimulation. A neurochronometrics of mind.* Cambridge, MA: MIT Press.

Windhorst, U., & Johansson, H. (Eds.). (1999). *Modern techniques in neuroscience research.* Berlin: Springer-Verlag.

Zatsiorsky, V. M. (1998). *Kinematics of human motion.* Champaign, IL: Human Kinetics.

Zatsiorsky, V. M. (2002). *Kinetics of human motion.* Champaign, IL: Human Kinetics.

Glossary

Abundance Availability of extra degrees-of-freedom in a multi-element system which afford the controller a rich repertoire of solutions.

    Principle of abundance Systems with more degrees-of-freedom than task constraints do not try to eliminate redundant degrees-of-freedom but organize them to produce flexible and stable task-specific behaviors.

Accelerometer A device that produces an electrical signal proportional to the acceleration of the device.

Action potential A relatively standard, short-lasting time profile of the transmembrane potential in muscle cells and neurons, which is generated when the membrane potential is brought to its threshold value.

    Complex An unusual action potential with multiple peaks; can be produced by Purkinje cells.

    Simple A typical action potential consisting of a single peak reaching a positive magnitude of the transmembrane potential followed by a period of hyperpolarization (lower potential as compared to the equilibrium potential).

Adaptation Changes in performance following practice of a novel task and/or in unusual external conditions and/or with unusual sensory input.

    After-effects Changes in performance seen after adaptation to a novel external force field or unusual sensory feedback seen after the novel conditions have been replaced by typical ones.

    To force field Changes in trajectories, torques, forces, patterns of muscle activation, and pattern of neuronal discharge after practice in a novel force field.

    To visual feedback Changes in trajectories, torques, forces, patterns of muscle activation, and pattern of neuronal discharge after practice with distorted visual feedback, for example while wearing glasses that rotate or flip the visual field.

Adequate language A small set of basic notions, specific for a class of problems, that allow research of those problems using the scientific method (formulating and testing hypotheses).

Afferent fibers (afferents) Axons of sensory neurons that carry sensory information from receptors to the central nervous system. More generally, fibers that carry information from a peripheral part of a system of interest into its more central part.

    Ia Afferents that deliver action potentials from the primary endings of muscle spindles; the fastest conducting afferents.

    Ib Afferents that deliver action potentials from the Golgi tendon organs.

    II Afferents that deliver action potentials from the secondary endings of muscle spindles.

All-or-none law The law according to which an excitable structure either generates a standard output (if brought to the threshold) or does not generate any output at all.

Angiography A method of visualizing blood vessels by injecting a contrast agent with an ability to absorb X-rays into the bloodstream.

Anticipatory postural adjustments (APAs) Changes in baseline activation of postural muscles in anticipation of an expected perturbation or an action triggering a postural perturbation.

Anticipatory synergy adjustments (ASAs) Changes in a synergy index in anticipation of an event that requires a quick change in the variable stabilized by the synergy.

Asynergia A clinical term synonymous with discoordination; originally used to describe a feature of motor disorders after an injury to (dysfunction of) the cerebellum.

Ataxia Loss of joint coordination during whole-body tasks typical of movement disorders after an injury to (dysfunction of) the cerebellum.

Attractor A point or trajectory towards which a dynamical system evolves over time.

>**Fixed point attractor** The final state that a dynamical system evolves towards.

>**Limit cycle attractor** A periodic orbit that a dynamical system evolves towards.

Basal ganglia A set of paired (left and right) subcortical nuclei involving the globus pallidus, caudate nucleus, putamen, substantia nigra, and the subthalamic nucleus.

>**Direct loop** A loop from the cortex through the striatum, internal part of the globus pallidus, thalamus, and back to cortex.

>**Disorders** Sensorimotor and cognitive disorders associated with impaired function of the basal ganglia; motor disorders include hypokinetic (e.g. Parkinson's disease) and hyperkinetic (e.g. dystonia, hemiballismus, and chorea) ones.

>>**Dystonia** A motor disorder characterized by clumsy postures and twisting component of involuntary movements.

>>**Hemiballismus** A disorder produced by an injury to a subthalamic nucleus. Leads to large-amplitude, poorly controlled movements on the side contralateral to the injury.

>>**Huntington's disease** A genetic disorder associated with degeneration of projections from the striatum to the external part of the globus pallidus. It leads to poorly coordinated excessive movements, in particular a dance-like gait (chorea).

>>**Parkinson's disease** A progressive disorder associated with death of dopamine-producing neurons in substantia nigra. Includes the following: *Bradykinesia*–Slowness in movement initiation and execution. *Gait freezing*–Episodes of inability to initiate a step. *Postural instability*–Poor balance associated with delayed and reduced anticipatory postural adjustments and poorly modulated, high-amplitude long-latency responses to perturbations. *Rigidity*–Increased resistance to externally imposed motion in a joint. *Tremor*–Involuntary cyclic movement associated with alternating activation bursts in the agonist and antagonist muscles. Parkinsonian tremor is typically postural; it may be alleviated by voluntary movement.

>**Indirect loop** A loop from the cortex through the striatum, external part of the globus pallidus, subthalamic nucleus, internal part of the globus pallidus, thalamus, and back to cortex.

Bernstein's problem The problem of finding a way to perform a motor action when the number of degrees-of-freedom (elemental variables) is larger than the number of constraints. Also known as the problem of motor redundancy.

Bernstein levels of movement construction Five levels: The paleokinetic level (A), the level of synergies (B), the level of the spatial field (C), the level of action (D), and the level of symbolic, highly coordinated action (E).

Center of pressure The point of application of the resultant force normal to the surface.

Center of gravity The point of application of the resultant force of gravity.

Central pattern generator (CPG) A structure in the central nervous system able to generate patterned activity without being subjected to a patterned input.

>**Half-center model** A simple CPG model with two groups of neurons inhibiting each other.

Cerebellum The "small brain." A brain structure located behind the brainstem with more neurons than the rest of the central nervous system.

    Cerebellar disorders Disorders associated with an injury to the cerebellum or to input pathways into the cerebellum.

        Dysmetria Movements over a wrong distance; can be hypometria (movements over a smaller distance) or hypermetria (movements over a larger distance).

        Tremor Involuntary cyclic movement associated with alternating activation bursts in the agonist and antagonist muscles. Cerebellar tremor has postural, kinetic, and intentional components.

    Cerebellar nuclei Three pairs of nuclei, the fastigious, the dentate, and the interpositus nuclei, which mediate the output of the cerebellum.

    Inputs Two pathways, the mossy fibers and the climbing fibers.

Clasp-knife phenomenon A phenomenon of increased resistance of a joint to external motion (via stretch reflex) followed by a quick collapse of the joint (due to reflex effects from Golgi tendon organs).

Coactivation Simultaneous activation.

    Alpha–gamma Parallel excitation of alpha- and gamma-motoneuronal pools by descending signals associated with an action.

    Agonist–antagonist Parallel changes (usually, parallel increase) in the levels of activation of two muscles with opposing actions (agonist–antagonist pair).

    Coactivation (c-) command One of the basic two commands to a joint within the equilibrium-point hypothesis. It leads to an increase in the joint angle range, within which both agonist and antagonist muscles are activated without a change in the mid-point of the range.

Coherence A property of waves. In movement studies, commonly, a measure of stability of the phase shift between pairs of signals, which is computed for each frequency separately.

Computational approach An approach to the central nervous system (brain) function that assumes computations performed by parts of the central nervous system.

Computer tomography A method using a sequence of two-dimensional X-ray images of an object to create its three-dimensional image.

Control theory An area of mathematics (engineering) that considers a system as composed of a controller and a controlled object. The controller manipulates the inputs to the controlled object to obtain the desired effect on its output.

    Control trajectory A time profile of a control variable.

    Control variable A time varying variable sent by a controller to a controlled object.

Convergence A pattern of distribution of neural signals from multiple sources to a single target.

    Cortex of large hemispheres The upper layer of the cerebrum.

    Anterior commissure One of the two major neural pathways that connect the two hemispheres directly, not via subcortical structures.

    Brodmann areas Common nomenclature of cortical areas.

    Corpus callosum One of the two major neural pathways that connect the two hemispheres directly, not via subcortical structures.

    Layers Neuroanatomical thin slices of cortical tissue parallel to its surface.

    Lobes The cortex consists of five lobes, frontal, parietal, temporal, occipital, and insular.

    Premotor area Lies anterior to the primary motor area (Brodmann area 6); implicated in sensory guidance of movements.

    Primary motor area, M1 An area in the posterior portion of the frontal lobe (Brodmann area 4); a source of the corticospinal tract.

Pyramidal cells Cortical neurons that make projections both within the cortex and to subcortical targets.

Stellate cells Interneurons within the cerebral cortex; their axons do not leave the cortex.

Supplementary motor area Located just in front of the primary motor cortex, in Brodmann area 6. Implicated in movement planning.

Cost function A function that is optimized (commonly, minimized or maximized) in the process of control.

Cross-bridge A molecular link between macromolecules in the muscle cell; the basic element of force production.

Cross-talk Recording of signals from an unintended source (e.g. a distant muscle) during electromyography.

Damping A feature of a mechanical system to dissipate kinetic energy, commonly by producing force against the vector of velocity.

Deafferentation Removal of sensory (afferent) signals into the central nervous system from parts of the body.

Decerebration Surgical procedure (typically performed in animals for research purposes) involving transection of the midbrain between the inferior and superior colliculi.

Degree of freedom A variable that can potentially be changed without changes in other variables at some selected level of analysis of a system (cf. elemental variable).

Diabetes A disorder associated with an impaired ability to metabolize glucose.

> **Sensorimotor consequences** Diabetes frequently leads to (partial) loss of sensory information from distal parts of the extremities resulting in poor postural control and motor coordination.

Direct perception A hypothesis within the ecological psychology approach that sensory signals could be coupled to motor commands directly without updating the picture of the world and one's own body.

Distributed processing module (DPM) A neural system that uses neurophysiological processes to link physical variables at the input and at the output of the system (cf. brain operator).

Divergence A pattern of distribution of neural signals from a single source to multiple targets.

Dualism (mind–body) A philosophical view positing that mind is a non-physical substance independent of the body.

Dual-strategy hypothesis A hypothesis on the origin of muscle activation patterns. It assumes that two classes of movement exist, those with intentional control over movement time and those without such control.

> **Excitation pulse** A hypothetical input into an alpha-motoneuronal pool modeled as a rectangular function with modifiable height and duration.

> **Speed-insensitive strategy** The subject is not trying to control movement time explicitly, the height of the excitation pulse is assumed constant, while its duration can be modified.

> **Speed-sensitive strategy** The subject is trying to control movement time explicitly, both the height and duration of the excitation pulse are modified.

Dynamical system Formalization for any system that follows a deterministic rule that describes the time transition of a system from a given state to another state.

> **Approach** An approach to biological systems that views them as dynamical systems that can potentially show loss of stability and qualitative changes in the patterns of variables that they produce.

Ecological psychology An area of psychology exploring interactions of a person (animal) with the environment, particularly those that occur under the action of the laws of nature without obligatory cognitive involvement.

Efferent (efference) copy (a) A copy of signals from motoneurons to muscles; or (b) a copy of neural signals associated with the generation of a motor action. Commonly, used for sensory purposes.

Efferent fibers Neural fibers from motoneurons to muscles. More general: neural fibers from a more central part of a system to its more peripheral part.

Eigenvector (of a square matrix) A non-zero vector that, after being multiplied by the matrix, remains parallel to the original vector.

Electroencephalography (EEG) A method of recording changes in the electrical field produced by neurons in the brain with electrodes placed on the skull. Characterized by poor spatial resolution and excellent temporal resolution.

    Brain waves 2–4 Hz delta rhythm; 4–8 Hz theta rhythm; 8–13 Hz alpha rhythm; 13–30 Hz beta rhythm; >30 Hz gamma rhythm.

Electromechanical delay A delay between a change in muscle activation and a change in a mechanical variable measured with an external sensor.

Electromyography (EMG) A method of recording muscle action potentials.

    Filtering A procedure that narrows the range of frequencies represented in the signal.

    Intramuscular EMG A method using thin electrodes placed inside the muscle of interest.

    Normalization A method of making signals comparable across persons, muscles, conditions, and trials. Frequently uses signals recorded in a standard task or in a maximal output task.

    Rectification A procedure that eliminates negative values in the signal.

    Surface EMG A method using pairs of electrodes placed on the skin over the muscle of interest.

Elemental variable A variable at a selected level of analysis that can potentially be changed without changes in other variables at that level.

Engram A term introduced by N. Bernstein meaning a pattern of a neural variable stored in memory and related to topological properties of a learned movement.

Equifinality Reaching the same final position despite possible transient changes in the external forces.

    Violations of equifinality Consistent effects of transient forces on the final position.

Equilibrium A state, at which the resultant force and moment of force acting on the mechanical system are zero.

    Stable The system returns to the original state after a transient perturbation.

    Unstable The system moves away from the original state after a transient perturbation.

Equilibrium-point hypothesis Voluntary movements are produced by neurophysiological signals that change the equilibrium states of the system "body plus external forces."

    Alpha-model The neurophysiological signal used by the central nervous system to produce movements is assumed to be at the level of activation of alpha-motoneuronal pools.

    Lambda-model The neurophysiological variable used by the central nervous system to produce movements is assumed to be the threshold of the tonic stretch reflex.

Equilibrium potential Electrical potential inside the membrane measured with respect to the extracellular space, at which there is no net charge movement across the membrane.

Error compensation If, within a multi-element system, one element introduces an error into the common output of the system, other elements adjust their outputs to reduce the error of the common output.

Evoked potentials Changes in a neurophysiological electrical signal associated with a sensory stimulus or an action that are time locked to the stimulus or action.

Excitation–contraction coupling A sequence of chemical and physical events transforming an electrical signal on the muscle membrane into force production by cross-bridges.

Feedback control A mode of control when the controller changes the control variables based of their effects on the state of the object.

> **Delay** The time interval between a sensory signal reflecting an error and the time when the correction takes place.

> **Gain** The ratio between the magnitude of a corrective vector and the magnitude of the original error vector.

Feed-forward control A mode of control when the controller does not change the control variables based of their effects on the state of the object.

Finger interaction Dependence of finger force on forces produced by other finger(s).

> **Enslaving (enslavement, lack of individuation)** Unintentional force production by a finger when another finger of the hand produces force intentionally.

> **Force deficit** A drop in the maximal force produced by a finger when it acts in a group of fingers as compared to a single-finger action.

> **Sharing** A pattern of percentage of force produced by each finger in multi-finger tasks.

Fitts' Law A logarithmic dependence of movement time on the ratio of movement distance to target size.

Force A variable that produces changes in the velocity vector of an object with mass.

> **Centripetal** Force acting on a rotating object proportional to its mass and tangential velocity squared and inversely proportional to the radius of rotation.

> **Coriolis** Force acting on a moving object in a rotating reference frame. It acts orthogonally to the object velocity vector. Its magnitude is proportional to object's speed in the rotating system of coordinates, its mass, and angular velocity of rotation of the reference frame.

> **Force sensor** A device that produces a signal (typically, electrical) proportional to the magnitude of force acting of the device.

> **Force platform** A relatively large force sensor that produces electrical signals proportional to the three force vector components and three moment of force vector components. Commonly used in studies of balance and gait.

> **Friction** Force due to molecular interaction between two objects; maximal friction force is commonly assumed to be proportional to the force normal to the surface of interaction.

> **Gravity** Force between two objects proportional to the product of the masses of the objects and the gravity constant and inversely proportional to the distance between the objects squared. On Earth, it is equal to the product of the object mass and acceleration of gravity, g.

> **Inertial** Force proportional to the acceleration and mass of the object (for rotational movement, the force is proportional to the rotational acceleration and moment of inertia).

> **Interaction** Forces acting on a body segment due to movement of another segment or to forces acting on the other segment.

> **Motion-dependent** Forces that depend on the kinematics of the object.

> **Reaction** Forces acting on an object from another object due to Newton's third law.

> **Shear** Forces tangential to the surface of an external object.

Force control An approach based on an assumption that there are neural structures that model interactions within the different structures of the body and between the body and the environments and use these models to pre-compute requisite force time profiles to fit specific motor tasks.

Goniometer A device that produces an electrical signal proportional to the joint angle.

Grip Finger forces acting on the grasped object that produce zero resultant force.

> **Aperture** Distance between the tips of the digits opposing each other while grasping an object.

> **Feed-forward control of grip force** Changes in the grip force in anticipation of or simultaneously with self-produced or predictable changes in inertial or other forces acting on the object.

Safety margin Proportion of extra normal force acting on the grasped object above the minimum required to prevent the object slipping.

Halen-Kelso-Bunz equation An equation that describes properties of relative phase between trajectories of two effectors, $d\phi/dt = -\sin\phi - 2k\sin2\phi$.

Hand muscles Extrinsic muscles (with the belly in the forearm) produce forces transmitted to all four fingers via tendons attached at the intermediate and distal phalanges; intrinsic muscles (with the belly in the hand) produce finger-specific forces at the proximal phalanges.

Extensor mechanism A connective tissue structure on the back of the digits that transmits forces produced by intrinsic muscles to more distal phalanges.

Hill equation The equation that links muscle force to velocity, $(F + a)V = b(F - F_0)$.

Homunculus (a) A "small man" in the brain making decisions; or (b) a distorted human-like figure drawn on the surface of an anatomical brain structure and representing sensory or motor projections.

Impedance Characteristic of a reaction of a system to a cyclic force input.

Control A view that the central nervous system modifies impedance of effectors to produce movements.

Inferior olives Paired structures in the medulla, the origin of the climbing fibers, one of the two major inputs into the cerebellum.

Interaction torque Component of joint torque that depends on movement in another joint(s).

Internal model (a) Any neurophysiological structure that participates in predictive behavior (synonymous with neural representation); or (b) a neural structure that computes/predicts effects of the interactions among parts of the body and between the body and the environment.

Direct A neural structure that computes/predicts effects of the current efferent command on the body motion and associated sensory signals. Commonly used within the force-control approach.

Inverse A neural structure that computes/predicts a requisite neural command based on a desired motor outcome. Commonly used within the force-control approach.

Interneurons Neurons within the central nervous system that project on other neurons.

Ia-interneurons Interneurons that receive excitatory projections from Ia-afferents and make inhibitory projections on alpha-motoneurons innervating the antagonist muscle (reciprocal inhibition).

Ib-interneurons Interneurons that receive excitatory projections from Ib-afferents and make inhibitory projection on alpha-motoneurons innervating the muscle of origin; in addition, Ib-interneurons contribute to facilitation of alpha-motoneurons innervating the antagonist muscle.

Renshaw cells Interneurons that receive excitatory projections from axons of alpha-motoneurons and make inhibitory projections on alpha-motoneurons of the same pool (recurrent inhibition) and on gamma-motoneurons innervating muscle spindles in the same muscle.

Inverse dynamics Computation of forces and moments of force based on kinematic variables.

Inverse kinematics Computation of kinematic variables at the level of joints based on kinematics of a specific point on the system, typically the endpoint of the extremity.

Inverse optimization A method that allows a cost function to be computed based on experimental observations.

Inverse problem A problem of defining a group of variables based on known values of another group of variables, which are a function of the first group.

Inverted pendulum model A model of postural control which considers the body as an inverted pendulum swinging about the ankle joints.

Jacobian A matrix that links small changes in the magnitudes of a set of variables to changes in another set of variables. Commonly, a matrix that links joint velocities to endpoint velocity for a multi-joint extremity.

Kimocyclography A method invented by Bernstein that allows trajectories of markers placed on the body to be recorded.

Kinesthetic illusion An erroneous perception of body location, configuration, or forces acting on or within the body.

Large fiber peripheral neuropathy A rare disorder characterized by selective loss of signal transmission along main groups of peripheral afferent fibers.

Leading-joint hypothesis A hypothesis from the force-control group that assumes that one joint plays a leading role and generates motion in all other joints with interaction torques; other joints are assumed to implement small torque adjustments.

Linear oscillator A system with a mass on a spring and a damping element.

> **Damping ratio** A dimensionless parameter characterizing transitions of a linear oscillator between equilibrium states.
>
> **Natural frequency** A parameter expressed in radians per second that characterizes the frequency at which the oscillator oscillates in the absence of external forces.
>
> **Overdamped** An oscillator with the damping ratio over unity. In the absence of external force shows no oscillations, but a smooth transition to the resting length of the spring.
>
> **Underdamped** An oscillator with the damping ratio under unity. In the absence of external force shows oscillations with an exponential drop in their amplitude.

Locomotion A motor activity associated with displacement of the whole body in the environment.

> **Corrective stumbling reaction** A phase-dependent, complex pre-programmed reaction that can be seen in leg muscles at a delay of 50–70 ms in response to foot stimulation, mechanical or electrical.
>
> **Gait** A pattern of leg motion characterized by a particular stable relative phase of homologous joint trajectories across limbs; for example, walking, trotting, and galloping.
>
> **Fictive locomotion** Phasic patterns of activity of alpha-motoneuronal pools that can be observed in a paralyzed animal.
>
> **Midbrain locomotor area** An area in the midbrain which, when electrically stimulated, leads to locomotion of the decerebrated animal.
>
> **Passive** Walking-like patterns demonstrated by inanimate objects, commonly under the action of gravity.

Long-term depression (LTD) A long-lasting decrease in the efficacy of a synaptic connection following a vigorous activation through that synapse or a particular combination of inputs into the target neuron.

Long-term potentiation (LTP) A long-lasting increase in efficacy of a synaptic connection following a vigorous activation through that synapse or a particular combination of inputs into the target neuron

Lumbar enlargement Part of the spinal cord at the level of vertebrae T12–L1 where many spinal segments are tightly packed.

Magnetic resonance imaging (MRI) A method of imaging internal body organs that uses a brief pulse of the electromagnetic field at a radio frequency to perturb the orientation of the spin axes of hydrogen atoms. Characteristics of the electromagnetic waves released while the spin axes return to their original orientation are analyzed.

> **Functional MRI** A method that uses two MRI examinations, before and after an action, and quantifies differences between the results of the two scans.

Magnetoencephalography A method of non-invasive recording and analysis of the magnetic fields produced by electrical currents in brain cells.

Mass A property of material objects, a coefficient that links force acting on an object and acceleration of the object.

Mass-spring models Simplified models that view muscles and moving body segments as inertial objects on springs with or without additional force-generating elements.

Membrane A biological structure built primarily from lipids that separates the cell from the environment.

    Channel Membrane sites specialized for transport of specific molecules across the membrane.

    Depolarization A decrease in the magnitude of the negative equilibrium potential inside the membrane that brings it closer to the threshold for action potential generation.

    Hyperpolarization An increase in the magnitude of the negative equilibrium potential inside the membrane that brings it further away from the threshold for action potential generation.

    Potential Electric potential inside the membrane as compared to the potential of the extracellular space.

    Threshold for activation Transmembrane potential, at which the cell generates an action potential.

Mirror neurons Cortical neurons that increase their activation level when an animal performs a particular action and when the animal observes another animal or a human performing this action.

Moment of inertia A coefficient that links moment of force to angular acceleration.

Motion analysis system A system that converts kinematic variables, in particular coordinates of special points on the body or on other objects into electrical signals.

    With active markers Systems that use markers (light-emitting diodes) connected to the main computer.

    With passive markers Systems that use infrared emitters, reflective markers, and cameras that record marker positions in space.

Motor control Area of science exploring natural laws that define how the nervous system interacts with other body parts and the environment to produce purposeful, coordinated movements.

Motoneuron A neuron that innervates (sends the axon to) muscle fibers.

    Alpha A motoneuron that innervates force-producing, extrafusal fibers.

    Gamma A motoneuron that innervates intrafusal fibers inside muscle spindles.

Motor evoked potential Muscle activation (EMG) signals time-locked to a stimulus.

Motor primitives (a) Hypothetical neural structures producing relatively simple blocks for complex actions; or (b) relatively simple patterns of mechanical variables that are used to construct complex actions.

Motor program An input into a subsystem within the neuromotor hierarchy expressed in neurophysiological variables and leading to actions produced by all the hierarchically lower subsystems.

    Generalized motor program A concept assuming that functions of control variables, directly related to forces and torques, are stored in the central nervous system and can be scaled in time and magnitude.

Motor redundancy Availability of more elemental variables than the number of constraints associated with typical motor tasks.

    Kinematic Availability of more joint-related kinematic variables (rotations and translations) as compared to the number of constraints associated with typical motor tasks.

    Kinetic Availability of more force and moment of force variables at the level of effectors (e.g. muscles, digits, etc.) as compared to the number of constraints associated with typical motor tasks.

Muscle Availability of more muscles as compared to the number of constraints associated with typical motor tasks.

Problem of motor redundancy The problem of finding solutions for a system with more elemental variables than constraints.

Motor unit An alpha-motoneuron and the group of muscle fibers innervated by that alpha-motoneuron.

Fast, fatiguable Large motoneurons innervating large groups of muscle fibers characterized by fast conduction velocities along the axon, large forces, high rates of force development, and a quick drop in force during maintained force production.

Fast, fatigue-resistant Medium-size motoneurons innervating medium-size groups of muscle fibers characterized by medium level forces, intermediate rates of force development, and resistance to fatigue.

Slow, fatigue-resistant Small motoneurons innervating small groups of muscle fibers characterized by slow conduction velocities along the axon, low forces, low rates of force development, and no signs of fatigue.

Muscle A biological structure that converts electrical signals into mechanical variables.

Agonist A muscle that produces force that contributes to desired (instructed) changes in a performance variable.

Antagonist A muscle that produces force that contributes to changes in a performance variable in a direction opposite to the desired (instructed) one.

Bi-articular A muscle with tendon attachments that span two adjacent joints.

Compartment A group of muscle fibers that shows anatomical and functional separation from other fibers within the same muscle.

Concentric contraction A contraction associated with shortening of the muscle.

Eccentric contraction A contraction associated with lengthening of the muscle.

Extrafusal fibers Muscle fibers that lead to tendon force production during contraction.

Extrinsic hand (muscles) Muscles with the belly in the forearm that have several tendons attached to different fingers of the hand.

Intrafusal fibers Muscle fibers inside muscle spindles. Have no direct effect on tendon forces.

Intrinsic hand (muscles) Muscles with the belly in the hand that produce finger-specific flexion action and contribute to the action of the extensor mechanism.

Invariant characteristic The dependence of active muscle force on muscle length; the term introduced within the equilibrium-point hypothesis.

Tetanic contraction Lasting contraction in response to a sequence of action potentials to muscle fibers.

Tone A poorly defined notion reflecting a feeling of resistance to an imposed motion in comparison to what is expected in a typical healthy person ("normal tone").

Twitch contraction Short-lasting contraction in response to a single volley of action potentials to muscle fibers.

Myelin A substance that covers neural fibers and increases the effective distance of local currents. This leads to higher speeds of action potential transmission.

Myelinated fibers Fibers covered with myelin. Characterized by high speeds of action potential transmission.

Neural maps Topographic patterns of neural activation over relatively large areas in brain structures associated with motor or sensory events.

Neural pathways Groups of axons traveling together within the central nervous system.

Non-negative matrix factorization (NNMF) A method of representing behavior of large groups of elemental variables that cannot have negative values with relatively few independent variables selected in an optimal way.

Occam razor A simpler explanation of a phenomenon should be preferred over a more complex one.

Operant conditioning Development of a behavior when the animal is allowed to explore the environment and gets a reward for certain types of action.

Optimal control A branch of mathematics developed to find ways to control a system, which changes in time, such that certain criteria of optimality are satisfied.

> **Optimal feedback control** An optimization method based on a cost function that combines a measure of internal effort spent on control and a measure of accuracy of performance.

Optimization An approach to controlling a redundant system by optimizing (typically, minimizing or maximizing) magnitude of a cost function.

> **Cost function** A function of elemental variables that is minimized or maximized by the controller.
>
> > **Minimal norm** Minimization of the Eucledian distance between the initial and final states in the multi-dimensional space of elemental variables
> >
> > **Minimum fatigue** The cost function is related to fatigue associated with actions.
> >
> > **Minimum jerk** The cost function represents the integral of jerk squared over movement time.
> >
> > **Minimum time** Performing the action within the shortest time.
> >
> > **Minimum torque-change** The cost function is the integral of torque derivative squared over movement time.
>
> **Direct** Assuming a cost function and computing values of elemental variables based on task constraints.
>
> **Inverse** Using observations to compute a cost function.

Pathways Groups of axons that travel together within the central nervous system.

> **Ascending** Pathways that carry sensory information in a rostral direction, from sensory neurons to structures within the central nervous system
>
> **Descending** Pathways that carry information in a caudal direction, related to a planned motor action
>
> > **Corticobulbar tract** A neural tract originating in the cortex and innervating the nuclei of the cranial nerves.
> >
> > **Corticospinal tract** A neural tract originating in the cortex and projecting on various spinal neurons.
> >
> > **Pyramidal tract** A neural tract from the cortical frontal motor areas with a contribution from neurons in the parietal somatosensory areas; it splits into the corticobulbar and corticospinal tracts.
>
> **Relay nuclei** Neuroanatomical formations that receive inputs from neural pathways and serve as outputs of other pathways.
>
> **Topographic organization** Preservation of topography: Neighboring original neurons project onto neighboring neurons in relay nuclei, which in turn project onto neighboring neurons in the target.

Perception-action coupling Coupling of sensory signals to motor commands directly without first using these signals to update the picture of the world and one's own body

Persistent inward currents Transmembrane currents that can modify the potential on the membrane and lead to an equilibrium potential above the threshold for action potential generation.

Phase portrait The dependence between object's velocity and coordinates.

Plasticity An ability of neural structures to change gains of synaptic connections and to establish new connections with practice or injury.

Population vector A vector (typically of a mechanical variable) representing activity within a large group of neurons.

Positron emission tomography (PET) A method of imaging internal body organs using a radioactive isotope incorporated into a molecule, which participates in biological processes within the body, injected into the bloodstream

Posture A combination of the relative positions of body segments and/or of the whole body with respect to a reference frame.

    Inverted pendulum model Analysis of vertical posture as the problem of balancing an inverted pendulum.

    Light touch effects Reduction of postural sway and other effects on posture by a light finger touch to an external object.

    Posture-movement paradox Posture-stabilizing mechanisms resist deviations produced by external forces but not those produced by voluntary movements.

    Posture-stabilizing mechanisms All the mechanisms that resist mechanical perturbations of posture, peripheral, reflex, pre-programmed, and voluntary.

        Ankle strategy A pattern of muscle activation that starts with major changes in the activation of muscles crossing the ankle joint and involves body motion mostly about the ankle joints.

        Hip strategy A pattern of muscle activation that starts with major changes in the activation of muscles crossing the hip joint and involves body motion mostly about the hip joints.

    Sway Involuntary changes in the coordinates of the center of pressure or the center of mass.

        Rambling A sway component representing an interpolation of the coordinates of instantaneous equilibrium points.

        Trembling A sway component representing the difference between the sway and rambling.

Preferred direction (of a neuron) The direction of a vector in the external space, which corresponds to the highest activity of the neuron.

Preflex The instantaneous reaction of a muscle to an external perturbation that depends on the muscle activation level and, hence, can be changed in advance.

Prehension The combined sensory-motor function of the grasping hand.

    Principle of superposition Elemental variables form relatively independent subgroups, which are used for the control of different performance variables such as the total force and the total moment of force.

    Synergy Co-varied adjustments of elemental variables produced by the digits that stabilize the mechanical action of the hand.

Pre-programmed reactions (M_{2-3}, triggered reactions) Reactions to perturbations that come at an intermediate latency, between spinal reflexes and voluntary reactions, and depend on the instruction to (intention of) the person.

Principal component analysis (PCA) A matrix factorization method that allows representing a multi-dimensional set of data with a smaller number of orthogonal principal components.

    Factor analysis An extension of PCA. It involves optimal rotation of the principal components.

Principle of mechanical advantage A principle according to which effectors with larger moment arms produce larger shares of the resultant moment of force.

Pseudo-inverse A particular solution for the problem of redundancy that minimizes the Euclidean distance between the initial and final state in the space of elemental variables.

Pulse-step model A model that assumes separate control over the movement trajectory (pulse) and over the final position (step). Typically, it assumes control with patterns of muscle activation.

Purkinje cells The largest cells in the cerebellum that produce output to the cerebellar nuclei.

Readiness potential (*Bereitschaftpotential*) A slow, gradual change of the brain potential, typically into negative values, seen in preparation to a voluntary action 1 s or more prior to movement initiation.

Reafference principle A principle of comparing afferent signals with a copy of efferent signals. As a result, afferent signals are interpreted as reporting deviations of the body from the referent coordinate, not from an absolute posture.

Receptor (a) A cell or subcellular structure (sensory ending) that converts physical variables into changes in the membrane potential; or (b) a molecular structure specialized for making chemical bonds with specific molecules.

> **Exteroceptors** Receptors sensitive to physical variables that carry information about events in the external world.

> **Interoceptors** Receptors sensitive to physical variables that carry information about events within the body.

> **Proprioceptors** Receptors sensitive to physical variables that carry information about contacts between the body and the external world, forces between body parts, and about the body configuration and its changes.

>> **Articular receptors** Sensory endings located in the joint capsule. They generate action potentials reflecting joint angle and joint capsule tension.

>> **Cutaneous receptors** Various receptors sensitive to skin deformation (pressure). They differ in size of the receptive field and rate of adaptation to maintained deformation.

>> **Golgi tendon organs** Sensory endings located at the junction between the muscle fibers and the tendon, sensitive to tendon force.

>> **Muscle spindle** A complex structure in the muscle that contains small muscle fibers (intrafusal fibers) and two types of sensory endings, primary and secondary. Connected to power producing muscle fibers by strands of connective tissue. Includes the following: *Primary endings*–Sensory endings sensitive to muscle length and velocity, innervated by Ia-afferents. *Secondary endings*–Sensory endings sensitive to muscle length, innervated by group II afferents.

Reciprocal inhibition An inhibitory reflex connection involving two synapses within the central nervous system from primary spindle endings mediated by Ia-interneurons to alpha-motoneurons innervating the antagonist muscle.

Reciprocal (r-) command One of the two basic commands within the equilibrium-point hypothesis. It leads to shifts of the mid-point of the joint angle range, within which both agonist and antagonist muscles are activated, without a change in the size of the range.

Recurrent inhibition Inhibition of alpha-motoneurons of a pool produced by small interneurons (Renshaw cells) that are excited by branches on the axons of the alpha-motoneurons of the same pool.

Red nucleus A small brain structure, the source of the rubrospinal tract. It receives an input from cerebellar nuclei.

Reflex A poorly defined notion. Typically, a quick reaction to a stimulus that is relatively stereotypical and does not depend on the instruction to the subject. It is frequently assumed that reflexes are mediated by spinal structures.

> **Autogenic** Reflexes seen in a muscle produced by sensory signals from receptors in the same muscle.

Conditioned Reflexes developed by repetitive simultaneous presentation of two stimuli with gradual substitution of a natural stimulus with a different one.

Crossed extensor Reflex contractions seen in many major extensor muscles of an extremity in response to stimulation of flexor reflex afferents in the contralateral extremity.

Flexor Reflex contractions seen in many major flexor muscles of an extremity in response to stimulation of flexor reflex afferents within the same extremity

H-reflex A monosynaptic reflex produced by electrical stimulation of Ia-afferents that make excitatory projections on alpha-motoneurons of the muscle from which the afferents originate.

Heterogenic Reflexes seen in a muscle produced by sensory signals from receptors located in another muscle.

Inborn Reflexes that are seen in newborn animals.

Latency Time delay between a stimulus and the initiation of the earliest response.

Long-loop A reflex response with a relatively long latency (on the order of 50–90 ms) that shows complex patterns of muscle activation that can change with action and instruction.

Monosynaptic Reflex response mediated by only one synapse within the central nervous system.

Oligosynaptic Reflex response mediated by a few (two to three) synapses within the central nervous system.

Phasic Transient, short-lasting, reacting to a change in the respective physical variable.

Polysynaptic Reflex response mediated by many (usually, an unknown number) synapses within the central nervous system.

Reversal Switching of reflex responses from a muscle to its antagonist with changes in the conditions such as body posture and/or contact forces with the environment.

Tonic Steady-state, reacting to magnitude of the respective physical variable.

Tonic stretch reflex A polysynaptic reflex that defines the dependence of active muscle force on muscle length.

Characteristic The dependence of active muscle force on muscle length.

Threshold The shortest muscle length, at which muscle activation is seen during a very slow stretch of the muscle.

Tonic vibration reflex Tonic muscle contraction seen in response to high-frequency, low-amplitude vibration applied to the muscle or its tendon (sometimes, seen in other muscles of the body).

Unloading reflex A short-latency change (usually, a decrease) in the muscle activation level in response to an unloading of the muscle leading to its quick shortening.

Vestibulo-ocular reflex Short-latency reflex eye rotation produced by sensory signals in the vestibular apparatus that helps keep the projection of an object of interest on the fovea.

Wiping reflex In some animals, a reflex action by an extremity wiping the irritating stimulus off the body.

Referent configuration (a) A body configuration at which all the muscles are at the threshold of activation via the tonic stretch reflex; or (b) a set of salient variables, for which referent values are set at a high level of the control hierarchy.

Refractory period A period of decreased or lacking response to stimulation.

Absolute The membrane does not generate an action potential even to a very strong stimulus.

Relative The membrane can generate an action potential but requires a stronger stimulus than usual.

Redundancy Availability of numerous (an infinite number of) solutions to motor tasks associated with a smaller number of constraints as compared to the number of degrees-of-freedom (elemental variables).

Renshaw cells Small interneurons located in the anterior horns of the spinal cord. They are excited by branches of the axons of alpha-motoneurons and inhibit alpha-motoneurons of the same pool as well as gamma-motoneurons innervating spindles within the same muscle.

Repetition without repetition A term coined by N. Bernstein that implies solving the same motor task with different neural and motor patterns.

Safety margin Extra gripping force above the minimal level necessary to avoid slippage of the hand-held object.

Scalar A physical variable characterized by magnitude but not by direction (e.g. mass, distance, temperature, and speed).

Secondary moment Moment of force that is not necessary for task execution.

   Minimization of secondary moments An optimization principle that posits that forces are selected to minimize secondary moments of force.

Sensory reweighting The importance of signals from different groups of receptors may be task specific and may also show changes with practice.

Servo-control A particular version of a feedback control system that acts to keep a variable at a level specified by a hierarchically higher system despite possible changes in the environment.

Servo-hypothesis A hypothesis on muscle control based on sending a signal to gamma-motoneurons to the muscle. This signal is viewed as setting a magnitude of muscle length that is kept constant with the help of the tonic stretch reflex viewed as a perfect servo.

Size (Henneman) principle The principle of orderly recruitment of motor units within a muscle, from the smaller ones to the larger ones. De-recruitment follows the opposite order.

Spasticity A clinical condition characterized by excessive involuntary muscle activation, spasms, and exaggerated reflex responses to peripheral stimuli.

   Negative signs Signs that are absent in a person with spasticity as compared to a healthy person (such as weakness, discoordination, and quick fatigueability).

   Positive signs Signs that are present in a person with spasticity but not in a healthy person.

      Clasp-knife phenomenon A specific pattern of joint reaction to an externally imposed motion: First, the joint resists the motion strongly, but at some point it collapses like a pocket-knife.

      Clonus Involuntary alternating activation of muscles within an agonist-antagonist muscle pair, typically at 6–8 Hz.

      Muscle tone A misnomer reflecting subjective impression that a clinician feels when trying to move a body segment while the subject tries to be relaxed.

      Spasms Involuntary brisk or long-lasting episodes of strong muscle contractions. Spasms can be local or involve large muscle groups (flexor spasms and extensor spasms).

Spectral analysis A method of signal processing that represents a signal as a superposition of sine waves at different frequencies and with different amplitudes.

Speed-accuracy trade-off When a person moves at different speeds to a visual target, movement time varies as a linear function of the ratio of distance to the standard deviation of the final position.

Speed–difficulty trade-off (Fitts' law) Under the instruction to be both fast and accurate, movement time shows a logarithmic dependence on the ratio of movement distance to target size.

Spinal cord The elongated structure within the central nervous system, from the medulla to the lumbar spinal vertebrae, which plays a major role in the sensorimotor function. It contains pathways that deliver sensory information to and neural commands from the brain, and interneurons that mediates reflexes and play a role in the control of certain movements.

    Roots Sites of entrance and exit of axons.

        Dorsal Sites of entrance of axons that carry sensory information into the spinal structures.

        Ventral Sites of exit of axons that carry signals from the spinal cord to peripheral structures such as muscles.

    Segments Each segment receives sensory information from a particular area of the body and innervates muscles in a more or less the same area of the body. There are 8 cervical segments, 12 thoracic segments, 5 lumbar segments, and 5 sacral segments.

Spinal ganglia Groups of neurons outside the spinal cord but in close proximity to it. Spinal ganglia contain bodies of proprioceptive neurons.

Stability A physical property of a system reflecting its ability to keep the current state or trajectory when subjected to a transient perturbation.

    Dynamic An ability to move towards the original trajectory after a transient perturbation.

    Postural An ability to maintain posture despite possible external perturbations.

    Static An ability to return to the same steady-state after a transient perturbation.

Stages of motor learning Three stages suggested by N. Bernstein: freezing redundant degrees-of-freedom, releasing those degrees-of-freedom, and utilizing external forces to one's advantage.

Stiffness A property of a certain group of physical objects (called "springs") that deform under the action of external force, generate force against deformation, and accumulate potential energy under deformation.

    Apparent stiffness A property of an object to show a dependence of force on length change or displacement.

    Joint stiffness A misnomer trying to represent joint mechanical behavior as that of a spring. "Apparent joint stiffness" is recommended.

    Limb stiffness A misnomer trying to represent limb mechanical behavior as that of a spring.

Synapse A structure consisting of a pre-synaptic membrane, a synaptic cleft, and a post-synaptic membrane that uses physical and chemical processes to enable transmission of excitation and inhibition between excitable cells.

    Excitatory A synapse that causes depolarization of the post-synaptic membrane, that is, brings its membrane potential closer to the threshold for action potential generation.

    Inhibitory A synapse that causes hyperpolarization of the post-synaptic membrane, that is, brings its membrane potential further away from the threshold for action potential generation.

    Neuromuscular A synapse between a terminal branch of the axon of a motoneuron and a muscle fiber.

    Non-obligatory A synapse that, when it acts alone, is unable to bring the post-synaptic membrane to the threshold for action potential generation. Neuro-neural synapses are typically non-obligatory.

    Obligatory A synapse that always brings the post-synaptic membrane to the threshold for action potential generation. Neuromuscular synapses are typically obligatory.

Synergy (a) A set of variables that show correlated changes in time or with changes in task parameters; or (b) a neural organization that shares performance among a redundant set of variables and ensures stability of performance variables by using flexible combinations of elemental variables.

Co-variation A feature of a synergy characterized by co-variation of elemental variables that helps maintain a desired value of a performance variable.

Linear torque synergy Linear scaling of joint torques during voluntary movement of a multi-joint chain.

Multi-muscle (a) A group of muscles that show correlated changes in activation levels over time or with changes in task parameters; or (b) a neural organization ensuring co-varied adjustments in muscle activation levels that keep a desired value or a desired time profile of a performance variable.

Sharing A feature of a synergy characterized by a pattern of relative involvement of elemental variables.

Tardive dyskinesia A neurological hyperkinetic disorder induced by long-term exposure to neuroleptic drugs.

Thalamus A brain structure that consists of a number of nuclei; it is part of several major loops that link the cortex of the large hemispheres, the basal ganglia, and the cerebellum, participating in the production of movement.

Tonic stretch reflex A reflex mechanism with an unknown neural path that links muscle length to active muscle force production.

Trajectory The time function of a physical variable.

Control The time function of a control variable.

Equilibrium The time function of variables characterizing equilibrium states of the system.

Virtual An imprecise term, used sometimes as a synonym of equilibrium trajectory and sometimes, as a trajectory that the system would have shown if the external load were zero.

Transcranial magnetic stimulation A method of non-invasive simulation of neural structures using eddy currents produced by a quickly changing magnetic field.

Tremor Involuntary cyclic movement associated with alternating activation bursts in the agonist and antagonist muscles.

Parkinsonian tremor is typically postural; it may be alleviated by voluntary movement.

Cerebellar tremor has postural, kinetic (increases during movement), and intentional (increases when the extremity approaches the target) components.

Tri-phasic activation pattern A muscle activation pattern consisting of an initial agonist burst accompanied by a low level of antagonist co-contraction, followed by an antagonist burst (during which the agonist is relatively quiescent), and ending with one more agonist burst.

Uncontrolled manifold A sub-space in the space of elemental variables corresponding to a fixed value of a performance variable; the controller does not have to exert control as long as the elemental variables stay within the uncontrolled manifold.

Hypothesis A hypothesis that the central nervous system organizes an uncontrolled manifold (UCM) corresponding to a desired value of a potentially important performance variable and then acts to keep the elemental variables within the UCM.

Variability A feature of motor performance reflecting different solutions for the same motor problems that are seen over time or during repetitive trials.

Variance A measure of variability equal to standard deviation squared.

"Good" variance A component of variance that does not affect a specific performance variable.

"Bad" variance A component of variance that affects a specific performance variable.

Vector (a) A physical variable characterized by both magnitude and direction (e.g. velocity, acceleration, force, and moment of force); or (b) a set of variables.

Vestibular apparatus Structures in the inner ear that contain vestibular receptors; these receptors convert linear and angular accelerations into sequences of action potentials.

    Vestibular nuclei Four paired nuclei located in the brainstem–the superior, lateral, medial, and inferior nuclei. They receive projections from the vestibular receptors and from other structures including the cerebellum.

    Vestibulospinal tracts The lateral vestibulospinal tract innervates antigravity muscles; the medial vestibulospinal tract innervates neck muscles that are responsible for stabilizing the head.

Vibration-induced falling (VIF) Violations of vertical posture produced by high-frequency, low-amplitude vibration applied to postural muscles (VIFs can also be induced by vibration applied to some of the other muscles).

Virtual finger An imaginary digit with the mechanical action equal to that of a set of fingers (commonly, the four fingers of a hand) combined.

Viscosity A property of liquids and gases to generate resistance to a moving object.

X-rays Electromagnetic radiation with the frequencies outside the visible range, between 10^{16} and 10^{19} Hz.

Index

Note: Page references followed by "f" indicate figure, and by "t" indicate table.